ABC OF MAJOR TRAUMA

Third edition

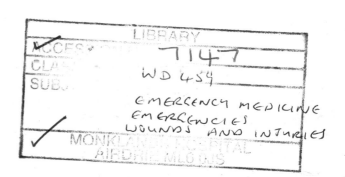

ABC OF MAJOR TRAUMA

Third edition

Edited by

PETER DRISCOLL
Consultant in Accident and Emergency Medicine, Hope Hospital, Salford

DAVID SKINNER
Consultant in Accident and Emergency Medicine, Oxford Radcliffe Hospital

RICHARD EARLAM
Consultant General Surgeon, Royal London Hospital

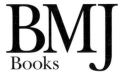

© BMJ Books 1991, 1996, 2000

BMJ Books is an imprint of the BMJ Publishing Group

First published 1991
by the BMJ Publishing Group,
BMA House, Tavistock Square
London WCIH 9JR

www.bmjbooks.com

Second edition 1996
Second impression 1996
Third edition 2000

British Library Cataloguing in Publication Data

A catalogue record for this book is available from the British Library

ISBN: 0-7279-1378-6

Colour reproduction by Tenon and Polert
Printed in China

Contents

Foreword

(to the second edition)

In December 1990 I wrote a foreword to the first edition of this book. At that time the Royal College of Surgeons of England's report on the management of major injuries, published in 1988, was beginning to have an impact on the way the seriously injured were managed in the United Kingdom. By 1990 its five major recommendations were at various stages of implementation. Training programmes for paramedics were under development and a pilot trauma centre was being established and evaluated at Stoke on Trent and compared with comparator centres in Preston and Hull. The Advanced Trauma Life Support programme was already well established by the Royal College at instructor and provider level and a national audit of the outcomes of serious injury, the Major Trauma Outcome Study, was funded by the Department of Health and subscribed to by an increasing number of hospitals. Many of those interested in the management of the seriously injured were meeting regularly under the auspices of the newly established British Trauma Society.

All these activities were evidence of an increased interest in the fate of the seriously injured, both in terms of the way they were managed and the outcomes that were achieved. At that time I hailed this book as a concise and readable reference book which would guide and stimulate those who were involved in the treatment of the injured, or who planned to make the management of trauma their lifetime career.

Five years later, where has all this activity got us? As one who has had a lifetime interest in trauma management, I am pleased to report that I believe there has been a radical change for the better. It is now generally accepted that concentration of the management of the seriously injured in the hands of those who are interested in the problem and who are willing to provide an immediate high quality service is in the best interests of the patient. Also it is now accepted that comparative audit can indicate variations in outcome and stimulate changes that will improve performance. ATLS training is now accepted and so valued that the Royal College is considering making it mandatory for all those who wish to take their examinations. The British Trauma Society is thriving.

The past five years have also seen the increasing influence of another report that was issued in 1988. That year the House of Lords committee on science and technology, in its report on priorities in medical research, proposed among other things, the evaluation of clinical practice and the dissemination and implementation of research results within the NHS. The NHS research and development directorate, which resulted from this report, has stimulated a move towards evidence based clinical practice. just as in 1990 we were in a period of change in the structure of trauma services, so now we are in the midst of a period of evaluation, not only of the treatments given, but the way services are provided. Evidence based medical practice research is assessing the process and outcome in areas of uncertainty such as the value of on site intravenous fluid administration to the seriously injured and the prevention of venous thromboembolism. This updated edition of the *ABC of Major Trauma* will continue to act as a valuable reference for those called on to treat the seriously injured. At the same time it recognises areas of uncertainty which need further research so that future editions of this book will be based on sound evidence of clinical effectiveness.

PROFESSOR SIR MILES IRVING
Professor of Surgery
Hope Hospital
University of Manchester

Preface to the first edition

The management of patients with major injuries in the UK has been the subject of much discussion and debate over the past 5 years. The report of the Royal College of Surgeons of England highlighted various areas where medical management was substantially suboptimal; patients who should have survived did not because of poor management. The report also emphasised that experienced consultants in various specialties must become more involved in emergency treatment.

The chapter on initial assessment gives a sequential method of management that can be followed by one doctor if he or she is unfortunate enough to be working in isolation. Recent evidence suggests that a "trauma team" approach provides more speedy diagnosis and resuscitation and decreases mortality and morbidity. The same tasks must be completed but they can be allocated to different members of the team in order that the initial assessment is more rapid. In the instructions on management we and many of the contributors have been influenced by the advanced trauma life support (ATLS) course, as originated by the American College of Surgeons and, more recently, run in the UK under the auspices of the Royal College of Surgeons of England. We believe that such a system will save lives and therefore have promoted a similar approach.

The various other chapters deal with specific problems related to one part of the body or with particular sorts of injuries, such as burns and blast injuries, or situations where large numbers of casualties are involved. We thank the authors for their efforts in producing a book which will, we hope, be of help to all those treating patients with major trauma. We also thank Fiona Whimster for encouragement and secretarial help.

DAVID SKINNER
PETER DRISCOLL
RICHARD EARLAM

Preface to the second edition

The past 5 years have seen significant changes in how injuries to separate and multiple body systems are managed. Furthermore, training in trauma care is now considered an integral part of a doctor's preparation for a career in anaesthetics, emergency medicine, or surgery. There has also been development of trauma training courses for nurses as well as staff working in the prehospital environment. Indeed many hospitals in the UK have incorporated several of these changes and developed multi-specialty trauma teams to optimise the care of the injured patient.

This second edition therefore provides a pertinent update on all the topics covered previously. Our aim, however, is to go further. We have taken the opportunity of incorporating several completely new aspects of trauma care. These include the management of medical problems in trauma patients, interhospital transfers, and trauma care in elderly people and hostile environments. The important role of the trauma nurse also forms an entirely new chapter.

We have endeavoured to ensure that this second edition remains relevant to all health care professionals involved in the chain of trauma care. If we have succeeded then it is in no small part due to the many people who have provided us with helpful advice over the past 5 years. Above all we are indebted to the authors of the individual chapters as well as to the continued support of the BMJ Publishing Group, and particularly to Deborah Reece. Without all their hard work and dedication this book could not have been written.

DAVID SKINNER
PETER DRISCOLL
RICHARD EARLAM

Preface to the third edition

The third edition of our text continues the objective of the first, namely to provide guidance to all members of the trauma team on the early management of patients with major injuries.

Clinicians involved in the delivery of this care in the UK continue to be influenced by the American College of Surgeons' Advanced Trauma Life Support course. We too support this approach and our text again follows this sequence.

Trauma care in the UK has almost certainly improved following the Royal College of Surgeons report on the management of patients with major injuries in 1988, particularly with regard to life-threatening conditions. The potential still exists however for considerable morbidity if the "secondary survey" is not conscientious and comprehensive. This third edition of the *ABC of Major Trauma* emphasises the importance of the secondary survey; individual chapters are allocated to different body areas, and there is an entirely new chapter on eye injuries.

Management of the psychological consequences of trauma is crucial to the surviving patient's well being—hence the inclusion in this edition of a helpful chapter by an experienced psychiatrist on the psychological problems faced by the trauma victim.

We hope that this book is useful to all colleagues, doctors, nurses and paramedics "in the front line", to whom we dedicate this third edition.

DAVID SKINNER
PETER DRISCOLL
RICHARD EARLAM

**This book is dedicated to Ian Haywood,
and to our colleagues "in the front line"
of trauma care**

Acknowledgments for illustrations

We should like to thank the following for permission to reproduce photographs: the American College of Surgeons' committee on trauma for photographs from the Advanced Trauma Life support™ slide set; the Resuscitation Council (UK) for photographs from slides used in the Resuscitation Council (UK) Advanced Life Support Course; the Department of Education and Medical Illustration Services, St Bartholomew's Hospital; the Department of Medical Illustration, Hope Hospital, Salford; and the Medical Illustration Department, Withington Hospital, Manchester. The line drawings were originally prepared by the Department of Education and Medical Illustration Services, St Bartholomew's Hospital; colour has been added and revisions done by Oxford Illustrators.

1 Initial assessment and management — I: the primary survey and resuscitation

Peter Driscoll, David Skinner

More than 90% of the injured patients seen in British emergency departments have been subjected to blunt trauma. These patients are often difficult to assess because many of their injuries are hidden. They should be managed using a team approach and a predetermined plan for the initial assessment and urgent resuscitation. All members of the team must be familiar with their own roles and those of their colleagues. These two essential elements will enable the members of the team to carry out their individual tasks simultaneously.[1,2]

The trauma team

Personnel—The trauma team should initially comprise four doctors, five nurses, and a radiographer. The medical team consists of a team leader, an "airway" doctor and two "circulation" doctors. The nursing team comprises a team leader, an "airway" nurse, two "circulation" nurses and a "relatives" nurse.

Team members' roles—Examples of paired roles and tasks are given on page 2, but assignments may vary among units depending on the resources available. To avoid chaos and disorganisation, no more than six people should be touching the patient. The other team members must keep well back.

Before the patient arrives

Many emergency departments are warned by the ambulance service of the impending arrival of a seriously injured patient. This communication system can also provide the trauma team with helpful information about the patient's condition and the paramedics' prehospital interventions.

After the warning, the team should assemble in the resuscitation room and put on protective clothing. The absolute minimum is rubber latex gloves, plastic aprons and eye protection because all blood and body fluids should be assumed to carry HIV and hepatitis viruses. Ideally, full protective clothing should be worn by each member of the team, and all must have been immunised against tetanus and the hepatitis B virus. Trauma patients often have sharp objects such as glass and other debris in their clothing, hair and on their skin. Ordinary surgical gloves give no protection against this, so the staff who undress the patient should initially wear more robust gloves.

While protective clothing is being put on, the team leaders need to brief the team, ensuring that each member knows the task for which he or she is responsible. A final check of the equipment by the appropriate team members can then be made. As the resuscitation room must be kept fully stocked and ready for use at any time, only minimum preparation should be necessary.

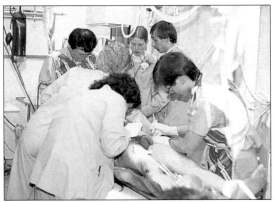

Trauma team in action.

Objectives of the trauma team

- Identify and correct life threatening injuries
- Resuscitate the patient and stabilise the vital signs
- Determine the nature and extent of other injuries
- Categorise the injuries in order of priority
- Prepare and transport the patient to a place of definitive care

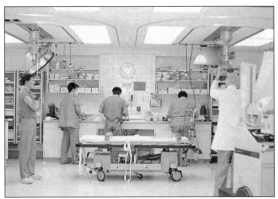

The resuscitation room: preparing for the patient's arrival.

Roles and tasks of the trauma team

Medical and other staff

Team leader

- Coordinates the medical team
- Assesses the patient's chest and, depending on the skill of the other team members, carries out particular procedures, such as pericardiocentesis.
- Assimilates information and lists the investigations and treatment in order of priority
- Liaises with other specialist personnel and questions the ambulance staff to ascertain the mechanism of injury, the prehospital findings, and the treatment given so far

Airway doctor

- Clears and secures the airway while taking appropriate cervical spine precautions
- Inserts central and arterial lines if required

Circulation doctors

- Assist in the removal of the patient's clothes
- Establish peripheral intravenous infusions and take blood samples for investigations
- Carry out certain procedures such as chest drain insertion, urinary catheterisation and splinting
- Carry out other procedures depending on their skill level

Radiographer

- Takes three standard *x* ray films on all patients subjected to blunt trauma—chest, pelvis, and lateral cervical spine. A more selective approach is used with victims of penetrating trauma

Nursing staff

Team leader

- Coordinates the nursing team
- Records clinical findings, laboratory results, intravenous fluid and drug infusion, and the vital signs as called out by the circulation nurse
- Prepares sterile packs for procedures
- Assists the circulation nurses and brings extra equipment as necessary

Airway nurse

- Assists in securing the airway and stabilising the cervical spine
- Establishes a rapport with the patient in the resuscitation room. Ideally all information should be fed through this nurse to the patient

Circulation nurses

- Assist in the removal of the patient's clothes
- Assist with starting intravenous infusions, chest drain insertion, and catheterisation. Monitor the fluid balance
- Assist in special procedures such as chest drain insertion
- Measure the vital signs and connect the patient to the monitors

Relatives' nurse

- Cares for the patient's relatives

Reception and transfer

If the ambulance bay is a long way from the resuscitation room, the staff in charge of the airway should assess the patient in the back of the ambulance. Provided there is no urgent airway problem requiring immediate intervention, the patient can be moved. Once the patient arrives in the resuscitation room, the nursing team leader should start the stop clock so that accurate times can be recorded.

The transfer of the patient from stretcher to trolley must be coordinated to avoid rotation of the spinal column or exacerbation of pre-existing injuries (see chapter 8). Team members should also check that lines and leads are free so that they do not become disconnected or snagged.

Primary survey and resuscitation

The objectives of this phase are to identify and treat any immediately life threatening condition. Each patient should be assessed in the same way, and the appropriate tasks performed automatically and simultaneously by the team. It is vital that problems are anticipated and prepared for, rather than reacted to. If the patient deteriorates at any stage, the medical team leader must reassess the patient, beginning again with the airway.

Essential prehospital information

- Nature of the incident
- Number, age and sex of the casualties
- The patient's complaints, priorities and injuries
- Airway, ventilatory, and circulatory status
- The conscious level
- The management plan and its effect
- Estimated time of arrival

- **Primary survey and resuscitation**

  Airway and cervical spine control

  Breathing

  Circulation and haemorrhage control

  Dysfunction of the central nervous system

  Exposure and environmental control

- **Secondary survey**

- **Definitive care**

Airway management, protecting the cervical spine

It is important to assume that the cervical spine has been damaged if there is suspicion of injury above the clavicles or if there is a history of a high speed impact. The doctor dealing with the airway should talk to the patient while the neck is kept manually in a neutral position by the airway nurse. If the patient replies in a normal voice, and gives logical answers to sensible questions, the airway is patent and the brain is being perfused adequately with oxygenated blood. If there is no reply, the patient's mouth should be opened and any solid foreign objects removed with Magill forceps and fluid sucked out.

The complications of alcohol ingestion and possible injuries of the chest and abdomen increase the chance of the patient vomiting. If the patient vomits, no attempt should be made to turn the patient's head to one side unless a cervical spine injury has been ruled out radiologically and clinically. If the patient is properly secured to a spinal (back) board, however, the whole body can be turned. In the absence of a spinal board the trolley should be tipped head down by 20° and the vomit sucked away with a rigid sucker as it appears in the mouth.

Chin lift or jaw thrust manoeuvres can be used to correct the position of the tongue, which often obstructs the airway in unconscious patients. Those with a gag reflex can maintain their own airway. As the use of Guedel airways in these patients can precipitate vomiting, cervical movement, and a rise in intracranial pressure, a nasopharyngeal airway is preferred provided that there is no evidence of a base of skull fracture.

If the patient is apnoeic, ventilation with a bag-valve-mask device may lead to gastric distension with air and can induce vomiting. Therefore patients without a gag reflex should be intubated so that ventilation can be carried out safely. Orotracheal intubation with in-line stabilisation of the neck is recommended, rather than nasotracheal intubation. If this proves impossible then a surgical airway must be provided.

Once the airway has been cleared and secured, every patient should receive 100% oxygen at a flow rate of 15 litres per minute. The neck must then be examined for wounds, tracheal position, venous distension, surgical emphysema and laryngeal crepitus. Consideration can now be given to securing the cervical spine so that the airway nurse can safely release the patient's head and neck. This is done with a semirigid collar, sand bags and tape, or a commercially available spine support. The only exception is the restless and thrashing patient. Here the cervical spine can be damaged by immobilising the head and neck while allowing the rest of the body to move. Suboptimal immobilisation with just a semirigid collar is therefore accepted.

Breathing

Listed in the box are five immediately life threatening thoracic conditions that must be urgently identified, and treated, during the primary survey and resuscitation phase (see chapter 4).

To see if any of these conditions is present, all the clothes covering the front and sides of the chest must be removed. The respiratory rate, effort and symmetry should then be recorded because these are sensitive indicators of underlying pulmonary contusion, haemothorax, pneumothorax and fractured ribs. At the same time, the medical team leader should visually examine both sides of the chest for bruising, abrasions, open wounds, and evidence of penetrating trauma. Cardiac tamponade after trauma is usually associated with a penetrating injury. The team leader should also remember that because of intercostal muscle spasm, paradoxical breathing is seen with a flail chest only if the segment is large, or central, or when the patient's muscles become fatigued. The patient with a flail chest usually has a rapid, shallow, symmetrical, respiratory pattern initially.

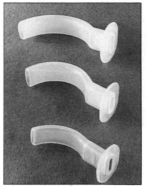
Guedal airway.

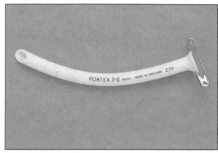
Nasopharyngeal airway.

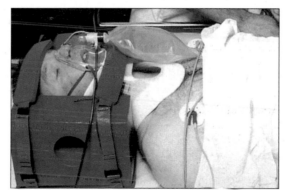
Patient with rigid collar in place.

Immediately life threatening thoracic conditions
- Tension pneumothorax
- Cardiac tamponade
- Open chest wound
- Massive haemothorax
- Flail chest

Common causes of inadequate ventilation
- Bilateral
  —obstruction of the upper respiratory tract
  — leak between the face and mask
- Unilateral
  —intubation of the right main bronchus
  —pneumothorax
  —haemothorax
  —foreign body in a main bronchus
  —significant lung contusion

After inspection, the chest should be auscultated and percussed to assess symmetry of ventilation and resonance. As listening over the anterior chest detects mainly air movement in the large airways, it is recommended that the medical team leader also listens over the axillae to gain a more accurate assessment of pulmonary ventilation. A tension pneumothorax or massive haemothorax can thus be identified. A tension pneumothorax should be relieved immediately by needle thoracocentesis and insertion of a chest drain. A pneumothorax or haemothorax should be treated by inserting a chest drain with a gauge of >28 in the fifth intercostal space just anterior to the mid-axillary line. This enables air and fluid to be drained but should always be preceded by intravenous lines. During examination of the chest the patient should be attached to a pulse oximeter.

Circulation and haemorrhage control

Having assessed the patient's breathing, the medical team leader should look for clinical signs of shock (see chapter 5), for which there is no specific test. In critical cases, when time and resources allow, plasma lactate can be recorded, and cardiac parameters measured by invasive monitors or ultrasound. More often the team leader will have to rely on routine physiological parameters. It is important to remember that up to 30% loss of blood volume produces tachycardia and reduces pulse pressure, but the blood pressure may stay within normal limits.

There is a consistent fall in the systolic blood pressure only when more than 30% of the blood volume has been lost. A urine output below 50 ml/h in an adult indicates poor renal perfusion, suggesting poor perfusion of the tissues in general.

While the assessment is in progress, the circulation doctor must control any major external haemorrhage by direct pressure. In addition, if there are no contraindications, the pneumatic antishock garment should be considered in shocked patients suspected of having fractures of the pelvis. Tourniquets are used only when the affected limb is deemed unsalvageable.

Two wide bore (gauge 14–16) peripheral lines must then be inserted, preferably in the antecubital fossae. If this is impossible, venous access should be gained by a venous cutdown or by inserting a short, wide bore, central line into the femoral or subclavian vein. If a subclavian approach is used and a chest drain is already in place, the central line must be inserted on the same side. As central vein cannulation can cause serious injury, it should be carried out only by experienced personnel.

Once the first cannula is in position 20 ml of blood should be drawn for group, type, or full cross match, full blood count, and measurement of urea and electrolyte concentrations. An arterial sample should also be taken for blood gas and pH analysis, but this can wait until the end of the primary survey. While venous access is being gained a circulation nurse must measure the blood pressure and record the rate, volume, and regularity of the pulse. An automatic blood pressure recorder and ECG monitor should also be attached to the patient. In seiously ill patients, palpating femoral and carotid pulses is a quick and reliable method of establishing that there is some cardiac output when no blood pressure can be recorded, either automatically or otherwise.

In the UK, the type of fluid initially given to injured patients to maintain fluid balance depends on departmental policy—some start with colloid while others use crystalloid such as physiological saline. It is therefore important for team leaders to know the local policy. The aim of fluid management in a hypotensive resuscitation should be to restore critical organ perfusion until haemorrhage that is amenable to surgery is stemmed. Therefore the initial approach in a standard adult trauma victim is to give 1 litre of warm colloid (or 2 litres of crystalloid) and then reassess the patient.[4]

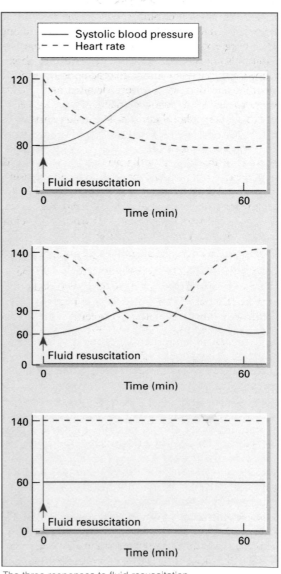

The three responses to fluid resuscitation.

When there is a limited response to the fluid bolus, or after a major injury, blood is required. To reduce the incidence of hypothermia, all fluids must be warmed before use.

In reassessing the circulatory state one of three responses may be seen:

(1) The vital signs return to normal after infusion of less than 1 litre of colloid solution (or 2 litres of physiological saline). In such cases patients have lost less than 20% of their blood volume and are not actively bleeding.

(2) The vital signs initially improve with the infusion but then deteriorate. These patients are actively bleeding and have usually lost more than 20% of their blood volume. They require transfusion with typed blood and the source of the bleeding must be controlled. This often requires an operation.

(3) The vital signs do not improve at all. This suggests either that the shock has not been caused by hypovolaemia or that the patient is bleeding faster than blood is being infused. History, mechanism of injury, and the physical findings will help to distinguish between these two possibilities. Measurement of the central venous pressure and, in particular, its change after a fluid bolus may assist in diagnosis.

Patients with hypovolaemia whose vital signs do not improve at all have lost more than 40% of their blood volume. The source of the bleeding requires immediate operation and is usually located in the thorax, abdomen, or pelvis.

Dysfunction of the central nervous system

A rapid assessment of brain and spinal cord function is made by assessing the pupillary reflexes and by asking patients to "put out your tongue", "wiggle your toes", and "squeeze my fingers". The patient must also be assessed on the AVPU scale (see box). Remember, however, that these quick manoeuvres will detect only gross neurological damage. A more detailed assessment, including assessment of the Glasgow coma scale, can be used if there is time, but is often delayed until the secondary survey.

Exposure

By this stage, all clothing impeding the primary survey should have been cut away with minimal patient movement, using large, sharp scissors. Remaining clothing should now be removed. To prevent patients subsequently becoming cold, they should be covered with warm blankets when not being examined and the resuscitation room kept warm.

By the end of the primary survey the medical team leader must make sure that all the allocated tasks have been completed. The vital signs should continue to be recorded every 5 minutes, to detect the patient's progress or deterioration. Only when all ventilatory and circulatory problems have been corrected can the team continue with the more detailed secondary survey. While the primary survey and resuscitation phase is underway, the relatives' nurse should greet any of the patient's friends or relatives who arrive. He or she can then take them to a private room that has all necessary facilities and stay there with them, providing support and information. Relatives should not be prevented from seeing the patient in the resuscitation room. However, they must be accompanied by the relatives' nurse so that they can be fully informed (see chapter 16).

Summary

Initial management of trauma victims requires a team approach in which each member carries out a specific task. Collectively, the team should aim to treat all the immediately life threatening conditions. The ABC approach provides an optimal system whereby the more urgent conditions are dealt with first.

Circulation and haemorrhage control

- Patients with hypovolaemia whose vital signs do not improve at all when fluid is administered have lost more than 40% of their blood volume.
- The source of the bleeding is usually in the thorax, abdomen, or pelvis, and requires immediate operation.

Conscious level can be assessed by the ATLS system of AVPU

A = **A**lert
V = Responds to **v**oice
P = Responds to **p**ain
U = **U**nconscious

References

1 Driscoll P, Vincent C. Variation in trauma resuscitation and its effects on outcome. *Injury* 1992; **23**: 111–5.

2 Driscoll P, Vincent C. Organising an efficient trauma team. *Injury* 1992; **23**: 107–10.

3 American College of Surgeons Committee on Trauma. *Advanced Trauma Life Support Course for Physicians*. Chicago: American College of Surgeons, 1997.

4 Bickles W, Wait M, Pepe P, et al. A comparison of immediate versus delayed fluid resuscitation for hypotensive patients with penetrating torso injury. *N Engl J Med* 1994; **331**: 1105–9.

2 Initial assessment and management — II: the secondary survey

Peter Driscoll, David Skinner

The objectives of the secondary survey[1] are listed opposite. In addition, radiography of the lateral cervical spine, chest, and pelvis should be standard practice in patients with blunt trauma. Protective lead aprons must therefore be worn by those staff who continue to manage the patient. One doctor, who may be the team leader, should ensure that the secondary survey is orderly and complete. He should hand over at the end of the emergency room phase to those who are in charge of the patient's subsequent care.

Head

Scalp

The scalp must be examined for lacerations, swellings, or depressions. Its entire surface needs to be inspected and palpated but examination of the occiput will have to wait until the patient is turned. Visual inspection may discover fractures in the base of the lacerations, but wounds must not be probed blindly as further damage to underlying structures can result. If there is major bleeding from the scalp, digital pressure or a self-retaining retractor should be used.

Neurological state

A "mini-neurological" examination of the patient can now be carried out. This comprises assessment of the conscious level using the Glasgow coma scale, the pupillary response and the presence of any lateralising signs (see chapter 6). A circulation nurse should continue to monitor these variables. If there is any deterioration, hypoxia or hypovolaemia must be ruled out before considering intracranial injury.

Base of the skull

Externally the base of the skull runs from the mastoid process to the orbit, so fractures of the base of the skull may produce signs along this line. When there is cerebrospinal fluid rhinorrhoea or otorrhoea, mixing of the fluid with the blood will delay the clotting of the blood and produce a double ring pattern if dropped on to a sheet. Examination with an auroscope may precipitate meningitis in patients with such problems and is therefore contraindicated.

Eyes

The eyes must be examined early, for pupil size and reactivity, before orbital swelling makes it impossible to do so. Retinal detachment, haemorrhages inside or outside the globe, foreign bodies under the lids, and evidence of penetrating injury must be noted. Visual acuity can be tested rapidly by asking the patient to read a nearby label. If the patient is unconscious the corneal reflex should be assessed.

Objectives of the secondary survey

- Examine the patient from head to toe and front to back
- Take a complete medical history
- Assimilate all clinical, laboratory and radiological information
- Formulate a management plan for the patient

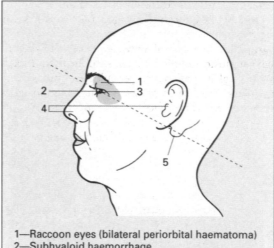

1—Raccoon eyes (bilateral periorbital haematoma)
2—Subhyaloid haemorrhage
3—Scleral haemorrhage without a posterior margin
4—Haemotympanium
 —Cerebrospinal fluid rhinorrhoea and otorroea
5—Battle's sign (bruising over the mastoid process)

Signs of a base of skull fracture.

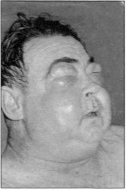

Extreme facial oedema.

Face

The face should be palpated symmetrically for deformities and tenderness. Nasal septal haematoma and loose or lost teeth must be identified. Instability of the maxilla can be assessed by traction on the upper incisors; instability suggests a middle third fracture of the facial skeleton. Although such injuries may be associated with fractures of the base of the skull, only those that are compromising the airway need immediate treatment. This usually entails pulling the fractured facial segment forwards to clear the airway. Mandibular fractures can also cause airway obstruction because of the loss of stability of the tongue. In these cases a traction suture is inserted into the tongue and the ends taped to the face or chest (see chapter 7).

Neck

With the patient's head held firmly by an assistant, the cervical immobilisation devices can be removed and the ears and neck examined. The ears should be checked for traumatic haematoma of the pinna, damage to the external auditory canal and perforation of the ear drum. If the patient is conscious, the clinician should then check that hearing is normal in both ears.

Once the features described previously for the neck have been reassessed, the cervical spinous processes need to be palpated for tenderness and deformities. The posterior cervical neck muscles should also be palpated for spasm and tenderness. A conscious patient can provide further help by telling if there is any pain in the neck and, if so, its location.

Lacerations must be inspected, but if a wound penetrates platysma it should be explored under general anaesthesia in the operating room.

A radiograph of the lateral cervical spine, showing all seven cervical vertebrae and the junction with the first thoracic vertebra, is essential in patients with multiple injuries. This view can still miss 15% of fractures, so an anteroposterior radiograph and odontoid peg views are required for a more complete evaluation of the cervical spine. These can be delayed until the secondary survey has been completed.

Thorax

The priority is to identify conditions that are potentially life threatening. In most cases this will require specialist investigation to confirm the team leader's initial suspicions, based on the mechanism of injury and the clinical findings.

Pulmonary and cardiac contusions are potentially life threatening and should be considered when the chest wall has received a severe direct blow. Cardiac arrhythmias or an infarct pattern on the ECG may reflect cardiac contusion. The thoracic aorta can be torn when the patient has been subjected to a rapid deceleration force, as experienced in a road traffic accident or fall from a height. A high index of suspicion, together with a thorough examination and a chest radiograph taken with the patient in the erect position are essential in these cases (see chapter 4). A ruptured diaphragm and perforated oesophagus can follow both blunt and penetrating trauma, and diagnosis is usually dependent on the appearance in the chest radiograph.

The chest wall must be re-inspected for bruising, signs of obstruction, asymmetry of movement and wounds. Acceleration and deceleration forces can produce extensive thoracic injuries; the marks invariably left on the chest wall should prompt the team to consider particular types of injury. For example, the bruise resulting from pressure exerted by a diagonal seat belt may overlay a fractured clavicle, a thoracic aortic tear, pulmonary contusion, or pancreatic laceration.

Facial injuries
- Maxillary fractures require immediate treatment only if they are compromising the airway
- Mandibular fractures can cause obstruction of the airway if stability of the tongue is lost

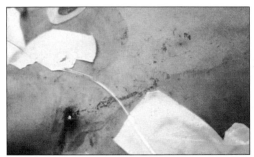
Gunshot wound to the neck.

Examination of the neck

A radiograph of the lateral cervical spine, showing all seven cervical vertebrae and the cervicothoracic junction, is essential in patients with multiple injuries

Potentially life threatening thoracic conditions
- Pulmonary contusion
- Cardiac contusion
- Ruptured diaphragm
- Aortic tear
- Oesophageal rupture
- Airway obstruction

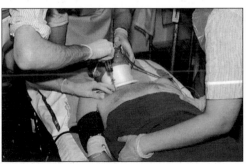
Needle aspiration of a tension pneumothorax.

The mark caused by impact with a steering wheel suggests a sternal fracture with cardiac contusion.

The clinician should then palpate the chest by feeling the ribs in the apices of both axillae and continuing caudally. The presence of crepitus, tenderness, and subcutaneous emphysema must be noted. Attention can then be directed to the anterior aspect of the chest by pressing on both clavicles, each rib, and the sternum. Palpation is completed by squeezing the chest in a lateral and anteroposterior plane to detect the presence of multiple rib fractures. Auscultation and percussion of the whole chest can then be carried out to check for asymmetry.

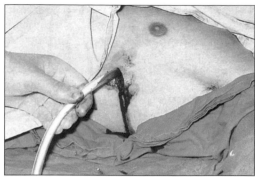

Chest drain in situ.

Abdomen

The team leader's aim in examining the abdomen is simply to decide if the patient requires a laparotomy. A precise diagnosis of which particular viscus has been injured is both time consuming and of little relevance at this stage.

A thorough examination of the whole abdomen is required, so the pelvis and the perineum must be assessed. All bruising, abnormal movement, signs of male urethral injury and wounds must be noted. Any exposed bowel should be covered with warm, saline-soaked swabs. Lacerations can then be inspected but not probed blindly as further damage may result. If a laceration extends into muscle, specialist advice is necessary because further investigations, including laparotomy, may be required (see chapter 9).

The abdomen must then be palpated and any signs of tenderness recorded. As squeezing the pelvis in two planes will detect only severe abnormalities, all patients with blunt trauma must undergo pelvic radiography. Finally, a rectal examination must be performed so that catheterisation can be carried out.

The catheter should be inserted so that the patient's rate of urine output can be measured. A perurethral approach can be used if there is no evidence of urethral injury. If an injury is suspected, however, a suprapubic catheter should be inserted and subsequently a retrograde urethrogram will be required. Irrespective of the catheterisation procedure, the urine must be tested for blood. A positive result supports the diagnosis of a renal injury and further investigations are required. A one-shot intravenous pyelogram can be taken in the resuscitation room and this will show if both kidneys are present, functioning and intact. This rapid investigation is commonly reserved for patients who require an urgent operation but in whom the presence of any major renal disease must be excluded. If there is no urgency, a definitive intravenous pyelogram and cystogram may be carried out at the end of the secondary survey. Urine should be saved for possible future microscopic examination and analysis of drug concentrations.

Pronounced gastric distension is common in crying children, adults with head or abdominal injuries, and patients who have been ventilated with a bag and mask. Insertion of a gastric tube decompresses the stomach, reduces the risks of aspiration, and facilitates abdominal examination.

An intra-abdominal bleed should be suspected if there are fractures of the ribs (5–11) that overlie the liver and spleen, the patient is haemodynamically unstable, or there are marks caused by seat belts or tyres over the abdomen. The detection of abdominal tenderness may be unreliable, particularly in patients with sensory defects caused by neurological damage or drugs, or if there are fractures of the lower ribs or pelvis. In these cases, CT, ultrasound or diagnostic peritoneal lavage (DPL) should be carried out to help rule out an intraperitoneal injury. Ideally DPL should be done by the general surgeon who will be responsible for any subsequent laparotomy.

Signs of urethral injury
- Blood at external urethral meatus
- Bruising of scrotum or perineum
- High riding prostate

Rectal examination
- Sphincter tone
- Presence of rectal damage
- Presence of pelvic fractures
- Prostate position
- Blood in the faecal residue

Signs of renal injury
- Flank pain
- Flank mass
- Flank bruising
- Haematuria

Indications of positive diagnostic peritoneal lavage
- >5 ml free blood aspirated from the peritoneal cavity
- Enteric contents aspirated from the peritoneal cavity
- Lavage fluid leaking into the chest drains or urinary catheter

In the lavage fluid
- >100 000 × 10⁹ red blood cells per litre
- Bile
- Food products
- Bacteria

Extremities

Each limb must be inspected for bruising, wounds, and deformities, and examined for vascular and neurological defects. The viability of the skin overlying fractures or dislocations must also be assessed before and after the deformity has been corrected. Using appropriate analgesia, this reduction should be carried out before radiography if the blood supply to the surrounding skin and soft tissues is compromised. Crepitus and instability can then be assessed by palpating and rotating all long bones. The level of active and passive movement must also be recorded.

The examiner must palpate all the bones in the limbs: metacarpal, metatarsal, and phalangeal fractures can easily be overlooked and may result in severe disability if left untreated.

Swabs should be taken for microbiological analysis from sites of open fractures. The wounds can then be covered with sterile dressings. Splinting of broken limbs is important because it reduces further damage to soft tissues, pain and possibly the production of fat emboli. A Polaroid picture or digital image taken before covering an open fracture will avoid the need for repeated inspection and reduce the risk of infection.

Spinal column

A detailed neurological examination is carried out at this stage to identify abnormalities in the peripheral nervous system. Sensory and motor defects, and evidence of priaprism, can help indicate the level and extent of the spinal injury. If the cord has been transected above the level of the sympathetic outflow, neurogenic shock results. This is manifested by hypotension without a corresponding tachycardia. The blood pressure falls as a consequence of vasodilation but its extent depends on how much sympathetic tone remains. For example, transection of the cervical spinal cord removes all vasoconstrictor tone and results in profound hypotension.

If a spinal injury is suspected, the patient should be moved only by a well coordinated "log rolling" technique. As the patient is turned away from the examiner, debris can be cleared away and the back examined from occiput to heels. Bruising and open wounds must be noted and the chest auscultated. The examiner's fingers should then palpate each spinous process in turn, so that any deformity or tenderness (in the conscious patient) can be detected. The paraspinal muscles are then similarly assessed. Finally the buttock cheeks must be separated so that any exit or entry wounds in this area are discovered. This is the ideal time to do a rectal examination, assessing the anal sphincter tone and that the prostate is in its correct position. The patient can then be "log rolled" back into the supine position.

In addition, the nursing team leader should make an initial assessment of the skin using a pressure sore scoring system—for example, the Waterlow system.[2] In elderly people and other high risk patients meticulous care must be taken to prevent the development of pressure sores.

Soft tissue injuries

A detailed inspection of the whole of the patient's skin will identify the number and extent of soft tissue injuries. Each breach in the skin should be inspected to ascertain its site, depth, and the presence of any underlying structural damage that will require surgical repair during the definitive care phase.

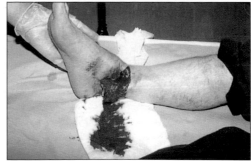
Open fracture and dislocation of the right ankle.

Signs of spinal injury
- Hypotension with relative bradycardia
- Decreased motor power and sensation below lesion
- Decreased anal sphincter tone
- Priapism

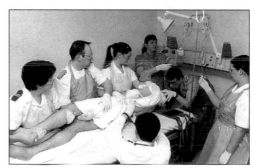
"Log rolling" a patient to allow examination of the back.

Injuries to the vertebral column are not always accompanied by physical signs on examination

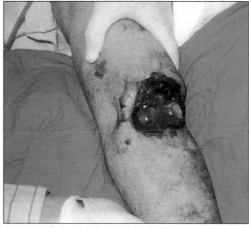
A deep soft tissue injury overlying the knee.

Once the patient is stable, however, superficial wounds can be cleaned, irrigated and dressed.

Medical history

This should be completed now. Information may be available from the patient, relatives and ambulance crew. A useful mnemonic is given in the box. It is crucial to find out the mechanism of the injury, as this gives invaluable information about the forces to which the patient was subjected and the direction of impact. Further help is provided by, for example, a description of damage to the car or details of the weapon used (see chapter 20).

Be aware that more than 30% of trauma victims in the UK have coexisting medical problems. These could impair the patient's response to the initial insult and to ongoing therapy.[2]

Reassessment

The team leader must constantly re-evaluate the response to resuscitation:

(1) Is the patient improving, deteriorating, or unchanged since resuscitation started? If the patient is not improving then the Airway, Breathing, Circulation, and Disability must be reassessed. As the patient's condition can change rapidly, repeated examination and constant monitoring are essential.

(2) What is the extent of the injuries and what are the priorities for treatment?

(3) Has an injury been missed? After blunt trauma, if no injury has been found in an area of the body between two injured sites, then the patient must be re-examined. Blunt trauma tends not to "skip" regions.

(4) Has analgesia been given? Victims of major trauma require pain relief. A mixture of 50% nitrous oxide and 50% oxygen (Entonox) may be given until completion of the secondary survey. Morphine can then be given intravenously, the dose being titrated against the patient's response.

(5) What is the patient's tetanus status and are antibiotics required?

(6) Are any further radiological investigations required? This depends on the condition of the patient. If he or she is hypoxic or haemodynamically unstable then these problems must be dealt with first. Once the condition stabilises, radiographs of particular sites of injury can be taken and other specialised investigations carried out. It is an important part of the team leader's responsibilities to assess the priorities of these investigations. Furthermore, adequate resuscitation equipment and monitors must be immediately available where these radiographs are taken.

The medical team leader is responsible for all documentation, which must be accurate and complete. The only one way to achieve this is to have one dedicated person recording the data and the exact times when the events occur. If a criminal cause for the injury is suspected all clothes, loose debris, bullets, and shrapnel must be collected, labelled and placed in bags, which must be signed for before release to the appropriate authorities according to local policy.

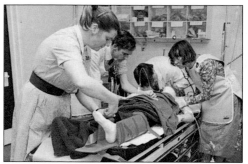

Medical history: AMPLE

A = Allergies
M = Medications
P = Past medical history
L = Last meal
E = Event leading to the injury, and the environment

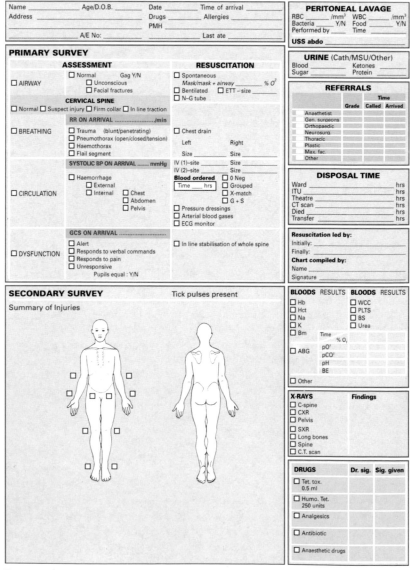

Trauma team in action during the secondary survey.

Trauma record sheet.

Responsibility for continuing care should be formally handed over, usually to the duty senior intensive care physician or surgeon, when the patient leaves the emergency department. The same level of care carried out in the resuscitation room must be maintained during the patient's transfer to the ward, theatre or specialist centre (see chapter 21). Finally, the nurse dealing with the patient's relatives and friends must inform them about the transfer. When the patient is to be moved to another hospital, this nurse should also help them to make their own transportation arrangements.

Summary

Once immediate life threatening conditions have been dealt with, the trauma patient requires a full assessment. This is best carried out head-to-toe, so that each body system is reviewed.

In addition, an AMPLE history needs to be taken so that appropriate investigations can be ordered and the correct management plan devised. Throughout the secondary survey, the patient requires continuous assessment so that the response to any therapy can be determined. If there is any deterioration, the primary survey should be repeated.

References

1 American College of Surgeons Committee on Trauma. *Advanced trauma life support course for physicians.* Chicago: American College of Surgeons, 1997.

2 Wardle T, Driscoll P, Oxbey C, Woodford M, Campbell F. Pre-existing medical conditions in trauma patients. In: *40th Annual Proceedings of the Association of Advanced Automotive Medicine* 1996; **40**: 351–61.

3 The upper airway

David Watson

First vital minutes

All severely injured patients experience hypoxaemia to some degree. As soon as medical help arrives the priority must be to ensure that the patient's airway is clear and ventilation is unimpaired. Immediate administration of supplementary oxygen to the unobstructed airway is of paramount importance.

Remember that in the first vital minutes the cervical spine of any patient with trauma should be considered broken until proved otherwise. The neck must be kept stabilised without traction (for example, by using a spinal board, sand bags, tape and a semirigid collar) at all times until the possibility of neck injury is excluded.

In an unconscious patient any obstruction to the airway must be removed under direct vision. The laryngeal and pharyngeal reflexes should then be assessed and respiratory performance examined. If protective reflexes are adequate—for example, the patient is coughing—retracting the tongue forward by employing the chin lift or jaw thrust manoeuvre or inserting an anaesthetic type airway or nasopharyngeal tube may suffice. If the reflexes are depressed or absent—that is, there is no gag reflex when oropharyngeal suction is attempted in an unconscious patient—the airway must be secured at the earliest opportunity by intubation with an appropriately sized endotracheal tube with a low pressure cuff. A laryngeal mask airway is not a substitute for a cuffed tube in the trachea, and is not yet proven effective in the emergency setting.

Ventilation and intubation

Patients with hypoxia or apnoea must be ventilated and oxygenated before intubation is attempted. Ventilation can be achieved with a mouth-to-face mask or bag-valve-face mask. Studies suggest that ventilation techniques with a bag-valve-face mask are less effective when performed by one person rather than two people, when one of the pair can use both hands to assure a good seal. When only one person is present to provide ventilation the method employing the mouth-to-face mask is preferred. During such manoeuvres the neck must be kept immobilised.

If intubation is performed a large bore gastric tube should also be passed. Nasal passage of a gastric tube is contra-indicated in patients with suspected basal skull fractures or injury to the cribriform plate.

Tracheostomy is rarely necessary as an emergency procedure. Severe distorting injury to the structures above or at the level of the larynx can render endotracheal intubation impossible, but cricothyroidotomy is preferred to emergency tracheostomy in such circumstances.

Signs and symptoms of upper airway obstruction

- Noisy breathing
- Effort of breathing: tracheal tugging; intercostal recession; abdominal see-saw movement
- Increased use of accessory muscles
- Apnoea (late)
- Cyanosis (late)

Indications for securing an airway with an endotracheal tube

- Apnoea
- Obstruction of upper airway
- Protection of lower airway from soiling with blood or vomitus
- Respiratory insufficiency
- Impending or potential compromise of airway (prophylactic intubation)—for example, after facial burns
- Raised intracranial pressure requiring hyperventilation

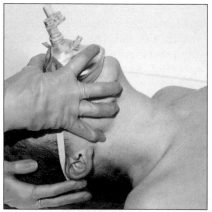

Mouth-to-face mask—preferred to a bag-valve-face mask when only one person is available to provide ventilation.

In patients with fractured ribs with or without a pneumo-thorax chest drainage on the side of the fractures is mandatory before artificial ventilation is undertaken. A tension pneumothorax should always be suspected when a patient with a recent crush injury has obvious respiratory distress or cyanosis. In patients with a chest injury complicated by pneumothorax an apical chest drain should be inserted through the space between the fifth and sixth ribs, just anterior to the mid-axillary line. If there is blood in the pleural cavity an additional basal drain may be required.

An open pneumothorax should be managed initially by inserting a chest tube to release any accumulated air and prevent the development of a tension pneumothorax. The opening can then be closed temporarily with a petroleum jelly gauze or other non-porous dressing.

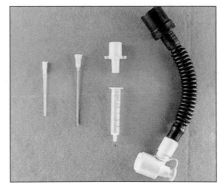

Apparatus for needle cricothyroidotomy. Modified large bore intravenous cannula and anaesthetic connections.

Indications for oxygenation and ventilation

Once the airway is secured the adequacy of respiratory gas exchange must be evaluated. The respiratory rate can be counted and respiratory effort assessed. Measurements of blood gas tensions should be undertaken as soon as is practicable.

Artificial ventilation in patients without respiratory failure must also be considered when there is coincidental head injury. Hypercapnia and hypoxaemia from asphyxia or inadequate ventilation with fluctuations in arterial blood pressure cause considerable deterioration in cerebral function. This is probably secondary to alterations in cerebral blood flow that adversely affect intracranial pressure.

- Ventilatory assistance is required when there is excessive respiratory work or obvious ventilatory insufficiency
- Failure of adequate oxygenation (PaO_2 <9 kPa) when the patient is breathing a high inspired oxygen concentration (6 l/min O_2 by facemask) demands endotracheal intubation and assisted positive pressure ventilation

Hospital management

An anaesthetist experienced in caring for victims of trauma should be available to examine the patient immediately on arrival at hospital. Evaluation of the patient's airway must proceed simultaneously with treatment. If the airway is satisfactory treatment may consist simply of increased oxygen delivery. If the airway is compromised or the patient needs ventilatory support a secure intratracheal airway, if not already in place, is required. Patients with hypoxia or apnoea must be ventilated and oxygenated before intubation is attempted.

The route of choice for securing the airway depends on several factors. Blunt trauma of the head and face is associated with an incidence of fractures of the cervical spine of 5–10%.[1] Patients with trauma should be assumed to have a cervical fracture until proved otherwise; manipulation of the neck is strictly contraindicated. Doctors in the United Kingdom generally accept that laryngoscopy and orotracheal intubation after induction of anaesthesia and muscle paralysis can be performed by a competent operator with minimal changes in the position of the cervical vertebrae while an assistant holds the patient's head.

Although optimum exposure of the larynx is not achievable under such conditions, experienced anaesthetists can intubate patients without clearly visualising the vocal cords. This may require aids such as the gum elastic bougie. Pressure on the cricoid must be provided by another skilled assistant to protect the patient from aspirating gastric contents.[2] The stomach may already have been emptied as much as possible by the passage of a nasogastric tube with the neck immobilised. Alternatively, if the patient's condition permits, fibreoptic endoscopy may facilitate difficult orotracheal or nasotracheal intubation.

Intubation of patients with head injuries
- Assume the patient has a cervical fracture
- An anaesthetist performs laryngoscopy while an assistant holds the patient's head
- Pressure on the cricoid must be provided by an assistant to prevent aspiration of gastric contents

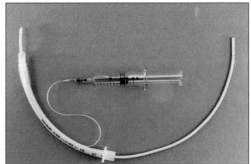

Gum elastic bougie and endotracheal tube.

Surgical cricothyroidotomy may be necessary for patients who cannot be intubated nasally or orally. Often these patients have massive facial trauma. Although surgical cricothyrodotomy can be performed through a small midline incision in the cricothyroid membrane, life saving oxygenation can also be provided by needle cricothyroidotomy with a cannula connected to wall oxygen at 15 l/minute with a Y connector or a side hole in the tubing attached between the oxygen source and the cannula. Spontaneous respiration after needle cricothyroidotomy, however, can be extremely difficult, requiring large pressure changes in the airway and considerable ventilatory effort. Intermittent insufflation (for which sedation and muscle paralysis are necessary) can be achieved by occluding the open end of the Y connector or the side hole of the oxygen tubing. The patient can be ventilated by this technique for only 30–45 minutes; this limits its usefulness, particularly in those with head injuries. Jet insufflation must also be used with caution when obstruction by a foreign body is suspected in the glottic area.

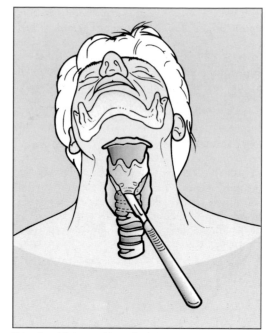

Cricothyroidotomy with scalpel.

Anaesthetic considerations

Anaesthetists caring for patients who are critically ill give reduced doses of all anaesthetics because hypovolaemia and hypotension alter the distribution and pharmacokinetics of drugs, thereby exaggerating their clinical effects. Intravenous opiates (morphine, pethidine, fentanyl or alfentanil) and anaesthetic induction agents (thiopentone, etomidate or propofol) are therefore given in smaller doses to avoid cardiovascular depression. Ketamine (1.0–2.0 mg/kg) is useful in trauma that is complicated by haemorrhagic shock. Ketamine and halogenated hydrocarbons such as halothane raise intracranial pressure and are therefore contraindicated in trauma of the head. Muscle relaxants given to facilitate[3] and maintain intubation include suxamethonium (1.0–2.0 mg/kg), rocuronium (0.6–0.9 mg/kg), pancuronium (0.1–0. 2 mg/kg), vecuronium (0.1–0. 2 mg/kg) or atracurium (0.4 mg/kg).

Rapid-sequence intubation with anaesthetic agents, neuromuscular blocking drugs and oesophageal occlusion by cricoid pressure should be performed only by those trained in their use, knowledgeable of their inherent complications and skilled in the techniques of airway maintenance, endotracheal intubation and assisted ventilation. In the UK this usually means anaesthetists.

Patients may have taken drugs such as opiates, cocaine, and marijuana before suffering trauma. These may interact with anaesthetics. Ethanol enhances the effect of anaesthetics and sedatives and reduces the minimum alveolar concentration of volatile general anaesthetics required.[4]

Before embarking on intubation an anaesthetist will check the equipment, including the suction and oxygen delivery apparatus. Anaesthetics should be ready in labelled syringes, and duplicate ampoules should be easily accessible. Vasoactive drugs such as atropine should also be ready in syringes in case untoward bradycardia complicates extended laryngoscopy. A skilled assistant must be at hand to apply pressure on the cricoid. The neck must be kept stabilised. Secure venous access is mandatory. Ideally a pulse oximeter should be attached to the patient's earlobe or finger to give a continuous display of the arterial haemoglobin oxygen saturation.

Anaesthesia is induced with the best possible monitoring available and only after administration of oxygen. Pressure on the cricoid is maintained by the assistant. Neuromuscular blockade is produced by suxamethonium, and intubation proceeds with the onset of paralysis and relaxation of the jaw.

Patients with responsive airway reflexes require induction of anaesthesia and muscle paralysis for the airway to be secured by

Drugs contraindicated in trauma

Head injuries
- Ketamine increases intracranial pressure
- Halothane and enflurane increase intracranial pressure

Burns and spinal cord injuries
- Suxamethonium is safe during the first 24 hours but subsequently it can cause potentially lethal hyperkalaemia

Eye injuries
- Suxamethonium is relatively contraindicated because it raises intraocular pressure

Essential equipment for endotracheal intubation
- Two laryngoscopes
- Endotracheal tube
- Connections
- Inflating bag (such as Ambu bag)
- 10 ml syringe for cuff inflation
- Suction apparatus
- Bougie or introducer catheter
- Magill curved forceps

an oral or a nasotracheal route. Deeply unconscious patients with head and brain injury should not be intubated without prior administration of a cerebral sedative and muscle relaxant, hence avoiding dangerous increases in cerebral blood volume and intracranial pressure during laryngoscopy. Nasotracheal intubation should not be undertaken if fractures of the base of the skull or of the cribriform plate are suspected.

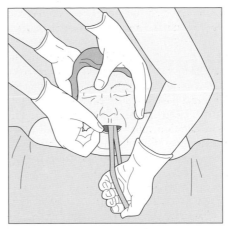

Inserting the laryngoscope.

Intubation technique

The anaesthetist takes the laryngoscope in his or her left hand and inserts it into the right hand side of the patient's mouth, thereby moving the tongue to the left. While carefully observing the back of the tongue he or she advances the curved blade of the laryngoscope until the epiglottis comes into view.

The tip of the blade is moved anterior to the epiglottis and the whole lower jaw lifted upwards, taking care not to move the neck. This should expose the arytenoid cartilages and vocal cords. The tracheal rings should be visible beyond. Under direct vision the anaesthetist advances a 60 cm gum elastic bougie or the endotracheal tube, aiming for the left vocal cord. If a gum elastic bougie is used a cut cuffed endotracheal tube of the appropriate size is subsequently "rail roaded" into the trachea. A size 8 tube is usually suitable for women and a size 9 for men. The cuff of the endotracheal tube is then inflated with air from a syringe until an airtight seal is secured.

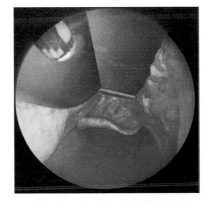

Lifting the root of the tongue.

The chest should be auscultated in both axillae to exclude intubation of the right main bronchus or oesophagus. An end tidal carbon dioxide monitor attached to the endotracheal tube between the adaptor and the ventilator device will rapidly confirm that the endotracheal tube is in the trachea. A disposable calorimetric carbon dioxide detector is commercially available. Pressure on the cricoid can only now be released and the tube secured with tapes.

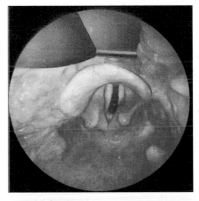

Direct visualisation of the glottis.

After intubation, oxygen-enriched ventilation should proceed with a tidal volume of about 10 ml/kg at a rate of about 10 breaths/minute. To facilitate ongoing respiratory support, sedation and analgesia may need to be maintained by intravenous administration of benzodiazepines (e.g. midazolam) or anaesthetic induction agents (e.g. propofol) and opiates (e.g. morphine, fentanyl or alfentanil) together with neuromuscular blocking drugs (e.g. atracurium, vecuronium, rocuronium or pancuronium) for muscle paralysis. Although capnography and pulse oximetry may provide immediate non-invasive assessment of oxygenation and the adequacy of ventilation, the arterial blood gas tensions should be analysed at the first opportunity. Radiography of the chest should also be performed routinely after endotracheal intubation to check the position of the endotracheal tube in the bronchial tree.

In conclusion, providing oxygen and ventilatory support as early as possible are prerequisites for successful resuscitation in victims of major trauma. Otherwise, as Haldane observed, hypoxia not only stops the machine but wrecks the machinery.

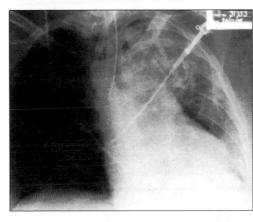

Chest radiograph showing inadvertent intubation of the right main bronchus.

References

1 McCabe JB, Angelos MG. Injury to the head and face in patients with cervical spine injury. *Am J Emerg Med* 1984; **2**: 333.

2 Sellick BA. Cricoid pressure to control regurgitation of stomach contents during induction of anaesthesia. *Lancet* 1961; **ii**: 404.

3 Scott RPF. Onset times and intubating conditions. *Br J Anaesth* 1998; **80**: 417–9.

4 Bruce DL. Alcoholism and anesthesia. *Anesth Analg* 1983; **62**: 84.

● Illustrations of the technique of intubation are reproduced from *A Systematic Guide to Intubation* (by P Lotz, FW Annefeld and WK Hirlinger) by kind permission of the publisher, Atelier Flad, Eckental, Germany.

4 Chest injuries

Stephen J Rooney, Jonathan A J Hyde, Timothy R Graham

There are more than 150,000 deaths from trauma in the United States each year, of which 25% are attributable to thoracic injuries. This percentage is mirrored in the United Kingdom, and thoracic injuries contribute significantly to a further 25% of trauma deaths. Many of these deaths are almost immediate; individuals who reach hospital are, therefore, a self selected group, most of whom should survive with appropriate early management. Less than 15% will require surgery. The remainder can be managed by simple measures such as intercostal drainage, adequate analgesia, and careful fluid management. Inappropriate management of these patients may cause unnecessary morbidity and even death, possibly during surgery for extra-thoracic injuries.

Patterns and pathophysiology of chest injury

The pattern of injury provides valuable information, and obtaining an accurate history may save time during later management. The broad categories of thoracic injury are direct injuries (penetrating, blunt and crush) and indirect injuries (deceleration or blast).

Major intrathoracic injuries can occur without obvious external damage, and more obvious injuries may delay the diagnosis of chest trauma. Diagnosis should depend upon prediction and exclusion rather than direct manifestation of injury, with a high index of suspicion for specific injuries. Distinct patterns of injury (high or low velocity, crush or penetrating trauma) are associated with differing thoracic and other injuries; predictors of thoracic injury include head and abdominal injuries; evidence of major haemorrhage in the absence of abdominal swelling or major bony injury; wounds, bruising, or seat-belt marks on the chest wall; and any degree of respiratory distress.

The main consequences of chest trauma result from its combined effects on respiratory and haemodynamic function. Blood loss, ventilatory failure, lung contusion or collapse, and displacement of mediastinal structures may cause hypoxia and subsequent acidosis, which rapidly compound the adverse effects of other injuries.

The aim of early intervention and resuscitation is to restore adequate delivery of oxygen to the tissues. Successful management of thoracic trauma is dependent, therefore, on effective cardiopulmonary resuscitation (CPR) and prevention of hypoxia, followed by the detection and rapid treatment of immediately life-threatening injuries.

Hypoxia
Hypoxia is the most common pathophysiological manifestation of any moderate to severe chest injury. Early

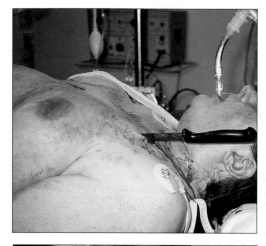

Knife wound to the upper left chest, traversing the lung and breaching the pericardium.

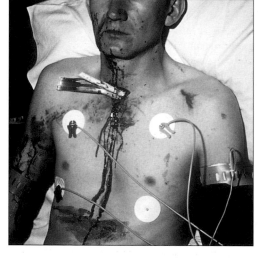

Industrial accident resulting in impalement injury to the neck and upper thorax.

Classification of thoracic injuries

Category	Mode	Common injuries
Direct	Penetrating	Laceration of heart, great vessels, intercostal bundle, lung parenchyma, airways, oesophagus, and diaphragm
	Blunt	Cardiac contusion, pulmonary contusion, rib and thoracic skeleton fractures
	Crush	Ruptured bronchus, ruptured oesophagus, cardiac contusion, pulmonary contusion
Indirect	Deceleration	Aortic disruption, major airway injury, ruptured diaphragm
	Blast	Massive pulmonary contusion, disruption to any intrathoracic organ

interventions are designed to ensure adequate oxygen delivery to all parts of the lung capable of normal ventilation and perfusion. Compromised respiratory function and hypoxia can arise from any of the following mechanisms: traumatic open pneumothorax, traumatic tension pneumothorax, or haemothorax.

A *traumatic open pneumothorax* usually occurs secondary to pulmonary parenchymal or tracheobronchial injury, and rarely as a result of oesophageal injury. When an associated chest wall injury creates a direct communication between the inner thoracic cavity and the external environment, an open pneumothorax (sucking chest wound) results. As air flows along the path of least resistance, there is preferential flux of air through the chest wall defect rather than through the tracheobronchial tree during inspiration and expiration. During expiration, the affected lung receives air from the unaffected one, which partially reverses the situation.

A *traumatic tension pneumothorax* is produced secondary to laceration of the lung or airway that allows escape of air into the pleural space. Airflow is unidirectional into the pleura on inspiration, but cannot escape during expiration because of the effective formation of a flap valve. The result is progressive accumulation of air in the pleura, with collapse of the ipsilateral lung, producing hypoxia, and shift of the mediastinum to the opposite side. This compresses the contralateral lung, further compromising ventilation, and the reduced venous return leads to low cardiac output. In advanced cases, hypoxia-induced myocardial failure may exacerbate low cardiac output.

Haemothorax after chest wall injury is often secondary to bleeding from intercostal vessels and less often to bleeding from the internal thoracic (internal mammary) vessels. A significant, life threatening haemothorax may follow major laceration of lung parenchyma, injury to the pulmonary hilum, aortic disruption or direct cardiac lacerations. A large haemothorax occupies space in the thoracic cavity normally occupied by lung; subsequent lung collapse will worsen hypoxia, triggering a progressive cycle of deterioration.

Impairment of gas exchange

Patients with a lung injury may experience major impairment of gas exchange because of diffuse interstitial and alveolar haemorrhage, as seen after pulmonary contusion. Pulmonary contusion is one of the main factors in the morbidity and mortality associated with chest trauma. Experimental and clinical studies have shown that the condition is progressive—initial haemorrhage and oedema are followed by interstitial fluid accumulation and decreased alveolar membrane diffusion. These changes produce relative hypoxaemia, increased pulmonary vascular resistance, decreased pulmonary vascular flow and reduced lung compliance.

In patients with impaired respiratory function because of pulmonary injury, the associated mediastinal shift secondary to haemothorax, pneumothorax or both may result in compression of the non-injured lung, further compromising ventilation. This ventilation-perfusion mismatch can lead to an intrapulmonary shunt of more than 30% that contributes significantly to hypoxaemia, especially in the period soon after injury. Later, this hypoxia-induced pulmonary vasoconstriction will divert the blood away from the non-ventilated alveoli, thus reducing the intrapulmonary shunt to about 5%.

Pathophysiology of life-threatening thoracic injuries

Process	Type	Example
Tissue hypoxia (inadequate oxygen delivery)	Hypovolaemic	Blood loss
	Ventilation–perfusion mismatch	Contusion or collapse
	Intrathoracic pressure changes	Tension or open pneumothorax
	Combination of above	Haemopneumothorax
Acidosis	Metabolic	Tissue hypoperfusion
	Respiratory (inadequate ventilation)	Airway obstruction or injury, intrathoracic pressure changes, or altered levels of consciousness
Low cardiac output	Hypovolaemic	Blood loss
	Mechanical	Cardiac tamponade
	Metabolic	

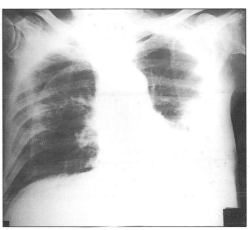

Plain chest radiograph showing a 50% right-sided pneumothorax as a result of blunt trauma.

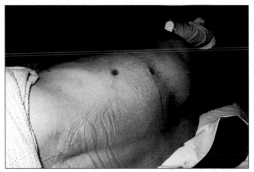

Patient with two posterolateral gunshot wounds (entry type) to the left chest.

Pulmonary contusion

- Pulmonary contusion is a major factor in the morbidity and mortality associated with chest trauma
- The condition is progressive. Initial haemorrhage and oedema are followed by interstitial fluid accumulation and decreased alveolar membrane diffusion

Hypovolaemia

Profound hypovolaemia can follow exsanguination in chest trauma. It is most often seen with aortic transection, great vessel rupture, pulmonary hilar injury or cardiac/pericardial laceration not producing tamponade. The result is a state of low cardiac output that compounds other consequences of chest injury such as hypoxaemia, cardiac tamponade, congestive cardiac failure and myocardial ischaemia and infarction.

Myocardial contusion

Myocardial contusion after blunt injury can reduce cardiac contractility and compliance of the ventricle, causing a low cardiac output state as a result of myocardial failure. Associated injury to coronary arteries or smaller vessels within the contused area can lead to tissue necrosis and infarction. When there is multiorgan trauma, with hypovolaemia and hypoxaemia, myocardial function is further compromised by reduced coronary perfusion, which ultimately leads to congestive cardiac failure. About 20% of patients with myocardial contusion experience arrhythmias. These arrhythmias vary widely, and include supraventricular tachycardia, including atrial fibrillation, ventricular ectopics, ventricular dysrhythmias, and sinus tachycardia. Conduction defects, ranging from bundle branch block to complete heart block, may also develop. Myocardial infarction as a result of coronary artery damage or occlusion or both can produce cardiogenic shock or myocardial failure.

Traumatic injury to the heart valves may result in acute volume overloading of the ventricles, and severe regurgitation may cause acute congestive cardiac failure and death. Acute insufficiency of any valve may go unnoticed in the presence of more obvious injuries. Hence, valve lesions are not often detected during the initial post-trauma survey and resuscitation phase; their recognition requires a high index of suspicion and further investigation (such as echocardiography).

Myocardial contusion can lead to:
• Low cardiac output because of myocardial failure
• Cardiac arrythmias
• Conduction defects

Heart valve lesions
• Can be fatal
• May be overlooked in the presence of other injuries
• Recognition of injury to the heart valves requires a high index of suspicion during the initial survey and resuscitation period, and further investigation, such as echocardiography

Primary survey and resuscitation

During the primary survey, simultaneous resuscitation and diagnosis of conditions that are an immediate threat to life are essential. Intervention is based upon the immediate clinical problems, but follows the "ABC" principles of resuscitation.

Airway

The priority is to assess patency of the airway, by listening for air movement at the nose and mouth, and looking for movement of the intercostal and supraclavicular muscles. Check the oropharynx for foreign body obstruction. Impending hypoxia is sometimes indicated by subtle changes in the breathing pattern, which may become shallow and tachypnoeic. Cyanosis is often a late sign resulting from peripheral hypoperfusion and blood loss. Securing an airway may be difficult and is potentially hazardous in patients who have received injuries to the neck or upper chest.

Breathing

The chest must be completely exposed to allow assessment of respiratory movement and quality of ventilation by observation, palpation, and auscultation. The mechanics of breathing can be disrupted by major airway obstruction, pain, haemothorax or pneumothorax, or pulmonary contusion.

Circulation

The pulse should be assessed for quality, rate, and regularity. The blood pressure and width of pulse pressure must be measured, as vasoconstriction can maintain a normal blood

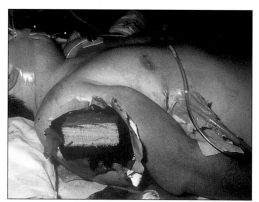

Severe impalement injury of the upper thorax following a motor cycle collision. The wooden stake completely traversed both lungs and the mediastinum, but there was no injury to the great vessels or the spine.

The ABC principles of resuscitation
• Establish a safe AIRWAY
• Restore the mechanics of BREATHING
• Maintain the CIRCULATION

pressure in spite of considerable blood loss. The peripheral circulation is assessed by skin colour and temperature. Venous distension in the neck may not always be present in a patient with cardiac tamponade who has hypovolaemia. An electrocardiograph should always be attached to the patient.

Resuscitation

Intubation and positive pressure ventilation may be necessary to establish an airway and restore the mechanics of breathing. If there is any doubt about the patency or adequacy of the airway, always take measures to establish a definitive one.

Once an airway has been secured, oxygen transport will be improved by maximising the inspired oxygen concentration. This can be achieved by giving high-flow 100% oxygen (about 15 litres/minute) via a face mask. It is pointless to restore a good circulating volume if the circulating fluid is not sufficiently oxygenated. Early correction of hypoxia and acidosis is vital, particularly in the presence of head injury to prevent secondary brain damage or when further surgery is to be undertaken. Measures taken must be based upon knowledge of arterial blood gas tensions and acid–base analyses.

The priority in treating haemorrhage remains control of the bleeding at source. Once bleeding has been stopped, or controlled as far as possible with available resources, the circulating blood volume can be increased.

The approach to circulatory management demonstrates the evolution of trauma care as a specialty. Until recently, the teaching has been to insert two large-bore cannulae and infuse volume rapidly. However, indiscriminate fluid replacement can be hazardous, particularly to patients with cardiac tamponade, traumatic aortic disruption or pulmonary contusion. If there is suspicion of these conditions, and no apparent massive haemorrhage, rapid volume infusion should be withheld.

Hypotensive or 'permissive' resuscitation is gaining acceptance as routine practice. There is good evidence, from studies in animals and clinical settings, that it is associated with improved outcome. The aim of hypotensive resuscitation is to restore the circulatory status of the hypovolaemic patient to the point of critical organ perfusion. This is the minimum systolic blood pressure required to ensure adequate perfusion of the distal vital organs, that is, heart, brain and kidneys. The next priority is improvement of peripheral perfusion and acid–base balance.

Hypotensive resuscitation fits well with the adoption of a 'scoop and run' approach to trauma, removing the need to spend valuable time at the scene attempting intravenous cannulation. Safe transfer usually requires only attention to airway and breathing and direct control of bleeding. Cannulation and necessary volume replacement can be performed in transit.

On arrival in the emergency room, it is prudent to continue with the policy until definitive diagnoses have been made. During this time, blood should be cross-matched and type specific Rhesus negative blood obtained if possible. Chest radiography and arterial blood gas tensions must be performed as part of the primary survey as soon as is appropriate after the patient's admission.

Base deficit is a sensitive indicator of oxygen debt and changes in oxygen delivery, and therefore reflects the adequacy of resuscitation. Patients with low cardiac output may benefit from the administration of calcium or inotropes, but these are useless without an adequate circulating volume.

Fatal haemorrhage can ensue from cardiac or vascular lesions arrested by tamponade, if such injuries are not identified before resuscitation raises the arterial and intracardiac pressures. Major injuries such as aortic transection and cardiac disruption, and major airway damage and diaphragmatic rupture, will be suggested from the plain chest radiograph.

Resuscitation

- Always ensure that the airway is patent and adequate
- Early correction of hypoxia and acidosis is vital
- It is pointless to restore a good circulating volume if the circulating fluid is not sufficiently oxygenated
- Control any haemorrhage at source as far as possible with available resources
- Consider the circulatory blood volume: avoid indiscriminate fluid replacement

Hypotensive resuscitation

- Hypotensive resuscitation aims to restore the circulatory status of the hypovolaemic patient to the point of critical organ perfusion
- Proponents of hypotensive resuscitation do not dispute that fluid treatment of shock usually benefits the patient. Evidence suggests, however, that withholding fluids, although not necessarily improving the clinical condition, does not worsen it; moreover, in some patients it may be of benefit
- Conditions in which indiscriminate fluid replacement can be hazardous include cardiac tamponade, traumatic aortic disruption, and pulmonary contusion

Fatal haemorrhage can ensue if cardiac or vascular lesions arrested by tamponade are not identified before resuscitation raises the arterial and intracardiac pressures

Immediately life-threatening chest injuries

Six specific thoracic injuries can be fatal if not recognised and treated immediately. These are airway obstruction (see chapter 3), tension pneumothorax, open pneumothorax, massive haemothorax, flail chest, and cardiac tamponade.

Tension pneumothorax

A tension pneumothorax is rapidly fatal unless decompressed. It is a clinical diagnosis — tension pneumothorax is recognised by respiratory distress, tracheal deviation away from the affected side, unilateral absence of breath sounds, and possibly distended neck veins.

The treatment is immediate decompression, which should not be delayed by performing a chest radiograph. Insertion of a needle into the second intercostal space in the midclavicular line confirms the diagnosis and temporarily decompresses the pleural space.

This life-saving procedure should always be performed unless the diagnosis can be excluded. The simple manoeuvre has few serious consequences, even in the absence of a tension pneumothorax. After decompression, obtain intravenous access and place a formal intercostal drain into the pleural cavity through the fifth intercostal space anterior to the mid-axillary line.

Open pneumothorax

Although penetrating injuries usually seal off, larger defects may remain open, causing a sucking chest wound. There is immediate equilibration between atmospheric and intrathoracic pressures, and if the defect is large enough air will pass preferentially through the defect with each respiratory effort, markedly reducing respiratory efficiency. The defect should be covered initially with an Asherman seal to act as a flutter valve, and an intercostal drain should then be placed away from the open wound. Surgical closure will be necessary later.

Massive haemothorax

Massive haemothorax is usually caused by penetrating injury but can result from blunt trauma. Penetrating wounds medial to the nipple or scapula suggest damage to the heart (with potential cardiac tamponade), great vessels, and the hilar structures.

In an adult, massive haemothorax is defined as loss of more than 1500 ml of blood into the chest cavity or drain, but adjustments must be made for body size. The signs are those of hypovolaemic shock associated with dullness to percussion and absent breath sounds on the affected side. The neck veins may be collapsed secondary to hypovolaemia, or dilated and full (because of associated tension pneumothorax or tamponade).

Massive haemothorax is managed by simultaneously decompressing the chest cavity and restoring the blood volume. Fluid is infused through large calibre intravenous lines, and changed to type specific blood (if available) or cross-matched blood as soon as this can be provided. A large bore intercostal drain (28 French gauge or larger) can then be inserted anterior to the midaxillary line through the fifth intercostal space.

Intravenous lines must be in place before insertion of the chest drain, as sudden decompression of a massive haemothorax may result in haemodynamic decompensation from the hypovolaemia, particularly if the source of bleeding is uncontrolled. Until a cardiac or vascular injury has been ruled out, the systemic pressure should not be allowed to rise uncontrollably as this may precipitate further bleeding and

---

Intercostal drainage

(1) Preferentially use the fourth or fifth intercostal space between the mid-and anterior axillary lines

(2) Surgically prepare the skin, drape the chest, and infiltrate the skin and periosteum with local anaesthetic. Advance the needle above the rib to infiltrate the pleura and then confirm the presence of air or blood on aspiration

(3) Incise the skin down to the rib, then develop the track above the rib by blunt dissection. This avoids damaging the the intercostal bundle

(4) Once the pleura is punctured, insert a gloved finger into the pleural cavity before any drain is placed, to ensure the incision is correctly placed and prevent damage to the lung or other organs

(5) Do not use the trocar to force the drain through the chest wall but introduce it with the tip of a large surgical artery forceps (for example, Roberts'). The drain should slide into position easily through the track already made, and be directed towards the apex of the chest cavity

(6) Attach the tube to an underwater seal drainage system

(7) When the drain is in position secure with zero gauge suture and insert a purse-string suture

(8) Check the position and efficacy of the drain on a chest x ray

(9) Do not clamp the tube after insertion

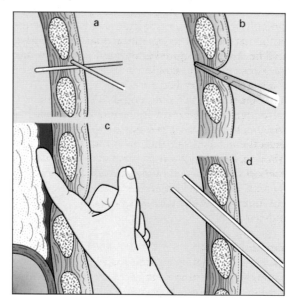

Chest drain insertion. (a) Penetration of the skin, muscle and pleura. (b) Blunt dissection of the parietal pleura. (c) Exploration of the pleural cavities. (d) Tube directed posteriorly and superiorly.

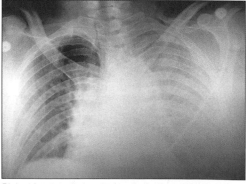

Plain chest radiograph (supine) demonstrating massive left-sided haemothorax as a result of blunt trauma.

cause death (hypotensive resuscitation). Continuing blood loss in excess of 200 ml/h indicates the need for surgical exploration. Placing a central venous line allows control of right-sided cardiac filling pressures and monitoring of the clinical response.

Flail chest

Severe crush injuries may cause extensive disruption of the chest wall with multiple rib and sternal fractures. When a segment of chest wall loses bony continuity with the thoracic cage it becomes flail and will move paradoxically on respiration, reducing tidal volume and compromising ventilation. In addition, rib fractures may be accompanied by significant blood loss. The principal cause of hypoxia after flail chest, however, is the accompanying severe pulmonary contusion.

Diagnosis is usually clinical, by observation of abnormal chest wall movement and the palpation of crepitus. The chest radiograph will not always reveal rib fractures or costochondral separation. Full lung expansion must be restored by intermittent positive pressure ventilation if required, and any haemopneumothoraces must be drained. Intercostal chest drains are almost always required.

The aim of further management is to preserve respiratory function. Pain reduces the tidal volume, and inadequate ventilation of the basal lung segments results in atelectasis. Pain also inhibits coughing, allowing secretions to obstruct bronchi and cause acute respiratory failure. Effective pain relief is required so that regular physiotherapy can be carried out with the patient's full co-operation. Careful management is essential because the injured lung is sensitive to inadequate perfusion subsequent to shock, and also to fluid overload (there is already capillary leakage).

A flail segment in itself does not justify mechanical ventilation, although elective intubation and ventilation is often appropriate. The degree of respiratory distress and hypoxia determines the need for ventilation, and it is important to be aware that pulmonary contusion may develop insidiously over a period of days. Functional, not physical, integrity is the main aim. Adequate analgesia and careful fluid management are essential. Operative stabilisation of fractures is rarely indicated.

Cardiac tamponade

Although penetrating injuries are usually responsible for cardiac tamponade, blunt trauma may damage the heart or great vessels and cause bleeding into the pericardium. Cardiac function is restricted by only a small amount of blood within the fixed, fibrous pericardium.

Beck's triad of elevated central venous pressure, hypotension, and muffled heart sounds may not be present; the neck veins in a hypovolaemic patient can be empty and the nature of the heart sounds may be difficult to assess in a noisy emergency room. Kussmaul's sign of paradoxical elevated venous pressure on inspiration associated with tamponade may also be seen.

Immediate pericardiocentesis is indicated in patients with suspected cardiac tamponade who have failed to respond to initial resuscitative measures. Removing as little as 20 ml of blood from the pericardial space can considerably improve the condition of a critically ill patient. Although pericardiocentesis may be life saving in certain circumstances, it has also caused death through cardiac laceration and should be performed with caution. In 25% of cases the blood within the pericardium has clotted and aspiration will not be possible. A fine balance between internal and external cardiac pressures may prevent exsanguination in cardiac tamponade, and

---

Flail chest

- The main cause of hypoxia after flail chest is the accompanying severe pulmonary contusion
- Provide effective pain relief to preserve respiratory function and permit regular physiotherapy
- Take care to avoid inadequate perfusion or fluid overload
- Operative fixation of fractures is rarely indicated

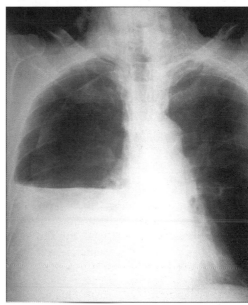

Plain chest radiograph (erect) demonstrating right-sided haemopneumothorax and, because the patient is upright, clearly showing the fluid level.

Pericardiocentesis

(1) Attach the patient to an electrocardiograph before starting. The vital signs and central venous pressure should also be monitored

(2) Prepare the skin surgically and infiltrate the sub xiphoid area with local anaesthetic

(3) Puncture the skin 1–2 cm inferior to the left xiphochondral junction with a wide bore plastic-sheathed needle (at least 15 cm in length). Initially at 45 degrees, the needle should then be aimed towards the tip of the left scapula—the base of the pericardium

(4) As the needle is advanced simultaneously aspirate until it fills easily with blood without ECG disturbance. Then aspirate as much blood as possible

(5) ECG changes such as widening/enlarging of the QRS complex or marked ST changes suggest that the needle is too far advanced and must be withdrawn. Serious damage to the heart is rare, though injury of the posterior descending branch of the right coronary artery is possible

(6) Positive pericardiocentesis must be followed by surgical exploration

aspiration of blood from the pericardium may contribute to fatal haemorrhage by reducing the external cardiac pressure and allowing a rise in intracardiac pressures.

If the patient is moribund pericardiocentesis should not be allowed to delay immediate thoracotomy. Patients with a positive pericardiocentesis must always undergo formal surgical exploration (in the operating theatre if possible) and inspection of the heart.

Emergency thoracotomy

We do not advocate indiscriminate emergency thoracotomy, as this major procedure is associated with a high mortality, and has the best chance of success if performed by an experienced surgeon. Rather, we intend to increase awareness of the limited indications for its use, and discuss the immediate surgical options that may be available in survivors of thoracic injury.

Resuscitative thoracotomy is controversial, and has often been attempted in hopeless situations. Thoracotomies performed anywhere outside the operating room, particularly those carried out by non-cardiothoracic surgeons, are associated with an extremely high mortality. Even in established trauma centres patients who require thoracotomy in the emergency room, for anything other than isolated penetrating heart injury, rarely survive. Outcome is even worse when the procedure is performed in the field.

Thoracotomy enables relief of tamponade, internal cardiac massage, and cross clamping of the aorta, which helps restore the perfusion pressure to the brain and the coronary arteries while reducing intra-abdominal haemorrhage. The emergency surgery may take the form of median sternotomy, anterolateral thoracotomy, or lateral thoracotomy depending upon the nature of the injury, the surgeon's experience, and the facilities available.

There are contraindications to emergency thoracotomy, and few specific, evidence-based indications. Attempts to perform the procedure outside established guidelines will almost inevitably end in failure. A thoracotomy should be considered only for those patients who have sustained certain injuries and fulfil specific criteria, and should be performed wherever possible in theatre by a cardiothoracic surgeon. Only if urgency absolutely dictates should the procedure be performed elsewhere.

It is important to realise that emergency thoracotomy is a controversial area, and the application of firm rules is not always appropriate.

Salvage thoracotomies for blunt trauma are almost always hopeless. In most patients in extremis with blunt chest trauma, the injuries discovered will be irreparable, the continued blood loss enormous, and the outcome fatal. There is often much venous bleeding, particularly from lacerated pulmonary veins, and posterior intercostal and lumbar vessels. Control of such large volume haemorrhage under suboptimal conditions is usually impossible. There may be pressure on the attending surgeon to "open the chest" as a last resort, but the outcome is seldom beneficial.

Emergency thoracotomy

Indications

- Penetrating trauma (cardiac tamponade diagnosed), with definite signs of life at the scene of the injury
- Uncontrollable life-threatening haemorrhage into the airways, and hilar clamping is required

Contraindications

- Blunt trauma with no signs of life at the scene of the injury
- Cardiopulmonary resuscitation (CPR) for more than 10 minutes

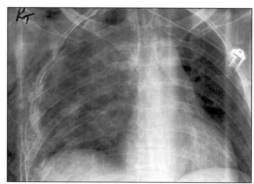

Plain chest radiograph demonstrating multiple right-sided rib fractures causing a flail segment, and underlying pulmonary contusion. Also present is considerable surgical emphysema

Salvage thoracotomies for blunt trauma are almost always hopeless

Secondary survey

Once immediately life-threatening conditions have been excluded or diagnosed and treated, the patient can be assessed thoroughly. This assessment includes a detailed history, full examination, chest radiograph, measurement of arterial blood gases and electrocardiograhy. A plain chest radiograph is the most important investigation in a patient with thoracic trauma, and should be performed with the patient erect if possible; in practice, when there is serious injury, it is often done with the patient supine or partially erect. An erect film allows the best assessment of lung expansion and free air or blood in the chest cavity. Widening and shift of the mediastinum and rib fractures may be evident.

Serious injuries such as cardiac tamponade, transected aorta, ruptured diaphragm, and major airway injury can usually be diagnosed from the chest radiograph. Multiple rib fractures, fractures of the first or second ribs, or scapular fractures indicate the delivery of severe force to the chest and its internal organs. Pneumomediastinum, pneumopericardium or air beneath the deep cervical fascia suggest tracheobronchial disruption. Surgical emphysema of the chest wall and haemopneumothorax are generally indicative of pulmonary laceration after fractures.

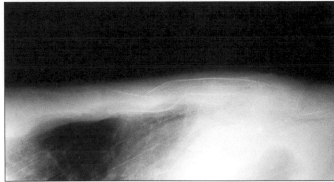
Lateral radiograph showing severe comminuted fracture of the sternum following a "steering-wheel" injury.

Potentially life-threatening chest injuries

The following injuries, which may be diagnosed during the primary or secondary survey of the patient, are not immediately life-threatening. They are, however, all serious and may cause death.

Pulmonary contusion
The insidious development of lung dysfunction mimicking adult respiratory distress syndrome (ARDS) as a result of pulmonary contusion makes this injury potentially lethal. There is associated atelectasis and shunting of blood, decreased lung compliance, and increased airway resistance. The resulting increase in the work of ventilation is in addition to that caused by injuries to the chest wall. Some patients may be managed without intubation and mechanical ventilation. There are situations (see box) when early intubation (within the first hour) must always be considered.

Myocardial contusion
Contusion of the heart is the most commonly undiagnosed fatal thoracic injury. It occurs when there is direct compression of the heart or rapid deceleration. It is often associated with sternal fractures; in such cases the right ventricle is more commonly damaged. Chest pain is usually assumed to be caused by chest wall contusion or rib fractures.

The diagnosis is established from the mechanism of injury, serial cardiac enzyme measurements, electrocardiographic changes, and two dimensional echocardiographic evidence of ventricular wall dysfunction and pericardial effusion. Sinus tachycardia, multiple ventricular ectopics, atrial fibrillation, non-specific ST segment and T wave changes, and conduction abnormalities such as right bundle branch block may all be seen. An area of contused myocardium behaves in the same way as an area of infarction, and the patient should be treated accordingly. The complications are those of myocardial infarction and should be managed similarly. Conduction defects may rarely require pacemaker insertion.

Cardiogenic shock is rare but some patients may need temporary intra-aortic counter pulsation balloon pumping to improve the perfusion of viable myocardium. Urgent surgical repair using cardiopulmonary bypass is sometimes necessary for cardiac rupture (particularly posterior), ventricular septal rupture, or valve damage.

Relative indications for early endotracheal intubation in cases of pulmonary contusion
- Hypoxia or worsening respiratory status
- Impaired level of consciousness
- The patient will be transferred to another hospital
- Pre-existing chronic pulmonary disease
- Surgery for abdominal or orthopaedic injuries is necessary
- Organ function failure in another system (such as ileus or renal failure)
- Extremes of age

Myocardial contusion
- Is the most commonly undiagnosed fatal thoracic injury
- The complications are those of myocardial infarction and should be managed similarly
- Urgent surgical repair is sometimes necessary

Traumatic disruption of the aorta

Tears of the aorta or pulmonary arteries are immediately fatal in about 90% of cases. They usually occur as a result of blunt or deceleration injuries, typically in a road traffic accident or fall from a height. The aorta may be completely or partially transected or may have a spiral tear. It is firmly fixed at three points: the aortic valve, the ligamentum arteriosum, and the hiatus of the diaphragm. Sudden deceleration will allow the mobile parts of the aorta to continue moving relative to the fixed parts.

The most common site of rupture is at the attachment of the ligamentum arteriosum, where the aorta remains tethered to the main pulmonary artery. The immediate survival of the patient depends on the development of a contained haematoma, maintained by the intact adventitia. The survival of patients after reaching hospital depends on early diagnosis followed by urgent surgical repair.

Any suspicion of aortic injury raised by the plain chest radiograph must prompt further investigation. No single radiographic sign absolutely predicts aortic rupture, but a widened mediastinum is the most consistent finding. If transfer is necessary the patient should be mechanically ventilated and the systolic blood pressure kept below 100 mm Hg using infusions of sodium nitroprusside or propanolol, or both. This is to prevent elevations of systemic blood pressure that may rupture the flimsy adventitial layer, causing fatal haemorrhage. Particular caution should, however, be taken in the use of these drugs in patients with myocardial contusion. A policy of "hypotensive" fluid resuscitation is also clearly prudent in such cases.

The treatment of traumatic aortic rupture is surgical repair, directly or by resection of the damaged segment and interposition of a vascular graft. This should take priority over other surgical procedures (except control of life-threatening haemorrhage). All clinical situations are different, and management needs to be tailored to the individual. Important caveats are in patients with simultaneous liver trauma or head injuries, where the systemic heparinisation required for cardiopulmonary bypass may be extremely dangerous.

Diaphragmatic rupture

Penetrating injuries cause small diaphragmatic perforations that are rarely of immediate significance. By contrast blunt trauma produces large radial tears of the diaphragm and easy herniation of abdominal viscera. The right hemidiaphragm is relatively protected by the liver and left sided ruptures are therefore more common; they are also more easily diagnosed because of the appearance of gut in the chest. Bilateral rupture is rare.

The chest radiograph can be misinterpreted as showing a raised hemidiaphragm, acute gastric dilatation, or a loculated pneumothorax. Contrast radiography, or locating an abnormal position of the stomach with plain radiography by passing and identifying the tip of a nasogastric tube, confirms the diagnosis. Unless intracranial injuries or potentially fatal haemorrhage require immediate surgery, repair of the diaphragm should not be delayed. This is often performed through a laparotomy for associated abdominal injuries.

Major airway injury

Extensive free air in the neck, mediastinum or chest wall should always raise suspicions of major airway damage. Laryngeal fractures are rare. They are indicated by hoarseness, subcutaneous emphysema, and palpable fracture crepitus. Attempted intubation is warranted if the airway is completely obstructed or there is severe respiratory distress. The airway may be hazardous to secure and require immediate tracheostomy followed by surgical repair.

Radiographic features suggestive of aortic disruption

- Mediastinal widening
- Loss of "aortic knuckle"
- Paratracheal stripe
- Pleural cap
- Right deviation of trachea or oesophagus (nasogastric tube)
- Elevation of right main bronchus
- Depression of left main bronchus
- Fractures of the first and second ribs

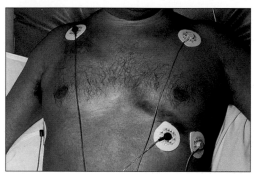

Seatbelt "tattoo" of the chest following a head-on automobile collision. The patient was kept under observation for 3 days because of a marked elevation of cardiac enzyme concentrations, but there was no residual myocardial damage.

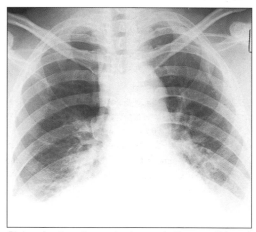

Plain chest radiograph demonstrating a widened mediastinum in a patient with traumatic aortic disruption. Other suggestive features present are right paratracheal stripe, bilateral apical pleural caps and right haemopneumothorax.

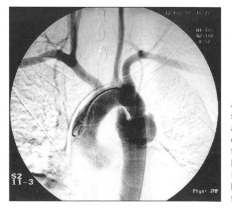

Arch aortogram of the same patient showing aortic disruption at the classical site close to the attachment of the ligamentum arteriosum. In addition, the haematoma formed by the leak is easily seen.

Transections of the trachea or bronchi proximal to the pleural reflection cause extensive deep cervical or mediastinal emphysema, which rapidly spreads to the subcutaneous tissues. Injuries distal to the pleural sheath result in pneumothoraces. Blunt tracheal injuries may not be obvious, particularly if the conscious level of the patient is depressed. Penetrating injuries are usually apparent and all require surgical repair. They may be associated with injury of adjacent structures, most commonly the oesophagus, carotid artery, or jugular vein. With missile injuries, there can be extensive tissue damage to the surrounding area because of the cavitation caused by the velocity of the projectile.

Laboured breathing may be the only sign of airway obstruction. Bronchoscopy, preferably rigid to improve airway clearance of blood and debris, confirms the diagnosis and early surgical repair is required. Injury to a major bronchus is usually the result of blunt trauma. There are often severe associated injuries and most victims die at the site of the accident; for those who reach hospital, mortality is at least 30%.

Signs of bronchial injury may include haemoptysis, subcutaneous emphysema, tension pneumothorax, and pneumothorax with a large, persisting air leak. Most bronchial injuries occur within 2.5 cm of the carina, and the diagnosis is confirmed by bronchoscopy. Mucosal oedema and debris can obscure the extent of a bronchial injury, so the site should be carefully inspected. Distortion of airway anatomy by adjacent haematomata makes management more difficult, and surgery is occasionally indicated. Bronchial tears must be repaired urgently through a formal thoracotomy performed in the operating theatre.

Oesophageal trauma

Damage to the oesophagus is usually caused by penetrating injury. Blunt oesophageal injury is rare, except when a severe blow to the upper abdomen causes sudden compression and a "burst" type of defect. Gastric contents are forced up into the oesophagus, producing a linear tear through which they can then leak. This is followed by mediastinitis, or rupture into the pleural space with empyema formation, or both. The clinical picture may be identical to that of spontaneous rupture of the oesophagus, but the diagnosis is often delayed.

The diagnosis is confirmed by cautious contrast study of the oesophagus, or by endoscopy. Treatment is by formal surgical repair in the operating theatre, and drainage of the pleural space or mediastinum or both.

Imaging in thoracic trauma

Imaging is essential to the accurate diagnosis of many conditions mentioned in this chapter. The plain chest radiograph remains fundamental; like the pelvic radiograph, it must be performed at the earliest possible stage in patients who have sustained major injury. Other thoracic imaging investigations can wait until the "secondary survey" stage.

Various imaging modalities are available to diagnose or eliminate most potentially life-threatening conditions. Portable ultrasound scanners are increasingly used; the quality of the images is operator dependent, but they can be useful in the diagnosis of pericardial and pleural fluid collections.

Computed tomography (CT) is widely available and useful in the diagnosis of aortic injuries. The gold standard for the diagnosis of aortic disruption is aortography. This can be performed in the radiology department, cardiac catheter laboratory, or possibly in the operating theatre, depending on the urgency of the situation.

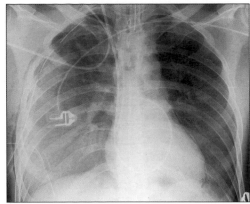

Plain chest radiograph of a patient following blunt chest injury and ruptured major airway, showing pneumopericardium. Right-sided chest tubes have been inserted to drain the haemopneumothorax also present.

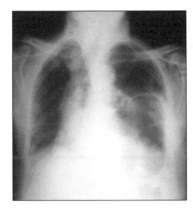

Plain chest radiograph demonstrating ruptured left hemidiaphragm. Abdominal viscera are clearly seen in the thoracic cavity, with associated mediastinal shift to the right.

Signs suggestive of oesophageal rupture

- Sharp, severe epigastric pain
- Shock disproportionate to the apparent injury
- Pneumomediastinum on the plain chest radiograph
- Left pneumothorax or haemothorax in the absence of rib fractures
- Gastric contents passing down the chest drain

The plain chest radiograph in thoracic trauma

- The single most important investigation for patients with thoracic trauma
- Should be performed as part of the primary survey (within 10 minutes of arrival in the emergency room)
- Allows diagnosis of free blood or air within the pleural space and/or mediastinum, relationships of vital structures, presence of foreign bodies (e.g. bullets), and confirmation of positioning of tubes and drains
- Enables decision-making for appropriate further investigations (e.g. CT scan or angiography if aortic disruption is suspected)
- An erect film is ideal, though not usually attainable

Analgesia

Analgesia for patients with chest injuries is an important part of their management and must not be underestimated. Concern about giving opiate drugs to hypoxic patients is well founded; however, if the cause of hypoxia proves to be reversible, such drugs can safely be used.

Most patients who have sustained thoracic trauma (particularly blunt trauma) will be in pain—usually there are fractures of the bony thoracic skeleton, regardless of the severity or absence of underlying injuries. In such patients, deep inspiration and expiration is extremely painful; the resulting shallow respiration will cause derangements in the acid–base status, often exacerbating other mechanisms of injury, such as hypoxia. It is vital, therefore, to maximise normal respiratory excursion by the judicious use of appropriate analgesic agents.

Analgesia can be given by several different routes. Oral compounds are clearly inappropriate if the patient requires imminent surgery or is unconscious. Intravenous and intramuscular agents, either opiates or non-steroidal anti-inflammatory drugs (NSAIDS) are most commonly used, the latter being particularly effective for musculoskeletal pain. Local anaesthetic administration, such as intercostal bupivacaine can be invaluable for extensive rib fractures, effectively blocking the neurovascular bundles in the spaces above and below the fracture sites.

Analgesia
- Thoracic trauma is painful and it is vital to maximise normal respiratory movement by providing effective analgesia
- Administration of local anaesthetic can be when there are extensive rib fractures

Stabilisation and transfer

Transfer from the emergency department must not be considered unless the patient is haemodynamically stable with secure respiratory function. This applies equally to internal transfer, perhaps for investigations in other departments, and external transfer to a specialist centre. As transfer for either reason may be essential for the patient's continuing welfare, the need for delay often creates a management dilemma. It must be clearly understood that transfer of an unstable or compromised patient is associated with an extremely high morbidity and mortality, and should not be undertaken unless there is no alternative. Most deaths occurring during transit from the emergency department or in other departments (e.g. radiology) may be avoidable.

Patient transfer
- Unless the patient is haemodynamically stable with secure respiratory function, transfer from the emergency room puts him or her at high risk
- This applies as much to internal transfer to another department as to external transfer to a specialist centre

Conclusion

Cardiothoracic trauma continues to be associated with a high mortality. The application of evidence-based medicine and updated management principles have resulted in improved outcome for a large group of patients who reach the hospital with intact vital signs.

Further reading

Driscoll PA, Skinner DV, eds. *Trauma care: beyond the resuscitation room*. London: BMJ Books, 1998.

Greaves I, Ryan JM, Porter KM, eds. *Trauma*. London: Arnold, 1998.

Westaby S, Odell JA, eds. *Cardiothoracic trauma*. London: Arnold, 1999.

5 Hypovolaemic shock

Peter J F Baskett, Jerry P Nolan

Hypovolaemic shock is a clinical state in which tissue perfusion is rendered relatively inadequate by loss of blood or plasma.

A reduction in blood volume causes a fall in systolic pressure, which triggers a sympathetic catecholamine response. This results in peripheral vasoconstriction, a rise in pulse rate, and a reduction in pulse pressure. The tachycardia and increased cardiac contractility raise the myocardial oxygen requirement.

Blood flow to the skin and peripheral tissues is reduced, in an effort to preserve reasonable perfusion of vital organs such as the brain, heart, liver and kidneys. Anaerobic metabolism, with the production of lactate, occurs in tissues that are inadequately perfused. If blood loss continues, the increasing metabolic acidosis will impair the function of vital organs. Further myocardial depression compounds the development of shock, and pain stimuli add to the sympathetic outburst.

Early symptoms and signs

The following are early symptoms and signs of hypovolaemic shock. They reflect the underlying pathophysiology.

- Tachycardia (caused by catecholamine release)
- Skin pallor (results from vasoconstriction caused by catecholamine release)
- Hypotension (caused by hypovolaemia, perhaps followed by myocardial insufficiency)
- Confusion, aggression, drowsiness, and coma (caused by cerebral hypoxia and acidosis)
- Tachypnoea (caused by hypoxia and acidosis)
- General weakness (caused by hypoxia and acidosis)
- Thirst (caused by hypovolaemia)
- Reduced urine output (caused by reduced perfusion)

In most cases signs and symptoms can be related to the amount of blood loss, which can be classed in four broad groups (classes I–IV).

Generally, losses up to 750 ml (class I) (15% of the circulating blood volume) generate no pronounced signs or symptoms. Further haemorrhage, up to 1.5 litres (class II), produces cardiovascular signs of catecholamine release, thirst, weakness, and tachypnoea. Systolic pressure begins to fall as blood loss mounts to 2 litres (class III) and often becomes unrecordable after 2.5–3.0 litres (class IV) have been lost.

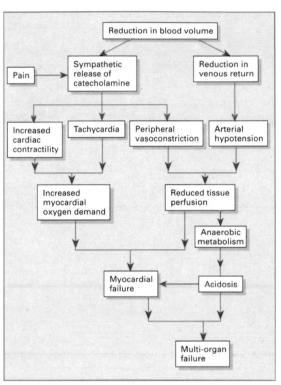

How blood loss can lead to multiorgan failure.

Classification of hypovolaemic shock by blood loss (adult)

	Class I	Class II	Class III	Class IV
Blood loss				
Percentage	<15	15–30	30–40	>40
Volume (ml)	750	800–1500	1500–2000	>2000
Blood pressure				
Systolic	Unchanged	Normal	Reduced	Very low
Diastolic	Unchanged	Raised	Reduced	Very low or unrecordable
Pulse (beats/min)	Slight tachycardia	100–120	120 (thready)	120 (very thready)
Capillary refill	Normal	Slow (>2 s)	Slow (>2 s)	Undetectable
Respiratory rate	Normal	Tachypnoea	Tachypnoea (>20/min)	Tachypnoea (>20/min)
Urinary flow rate (ml/h)	>30	20–30	10–20	0–10
Extremities	Colour normal	Pale	Pale	Pale, clammy, and cold
Complexion	Normal	Pale	Pale	Ashen
Mental state	Alert	Anxious or aggressive	Anxious, aggressive, drowsy	Drowsy, confused, or unconscious

Previously healthy young adults have remarkable compensatory capabilities and systolic pressure is often preserved in spite of quite appreciable blood loss (1.5–2.0 litres). A narrowed pulse pressure is often the earliest sign. Eventually, however, there is a precipitous fall as the myocardium suddenly fails because of hypoxia and acidosis. Conversely, patients with coronary arterial disease may become hypotensive because of myocardial insufficiency after only modest blood losses of up to 1.5 litres.

Factors affecting response to blood loss

Patients receiving certain drugs (for example, β blockers) may be unable to produce an appropriate sympathetic response and may also become hypotensive after modest blood loss.

Other factors that can modify the response to blood loss include the patient's age, the extent of tissue damage, and the period of time between injury and examination.

In children, normal haemodynamic values are maintained until blood loss is relatively great. Tachycardia and skin pallor are the earliest signs, and hypotension indicates uncompensated shock with severe blood loss and inadequate resuscitation. As a rule, a child's systolic blood pressure is 80 mm Hg plus twice the age in years. The diastolic pressure is about two thirds of the systolic pressure. A systolic pressure of 70 mm Hg or less in a child therefore indicates serious cardiovascular decompensation.

In elderly patients, hypotension may be an early sign of blood loss. Their physiological reserves are reduced and they are less able to respond to release of catecholamines by tachycardia. The ensuing hypotension may result in early organ failure because of hypoperfusion, and this is exaggerated in normally hypertensive patients.

Extensive tissue damage from major limb injuries is associated with early cardiovascular decompensation, not only because of blood loss and haematoma formation but also because of extravasation of fluid while oedema is developing. About a quarter of the volume of oedema fluid is contributed by lost plasma volume, and this may amount to 20–30% of the overt blood loss. Clearly, oedema formation increase with time and this becomes more important as the time between injury and examination increases.

The objective of the management of hypovolaemic shock is to maintain tissue oxygenation and restore it to normal values. This entails applying the basic principles of resuscitation of patients with trauma. Resuscitation is followed by definitive treatment (including surgery).

Pulmonary oxygenation

To ensure optimal pulmonary oxygenation, patients with hypovolaemic shock should have a clear airway and adequate ventilation with oxygen at a high inspired concentration. Unconscious patients with severe shock should be intubated and will require positive pressure ventilation. A pneumothorax, haemothorax, or significant gastric distension will impair ventilation and should be treated immediately.

Control of haemorrhage

Peripheral haemorrhage should be controlled with firm pressure and, where possible, by elevation of the injured part.

Symptoms of hypovolaemia according to blood loss*

Blood loss (ml)	Class	Symptoms
<750	I	None
Up to 1500	II	Cardiovascular signs caused by catecholamine release: thirst, weakness, tachypnoea
Up to 2000	III	Systolic pressure falls
>2000	IV	Systolic pressure becomes unreadable

*Assuming a 70 kg patient

Resuscitation of patients with trauma

(1) Adequate pulmonary oxygenation
(2) Control of haemorrhage
(3) Replacement of lost volume
(4) Monitoring the effects of (1), (2), and (3)
(5) Support of myocardial contractility
(6) Relief of pain

Pulmonary oxygenation in patients with hypovolaemic shock

- Ensure a clear airway and adequate ventilation with oxygen at a high inspired concentration
- Intubate patients with severe shock and use positive pressure ventilation

Peripheral haemorrhage

- Control with firm pressure and, where possible, by elevation of the injured part

Replacement of blood loss

In most cases blood loss should be replaced intravenously in the pre-hospital phase, in response to the patient's clinical signs and symptoms.

In all patients with blunt trauma and an anticipated transit time to hospital of more than 15 minutes, intravenous replacement should be started without delay. However, in patients with penetrating torso injury, particularly if the anticipated transit time is short, it is reasonable not to infuse fluid in an attempt to maintain normotension. Aggressive transfusion in such cases may dislodge existing blood clots and will enhance haemorrhage. There will be loss of oxygen carrying capacity and dilution of clotting factors. As there is no prospect of arresting haemorrhage in the field in penetrating torso injury, the priority must be to transport the patient for definitive surgical care without delay. Exceptions to the rule include:

- the entrapped patient, where efforts must be made to achieve a systolic blood pressure of 80 mm Hg during release, and
- patients with head injury, where the priority is to maintain a well oxygenated cerebral perfusion (see chapter 6).

In all patients with blunt trauma estimated to have lost more than 750 ml of blood, the loss should be replaced with intravenous fluid.

Intravenous cannulation

Two short, large bore intravenous cannulae (14 gauge or larger) should be inserted. Blood samples for full blood count, urea and electrolytes, and cross match can be taken from the first cannula.

Easiest access is usually at the antecubital fossa, but anywhere on the upper limb is acceptable. The long saphenous vein at the ankle or the femoral vein in the groin can be used, but these are not ideal if the patient has pelvic or intra-abdominal injuries. If peripheral access is impossible percutaneously, other options include cut down on a peripheral vein, central venous cannulation or the intraosseous route. A cut down has few complications and can be performed quickly with minimal training. Standard large bore cannulae can be inserted by cut down. Possible cut down sites are the antecubital fossa, the saphenous vein at the ankle, and the proximal saphenous vein.

Central venous access may not be easy in the hypovolaemic patient and there is a risk of creating a pneumothorax. Successful central venous cannulation will depend largely on the skill and experience of the operator. If the central route is to be used for rapid fluid resuscitation a relatively short large bore catheter (e.g., 8.5 F pulmonary artery introducer sheath) should be used. In the hypovolaemic patient, central venous pressure monitoring will often be required after the initial fluid challenge; this is best displayed continuously, via a transducer.

The intraosseous route (usually the proximal tibia) is useful in children but will not allow high enough flow rates for effective fluid resuscitation in adults.

A sample for arterial blood gas analysis should be obtained at an early stage. Severely injured patients will have a marked lactic acidosis that will be reflected by a significant base deficit and high plasma lactate (often > 2 mmol per litre). Reversal of the base deficit is an indicator of adequate resuscitation. Insertion of an arterial cannula (radial, brachial, or femoral) will allow continuous direct blood pressure monitoring and is convenient for repeated blood gas sampling. Patients with major injuries are critically ill and warrant invasive monitoring at the earliest opportunity.

Hypotensive resuscitation

- Patients with penetrating torso trauma should be transported to definitive surgical care without delay
- Vigorous fluid infusion to maintain normotension may increase bleeding and cause haemodilution

Intravenous fluid replacement in haemorrhagic shock

Class I haemorrhage <750 ml (15%)	2.5 l Ringer-lactate solution or 1.0 l gelatin solution (or 0.75 l 6% starch)
Class II haemorrhage 750–1500 ml (15–30%)	1.5 l gelatin solution (or 1.5 l 6% starch), plus 1.0 l Ringer-lactate solution
Class III haemorrhage 1500–2000 ml (30–40%)	1.5 l gelatin solution (or 1.5 l 6% starch), plus 1.0 l Ringer-lactate solution and red cells
Class IV haemorrhage >2000 ml (40%)	1.5 l gelatin solution (or 1.5 l 6% starch), plus 1.0 l Ringer-lactate solution and red cells

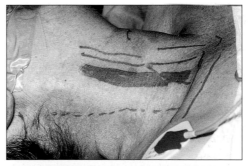

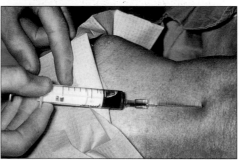

Cannulation of the internal jugular vein. Remember that the neck should not be turned until injury to the cervical spine has been excluded radiologically and clinically.

Choice of intravenous fluid

Principles of fluid management emphasise fast and efficient restoration of intravascular volume. As anaemia is better tolerated than hypovolaemia, fluid resuscitation can initially be with non-blood agents such as a crystalloid (e.g., sodium chloride or Hartmann's solution) or a colloid (e.g., a gelatin or starch solution). Colloids are more efficient, in that equivalent intravascular volume expansion will be achieved with less colloid. However, crystalloids are cheaper than colloids and carry no risk of causing anaphylaxis. Fluid overload is bad for the patient whatever type of fluid is used, and interstitial oedema has several adverse effects (see box).

No prospective, randomised trials have clearly shown that colloids are superior to crystalloids for trauma resuscitation, although a recent meta-analysis purports to show increased mortality with colloids. Double blind studies with the power to define the relative merits of colloids and crystalloids in fluid replacement are unlikely to be carried out, given the complexity of trauma cases and difficulty in establishing matched controls.

Crystalloid solutions—The American College of Surgeons' ATLS committee recommends the use of Hartmann's solution for the initial resuscitation of severely injured patients. Part of the rationale for using crystalloids is that trauma patients will have sustained considerable interstitial fluid losses as well as intravascular loss. Replacement volumes should be three to four times the estimated intravascular loss.

Colloid solutions—Gelatins are the only cheap colloids available that can be infused in relatively unrestricted volumes. They have no effects on the cross matching of blood and act as an osmotic diuretic. It has been suggested that bleeding time is prolonged after the use of gelatin solution for fluid resuscitation, compared with that seen after the use of saline. However, the case is far from proven and further study is required. In comparison with that of other colloids, the intravascular half-life of gelatins is relatively short (approximately 2 hours).

Hydroxyethyl starch solutions—Hydroxyethyl starch (HES) solutions are synthetic polymers derived from amylopectin. The properties of HES solutions vary according to the degree of substitution of hydroxyethyl groups for glucose.

Hetastarch (HES 450/0.7) has an average molecular weight of 450 000 Da. Its high molar substitution ratio (0.7) makes it relatively resistant to breakdown by amylase. This solution has a long half-life (more than 24 hours) and the larger starch molecules tend to accumulate in the reticuloendothelial system. It also causes a coagulopathy via an effect on factor VIII and von Willebrand factor. For these reasons the maximum dose of high molecular weight HES is restricted to 20 ml per kg per day and it cannot be recommended for the resuscitation of trauma patients.

The starches of medium molecular weight (200 000 Da), such as Pentastarch or HAES-Steril (HES 200/0.5) have an intravascular half-life of about 6 hours. The maximum recommended dose for these solutions is 33 ml per kg per day. There is some evidence that 10% HES (200/0.5) results in significantly better systemic haemodynamics and splanchnic perfusion than volume replacement with 20% human albumin. The medium molecular weight starches may reduce capillary leak after trauma.

Hypertonic saline solutions—Hypertonic crystalloid solutions provide small volume resuscitation and rapid restoration of haemodynamics, with laboratory evidence of improved

Adverse effects of interstitial oedema
- Cerebral: reduced conscious level
- Pulmonary: impaired gas exchange
- Myocardial: reduced compliance
- Tissue: impaired wound healing
- Gut: reduced absorption and enhanced bacterial translocation

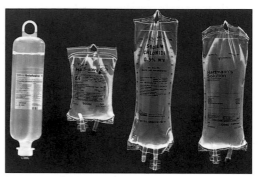

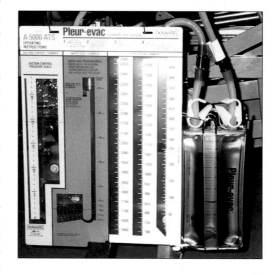

Intravenous fluids.

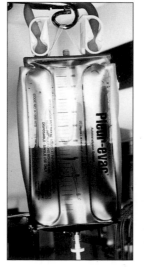

Pleurevac chest drain system, which allows reinfusion of blood drained from the pleural cavity.

microcirculatory haemodynamics. They exert their effect by recruitment of interstitial volume, thus increasing circulating volume and increasing blood pressure. However, raising the blood pressure may not always be an ideal goal, and the role of hypertonic solutions in trauma resuscitation has yet to be defined. Head-injured patients with a score of less than 9 on the Glasgow Coma Scale may benefit from hypertonic saline.

Blood and haemoglobin solutions—Once a patient has lost more than 30–40% of his or her blood volume a resuscitation fluid with good oxygen-carrying capability will become necessary. Currently, this implies the need for a blood transfusion, which unfortunately has several disadvantages (see box).

Several haemoglobin solutions are at an advanced stage of development; problems related to toxic stroma, short intravascular half-life, and high colloid osmotic pressure have been overcome. An increase in mean arterial pressure (an effect related partly to binding of nitric oxide), and decreased viscosity of the haemoglobin solutions, may result in significantly better oxygen delivery to vital organs. However, some clinical studies of haemoglobin solutions have been stopped prematurely because of side effects in the study group. Furthermore, the long term safety of massive transfusion with haemoglobin solutions in humans has yet to be demonstrated.

What is the optimal haematocrit in the acute trauma patient?

Hypovolaemia is tolerated considerably less well than anaemia. Traditional teaching is that all patients require a haematocrit of 30% or a haemoglobin of 10 g per dl for optimal oxygen delivery. However, normovolaemic patients with good cardiopulmonary function will tolerate haemoglobin levels down to at least 7 g per dl. As long as normovolaemia is achieved the reduction in viscosity results in a significant increase in cardiac output and tends to improve tissue oxygenation.

The problem is that a history of ischaemic heart disease or significant respiratory disease may not be available during resuscitation of the acute trauma patient. Furthermore, the haemoglobin concentration of a haemorrhaging patient undergoing resuscitation will be changing rapidly. Under these conditions the margin of safety is small if the haemoglobin concentration is reduced as low as 7 g per dl. Until more data are available, the target haemoglobin concentration of a severely injured patient should be around 10 g per dl.

Fluid warming

All intravenous fluids should be properly warmed. A high capacity fluid warmer, such as the Level 1 (Level 1 HI000, Sims Level 1 Inc, Rockland, MA, USA), will be required to cope with the rapid infusion rates used during resuscitation of a trauma patient. Hypothermia (core temperature below 35°C) is a serious complication of severe trauma and haemorrhage. The causes of hypothermia in a patient requiring massive transfusion include exposure, tissue hypoperfusion, and infusion of inadequately warmed fluids. Hypothermia has several adverse effects (see box), and in trauma patients is an independent predictor of survival.

Monitoring progress and treatment

The volume status of the patient is best determined by observing the vital signs and other monitored variables (see box) after a reasonably large fluid challenge (such as 2 litres of

Disadvantages of blood transfusion

- Blood is antigenic and cross matching takes considerable time
- Blood is expensive and in relatively short supply. The requirement for leucodepletion will increase cost
- Blood has a limited shelf life and requires a storage facility
- Transfusion carries a small but significant risk of disease transmission
- Blood transfusion has an immunosuppressive effect

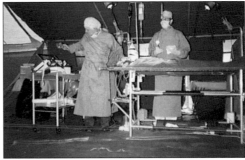

Intravenous infusion in military surgery.

Adverse effects of hypothermia

- A gradual decline in heart rate and cardiac output and increased chance of myocardial dysrhythmias and other morbid cardiac events
- A shift to the left of the oxyhaemoglobin dissociation curve, impairing peripheral oxygen delivery
- Shivering, which may compound the lactic acidosis that typically accompanies hypovolaemia
- Hypothermia contributes to the coagulopathy accompanying massive transfusion
- Mild hypothermia increases the incidence of wound infection

Hartmann's solution or 1 litre of gelatin solution). Fluid resuscitation should be continued to produce an adequate arterial pressure, a urine flow of at least 1 ml per kg per min, and a central venous pressure that responds to a rapid infusion of 200 ml by a sustained rise of more than 3 cm H_2O over the previous value.

Lack of improvement in the patient's vital signs after fluid replacement suggests exsanguinating haemorrhage (associated with major thoracic, abdominal, or pelvic injuries) and the need for immediate surgical intervention and transfusion of blood. Group O blood can be obtained immediately in the emergency room, group confirmed blood can be issued in 10 min, and a full cross match will take 45 min.

A transient response to the initial fluid challenge suggests that the patient may have lost 20–40% of his or her circulating blood volume and has ongoing bleeding; immediate surgical assessment is required and the patient is likely to need blood.

A sustained reduction in heart rate and increase in blood pressure suggests only moderate blood loss (less than 20% of the circulating volume). In the absence of ongoing bleeding, such patients can be effectively resuscitated with clear fluids only.

A rising central venous pressure associated with a low blood pressure, tachycardia, and a reduced urine output indicates tension pneumothorax, cardiac tamponade, or cardiac failure (secondary to cardiac contusion or ischaemic heart disease). Cardiac tamponade is treated by thoracotomy, sometimes preceded by rapid needle pericardiocentesis. Cardiac failure can be confirmed by echocardiography, which will demonstrate a poorly contracting myocardium. The insertion of a pulmonary artery catheter may help to optimise volume replacement. These patients may require inotropic drugs such as dobutamine or adrenaline.

Resuscitation end-points

Some investigators have questioned whether the return to normal of heart rate, blood pressure, and urine output is a suitable resuscitation end-point for the trauma patient. Once bleeding has been controlled and the patient admitted to an intensive care unit, goal directed therapy (increasing oxygen delivery and oxygen consumption to empirically derived values) might increase survival following severe trauma. This approach is highly controversial and requires the early insertion of a pulmonary artery floatation catheter. Most intensive care specialists will use the serum lactate or base deficit as an indicator of adequate oxygen delivery.

Pain relief

Pain relief is essential, not only for compassionate reasons but also because it influences the pathophysiology of hypovolaemic shock by reducing catecholamine secretion. Giving a mixture of 50% nitrous oxide and 50% oxygen (Entonox) before the patient reaches hospital is of value. This should be supplemented with intravenous opioid given in increments (e.g., morphine 5 mg or fentanyl 50 micrograms) and titrated to effect. An antiemetic drug should be given intravenously if an opioid is given.

Communication with the specialist

Most patients with hypovolaemic shock will require surgical control of bleeding. It is good practice to call the surgical specialist(s) to the emergency department at the earliest opportunity, so that priorities can be assessed and arrangements made for definitive care. Chest radiograph, abdominal

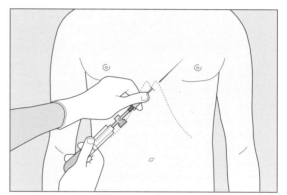

Variables to monitor during fluid replacement
- Peripheral oxygen saturation
- Respiration rate
- Pulse rate
- Arterial pressure
- Pulse pressure
- Central venous pressure
- Urinary output
- Base deficit or lactate
- Temperature
- End tidal carbon dioxide levels
- Mental state
- Changes in the electrocardiogram

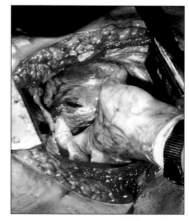

Needle pericardiocentesis.

Resuscitative thoracotomy for cardiac tamponade caused by a stab wound.

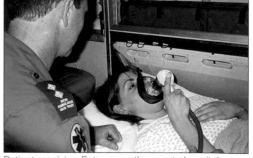

Patient receiving Entonox on the way to hospital.

ultrasound or diagnostic peritoneal lavage, urinary or gastric catheterisation, computed tomography or arterial angiography, as indicated, may help to determine the likely source of haemorrhage. However, patients with severe haemodynamic compromise require immediate surgical intervention on clinical grounds alone.

Summary

Many patients die of hypovolaemic shock, even though the principles of management and treatment are well known and understood. Too often, however, too little clinical treatment is given too late, allowing a malignant, irreversible cycle of pathophysiological changes to be established. Early, aggressive treatment offers the best results in most cases. Reliable intravenous access should be established in accordance with the expertise and experience of the attending clinician. Achieving restoration of tissue perfusion and oxygenation using an appropriate volume of fluid is more important than the choice of intravenous fluid. Fluid resuscitation should be guided by haemodynamic variables, urine output, and serum lactate or base deficit or both.

Early surgery offers the best chance to control ongoing bleeding and an opportunity to correct abnormal physiology. This is particularly important in penetrating torso trauma, where controlled hypotension is acceptable until haemorrhage is arrested.

6 Head injuries

Ross Bullock, Graham Teasdale, Ian Swann

Staff in an accident and emergency department serving a population of 250 000 people can expect each year to treat about 5000 patients who have suffered a head injury—10% of their work. Most attenders are only mildly injured, but head injuries have a reputation for being treacherous. A traumatic intracranial haematoma will develop in fewer than 12 patients each year but can transform an initially mild injury into a life threatening emergency.

In the few patients (less than 5%) who present with persistent impaired consciousness, correct diagnosis and assignment of priorities can be life saving. The limited availability of specialist neurosurgical facilities in the United Kingdom means that only 1% of patients with head injuries who attend hospital are admitted to a neurosurgical unit.

Management guidelines

In recent years the development of agreed guidelines for the management of head injury has simplified the task for staff in accident and emergency departments. These guidelines reflect increased knowledge of the mechanisms of head injury, improved methods of assessment and diagnosis, and more accurate identification of those patients who are at risk of brain damage.

However, while there is a sound body of evidence for a rational approach to the management of head injuries, few key aspects of management have been, or even could be, the subject of randomised prospective controlled trials. As a result, several sets of guidelines have been produced in the United Kingdom and in other countries. All share common principles and approaches, and staff in each accident and emergency department should determine the specific application of the chosen guidelines in their own circumstances, in consultation with colleagues in other specialties such as neurosurgery.

Advice given in this article accords with guidelines recommended by the Society of British Neurological Surgeons[1] that were included in a report from a Working Party of the Royal College of Surgeons of England on the management of patients with head injuries.[2]

Principal aims of management

The two main aims of management of patients with head injuries are:
● to provide the best conditions for recovery from any brain damage already sustained; and
● to prevent or treat complications leading to secondary brain damage.

Head injury patients and common causes of injury

Characteristics of patients with head injuries attending accident and emergency departments in Scotland. Numbers are percentages of patients

Male	70
Adult	60
Child	40
Recently drunk alcohol	25
Type of injury	
Scalp laceration	40
Skull fracture	2
Conscious level	
Never unconscious	80
Recovered from amnesia	15
Impaired	3.5
Cause of injury	
Fall	14
Assault	16
Road traffic accident	18
Domestic	18
Sport	12
Work	8

Role of accident and emergency and trauma staff in management of head injuries

● Resuscitate, diagnose, and record
● Detect or exclude other injuries
● Request, supervise, and interpret results of radiography and other initial investigations
● Decide if admission is needed and if so, where
● Liaise with other specialties—for example, neurosurgery—about serious cases
● Ensure adequate arrangements for observing and maintaining patient's condition during transfer to other departments or hospitals
● Observe progress of patients with minor injuries, who should be admitted to short stay beds
● Ensure adequate arrangements for follow up

Mechanisms of brain damage

Immediate damage to the brain as a result of severe head injury may be diffuse or focal, and damage can also ensue because of hypoxia, ischaemia and raised intracranial pressure.

Diffuse damage

The brain is poorly anchored within the skull and its soft consistency renders it liable to move within the skull in response to acceleration or deceleration.

Contact between the surface of the brain and the interior skull causes bruising (contusions), particularly at the frontal and temporal poles. Distortion of the brain caused by internal shearing forces leads to stretching and tearing of axonal tracts within the white matter. Such diffuse axonal injury manifests itself as microscopic retraction balls at the site of damaged fibres; these are widespread in severe injuries, but mild stretch injury with reversible loss of function is also responsible for the transient disturbance of consciousness known as "concussion".

Focal impact damage

Skull fracture—At the point of impact the skull deforms inwards and fracture may occur. Such fractures are less common in children than in adults because of their more elastic skulls.

A compound depressed fracture results when a violent sharp blow lacerates the scalp and drives bone fragments into the intracranial cavity, sometimes tearing the dura mater and exposing the surface of the brain. An injury of this type is an important source of intracranial infection and requires prompt surgical elevation and debridement. A depressed fracture is also a powerful cause of epilepsy, but the risk of this complication is not influenced by surgical treatment.

A linear fracture is important chiefly as an indicator of potential secondary intracranial bleeding.

Extradural haematoma—Inbending of the skull may strip off underlying dura and create a space in which an extradural haematoma develops. This can be associated with little primary brain damage, and optimal management should minimise mortality and morbidity caused by secondary cerebral compression. Delay in treatment can cause irreversible cerebral damage.

Intradural haematoma—Subdural and intracerebral bleeding are four times more common than extradural haematoma. They result from tearing of cerebral veins or from laceration of the brain's surface, or both. An association with primary brain damage is common, but the outcome may

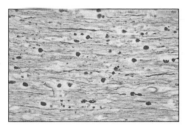

Causes of brain damage after severe head injury.

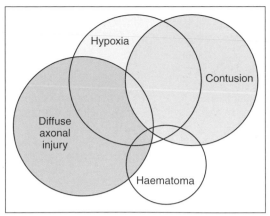

Retraction balls—the microscopic feature of diffuse axonal injury.

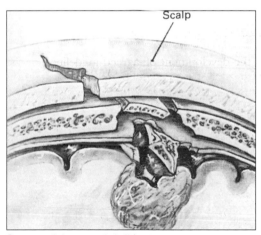

Compound depressed skull fracture.

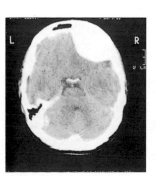

Moderate sized right frontal extradural haematoma.

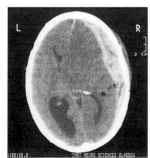

Large right subdural haematoma with pronounced midline shift and contralateral ventricular dilation.

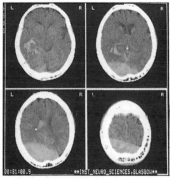

Large occipital extradural haematoma overlying confluence of intracranial venous sinuses with left temporal contusion.

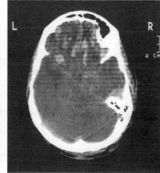

Multiple bifrontal cerebral contusion caused by a fall on to the occiput.

nevertheless be good if an operation is performed promptly. Contusions may coalesce and swell into a space-occupying volume that may need excision. The removal of intradural haematomas requires the facilities and expertise of a neurosurgical unit.

Hypoxia and ischaemia

The brain requires continuous perfusion with well oxygenated blood. Permanent ischaemic neuronal damage occurs within a few minutes if perfusion is reduced below a critical threshold. The brain regulates its own blood supply to maintain constant perfusion, despite variations in systemic blood pressure, but when injured it loses this capacity and so is particularly vulnerable to ischaemic damage when hypotension or hypoxia occur. A mean arterial blood pressure below 60–80 mm Hg, particularly when intracranial pressure is raised, may cause ischaemic neuronal damage if sustained for more than a few minutes.

Multiply injured patients may become severely shocked. When a severe head injury causes unconsciousness the airway is often compromised because of mechanical obstruction or loss of protective reflexes. Early respiratory disorders and bradycardia occur and are a potent cause of ischaemic damage.

Raised intracranial pressure

About 70% of patients persistently in coma after severe head injury have raised intracranial pressure. This jeopardises cerebral perfusion because cerebral perfusion pressure is equal to mean arterial blood pressure minus intracranial pressure.

As intracranial pressure rises cerebrospinal fluid is driven out of the intracranial compartment—the first stage in compensation. As the pressure continues to rise brain shifts occur within the cranial cavity. The most important of these brain shifts is uncal transtentorial herniation or "coning". This causes impairment of conscious level, development of a fixed dilated pupil, and brain stem compression with cardiovascular and respiratory abnormalities.

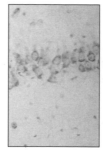
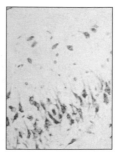

Normal hippocampal neurones (left); shrunken, pyknotic hippocampal neurones irreversibly damaged by ischaemia or hypoxia (right).

Causes of raised intracranial pressure after head injury

- Haematoma
- Focal cerebral oedema related to a contusion or haematoma
- Diffuse oedema after ischaemia (cytotoxic)
- Diffuse brain swelling ("brain engorgement")
- Obstruction of cerebrospinal fluid pathway (this is rare)

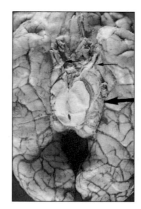

Midbrain sectioned at level of third cranial nerves shows uncal transtentorial herniation or "coning" (large arrow). Note bilateral "notching" of third nerves due to compression against tentorium (small arrows).

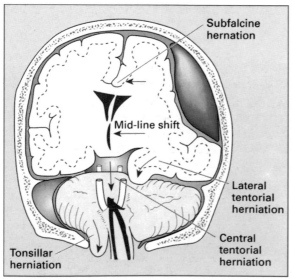

Intracranial contents within closed skull show shifts in response to haematoma.

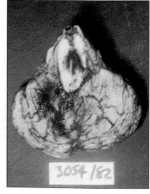

Consequences of unrelieved brainstem compression: "flame shaped" brainstem haemorrhage with irreversible damage to vital centres.

Management of head injuries

For patients with a depressed conscious level the priorities are to establish a clear airway, provide neck control, and stabilise respiration and circulation to prevent further cerebral damage. The risks of secondary complications then need to be assessed and a decision made regarding transfer to a neurosurgical centre.

All patients require ongoing recording of conscious level (by the Glasgow coma scale; see chart)—the best motor response should be used. To exclude traumatic tetraplegia the response to painful stimuli should be tested by supraorbital nerve compression if limb responses are absent. Observation of the patient may be in hospital or, in certain cases, at home, provided that he or she can be discharged into the care of a responsible adult.

Priorities for management depend on whether the patient can talk. If he or she cannot do so, intracranial and extracranial complications are more likely. Life threatening airway, respiratory and circulatory conditions should be treated as soon as they are identified. Urgent blood tests include blood glucose, arterial blood gas analysis and a coagulation screen.

In patients who can talk, document their history, duration of amnesia after trauma, mechanism of injury, previous medical and surgical history, and previous intake of drugs and alcohol.

When the secondary survey has been completed, give tetanus prophylaxis when indicated.

Guidelines for endotracheal intubation

If injury of the cervical spine has not been excluded, intubate the patient with the neck stabilised by an assistant or by using sandbags and forehead tape. Always assume a full stomach and use a rapid sequence of induction, with cricoid compression. Not all intubated patients need artificial ventilation.

Short acting drugs (e.g. thiopentone, etomidate, propofol, and suxamethonium, atracurium, and vecuronium) should be used to facilitate intubation, which should be performed by an experienced person (usually an anaesthetist).

A cuffed endotracheal tube should be used, except in young children, and securely fixed to the patient with a neck halter and adhesive strapping. After intubation adjust the position of the tube to ensure air entry in both lungs—intubation of the right main bronchus is common. An anaesthetist (or other experienced person) should accompany an intubated patient during transfer within the hospital or between hospitals.

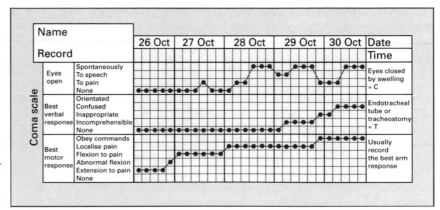

Name Record		26 Oct	27 Oct	28 Oct	29 Oct	30 Oct	Date Time
Eyes open	Spontaneously / To speech / To pain / None						Eyes closed by swelling = C
Best verbal response	Orientated / Confused / Inappropriate / Incomprehensible / None						Endotracheal tube or tracheostomy = T
Best motor response	Obey commands / Localise pain / Flexion to pain / Abnormal flexion / Extension to pain / None						Usually record the best arm response

(Coma scale)

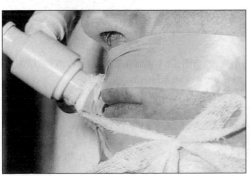

Intubated patient with head injury. Note secure fixation of endotracheal tube.

Additional factors to record

In addition to the factors recorded on the Glasgow coma chart the following should be recorded:

- Pupil diameter and reaction to light
- Pulse and blood pressure
- Temperature and respiration
- Movement of all limbs

Management of patients who cannot talk

- **Airway with cervical spine control**—Definitive control of airway; immobilise cervical spine
- **Breathing**—Analysis of blood gas tensions (PO_2 >13 kPa (100 mm Hg) and PCO_2 <5.3 kPa (40 mm Hg) is acceptable)
- **Circulation**—Restore haemodynamic stability
- **Dysfunction of central nervous system**—Check responses on coma scale, pupils, limb movements
- **Exposure and radiographs**—Remove all clothing and examine "head to toe" (as described in chapter 2). Obtain chest, pelvis and cervical spine radiographs rapidly. If the C7/T1 junction is not visualised, a computed tomogram of the cervical spine can be obtained when CT scanning of the brain is performed

---

Indications for endotracheal intubation in patients with severe head injuries

- Absent gag reflex when oropharyngeal suction is attempted in unconscious patients
- When airway protection is needed—for example, when there is oropharyngeal bleeding, facial fracture, or vomitus that cannot be easily cleared by the patient
- When ventilation or blood gas tensions, or both, are too poor to allow spontaneous ventilation (PaO_2 <9 kPa breathing air or <13 kPa when receiving supplemental oxygen; $PaCO_2$ >5.3 kPa). Exclude pneumothorax on the basis of the chest radiograph
- To allow hyperventilation when a patient's condition is deteriorating because of raised intracranial pressure (discuss with a neurosurgeon)

Indications for skull radiography

If any of the following are present in a fully orientated patient with a head injury, skull radiography should be performed:
- Loss of consciousness, amnesia or vague history of event
- Mechanism of injury implying a strong force of impact
- Symptoms at the time of examination, e.g. severe or generalised headache, nausea or dizziness
- Vomiting
- Suspected skull vault penetration or foreign body injury.

Skull radiography is unnecessary if computed tomography is indicated, for example because of signs of basal skull fracture, depressed fracture evident in a wound, confusion with no other cause such as hypoxia, alcohol/drug intoxication or acute neurological signs.

Computed tomography

Increasing numbers of emergency departments have access to computed tomography for patients with head injuries. The aim should be for every department to have such a scanner and ideally these machines should be of the fast spiral variety. CT scans should be performed urgently within 2–4 hours of admission and the service should be available day and night. If there is doubt about the interpretation of CT scans a neurosurgical opinion should be obtained. The technology to transfer these images electronically exists and should be used if available.

The indications for urgent CT scan are the presence of any of the following factors:[1]
- Coma persisting after resuscitation
- Deteriorating consciousness or progressive neurological signs
- Fracture of the skull with any of the following:
  —confusion or worse impairment of consciousness
  —epileptic seizure
  —neurological symptoms or signs
- Open injury:
  —depressed compound fracture of the skull vault
  —fracture of the base of the skull
  —penetrating injury.

Additional indications for computed tomography in a general hospital are the following:[1]
- Skull fracture, or after a fit
- Confusion or neurological signs persisting after initial assessment and resuscitation
- Unstable systemic state precluding transfer to neurosurgery
- Uncertain diagnosis
- Tense fontanelle or suture diastasis in a child.

Hospital admission and discharge from the emergency department

The following list of indications for admission of patients with head injuries should be displayed in emergency departments.

A. Orientated patient
- Skull fracture or suture diastasis
- Persisting neurological symptoms or signs
- Difficulty in assessment (e.g. suspected use of drugs or alcohol, non-accidental injury, epilepsy, attempted suicide)
- Lack of responsible adult to supervise patient
- Other medical condition-for example, coagulation disorder

B. All patients with impaired consciousness
Note: transient unconsciousness or amnesia with full recovery in an adult is not necessarily an indication to admit but may be in a child.

If the patient is to be observed outside hospital he or she

Indications for referral to a neurosurgical unit after CT in a district general hospital[1]
- Abnormal CT scan
  —high or mixed density intracranial lesion (size and site)
  —shift of midline
  —obliteration of III ventricle
  —relative dilation of a lateral ventricle(s)
  —obliteration of basal cisterns
  —intracranial air
  —subarachnoid or intraventricular haemorrhage
- CT scan normal, but clinical progress unsatisfactory

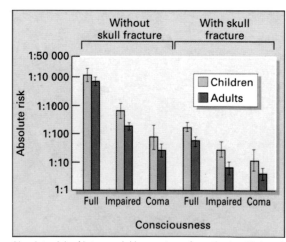

Absolute risk of intracranial haematoma in patients with head injury.

should be discharged with a head injury "warning card" into the care of a responsible person.

The aims of hospital admission are to provide optimal conditions for recovery of the brain and to detect complications before they cause secondary brain damage. The mainstay of admission is neurological observation, which should be hourly for at least the first 24 hours. If the patient has had an abnormal CT scan, but not an operation, repeat scanning is also valuable because worsening in appearances is common.

Drugs in acute head injury

Sedation and analgesia
Sedation and analgesia for patients with head injuries are often a problem; they may be in pain and nauseous, yet strong opiate analgesics and drugs with respiratory depressant effects must be avoided as they may cause iatrogenic deterioration in conscious level and respiratory depression. For adults give paracetamol 250–500 mg every 6 hours or dihydrocodeine preparations such as DF118, or Cocodamol one to two tablets every 4–6 hours. If given parenterally DF118, 30 mg every 6 hours is usually safe and effective. Give metoclopramide 10 mg up to every 8 hours for nausea intravenously or orally. For children paracetamol suspension 125–250 mg every 6 hours is suitable.

Antibiotics
The choice of antibiotic for an established infection—for example, hypostatic pneumonia, wound or intracranial infection—should be guided by identification of the causative organism and its sensitivity. The value of prophylactic antibiotics is controversial because of the risk of developing resistant infection. It is essential to seek advice from the local neurosurgeon.

Mannitol
Mannitol is a powerful osmotic diuretic and may be life saving, but it carries dangers. Use it, in consultation with a neurosurgeon, to "buy time" while the patient is prepared for transfer to the nearest neurosurgical centre. Give 0.5–1 g/kg as a bolus over 10–30 minutes (for adults, usually 250–400 ml of a 20% solution). A catheter should be inserted into the bladder.

Steroids
Several trials have shown no clear benefit from steroids, even at high doses.

Management of seizures
Seizures within the first week carry a low risk of future epilepsy but may cause severe hypoxic brain damage. Prevent further seizures with phenytoin as a loading dose of a 10–15 mg/kg bolus given intravenously over 20 min (with electrocardiography) then intravenous infusion of 250–500 mg over 4 hours. Thereafter give 100 mg every 8 hours intravenously or orally.

If seizures persist after phenytoin loading give clonazepam 0.25 mg intravenously incrementally after each seizure. Be prepared to ventilate the patient in an intensive care unit. Intravenous diazepam 5–10 mg may be used if seizures still persist but may cause respiratory depression.

Restlessness
In patients with head injury restlessness is often a warning sign. Do not sedate restless patients without excluding hypoxia, hypotension, metabolic derangement, a full bladder, or pain from other injuries. Consider the "checklist" for secondary deterioration (below) before sedation is prescribed.

HEAD INJURY WARNING CARD

(Accident and Emergency Dept telephone no ....)

This person has recently sustained a head injury and should be kept under regular observation every 2 hours for the first 24 hours. The person should be asked to tell you his or her name, where he or she is, the year, and who you are and should show you that he or she can move all four limbs normally. If asleep, the person should be wakened to do these tests. If the person develops any of the following problems, he or she should be brought back to hospital without delay:

(1) Drowsiness or excessive sleepiness

(2) Confusion or disorientation

(3) Severe headaches, vomiting, or fever

(4) Weakness of any limbs or double vision

(5) Convulsion, seizure, or passing out

(6) Discharge of blood or fluid from ears or nose

Antibiotics in head injury

Indications
- Basal fracture
- Open vault fracture
- Suspected or proven meningitis

Suitable agents
- Benzylpenicillin 1 million units intravenously every 6 hours for 7 days or phenoxymethylpenicillin orally 500 mg every 6 hours (children 10–20 mg/kg/day)
- For patients with penicillin allergy give oral co-trimoxazole 960 mg twice daily

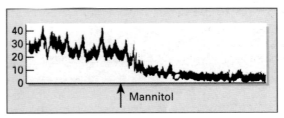

The effect of mannitol in a patient with raised intracranial pressure after severe focal brain injury.

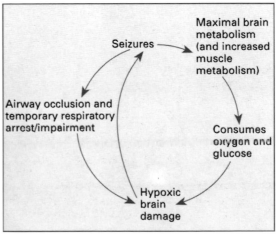

The consequences of uncontrolled seizures.

Secondary deterioration in conscious level

If deterioration in conscious level is apparent the following possibilities should be investigated.

Hypoxia—Assess airway patency and respiration and start or continue treatment with oxygen. Check arterial blood gas tensions and chest radiographs.

Ischaemia—Check pulse, blood pressure, electrocardiogram, and full blood count, particularly if there has been a substantial delay between the patient sustaining the head injury and assessment. Exclude intra-abdominal bleeding (consider peritoneal lavage, CT or ultrasound investigation).

Metabolic derangement—Exclude dehydration and check urea, electrolyte, and blood glucose concentrations.

Missed intracranial haematoma—If hypoxia, ischaemia, and metabolic derangement have been excluded repeat computed tomography urgently.

Seizures—Seizures may not have been witnessed. Control them with drugs. Consult a neurosurgeon.

Meningitis—If meningitis is suspected obtain a computed tomogram to exclude presence of a haematoma, which may cause neck stiffness. Start treatment with high doses of antibiotics immediately. Perform lumbar puncture only after computed tomography has excluded raised intracranial pressure. (Appropriate antibiotic treatment is i.v. penicillin 5 million units every 6 hours and i.v. chloramphenicol 1–2 g every 6 hours.)

Exploratory burr holes

The use of exploratory burr holes in modern management of head injury is extremely limited. Even experienced neurosurgeons miss one third of intracranial haematomas and may start bleeding and worsen brain damage. Use of burr holes may be indicated if a capable surgeon is available and a previously alert patient rapidly deteriorates and develops a fixed dilated pupil that is ipsilateral to a skull fracture and in patients whose transfer to a neurological centre is likely to take 2 hours or more.

Interhospital transfer

It is not feasible for all patients with head injury to be admitted in the first instance to a neurosurgical centre. The district general hospital, ideally equipped with a fast spiral CT scanner, therefore acts as the receiving hospital to diagnose and treat these patients, managing their other injuries and sifting out those who require neurosurgical expertise. The application of current guidelines should indicate appropriate management for most patients, and identify at an early stage the minority who require transfer to a neurosurgical unit. Telephone consultation, supplemented by image transfer, should precede transfer of the patient and help decision making if there is uncertainty.

The events associated with interhospital transfer are a potent cause of avoidable mortality and morbidity after head injury. Problems are caused by:

- Delay in arranging transfer
- Inadequate resuscitation before transfer
- Inadequate preparation for journey
- Inadequate care during the journey.

Hypovolaemic patients not fully resuscitated may develop profound hypotension on an ambulance journey. A patient in a coma should be intubated and accompanied by a doctor with the necessary experience and equipment to cope with any eventuality.

Guide to siting of exploratory burr holes (after discussion with neurosurgeon)

(1) Give 0.5 g/kg of 20% mannitol solution intravenously over 15 minutes while the theatre is prepared

(2) Perform the procedure with the patient intubated and under general anaesthesia. Blood should be cross matched and an intravenous line (preferably plus a central venous line) established

(3) Shave, prepare, and drape the patient for "whole head" access

(4) Place the first burr hole adjacent to the fracture, ipsilateral to the first pupil to dilate or, in the absence of a fracture, in the temporal region (2.5 cm above the zygoma and 2.5 cm behind the zygomaticofrontal ridge)

(5) If an extradural clot is found enlarge the hole, following the clot

(6) If the underlying dura is blue and tense enlarge the burr hole to 5–8 cm in diameter and open the dura and evacuate as much clot as possible.

(7) If no clot is seen beneath the dura make frontal and parietal burr holes ipsilateral to the first dilated pupil

(8) If no haematoma is found, needling the brain is unlikely to be useful. Close the burr holes and transfer the patient to the neurosurgical centre

---

Checklist for interhospital transfer

Airway with cervical spine control—Use an endotracheal tube, or Guedel airway if intubation is inappropriate. Give oxygen by a mask or T piece. Immobilise the neck

Breathing—Give oxygen. Use an Ambu bag and appropriate connectors or portable ventilator (e.g. Oxylog)

Circulation—Once intravenous infusion is established give plasma, Hartmann's solution, or Ringer's solution to maintain haemodynamic stability

Dysfunction of central nervous system—Send with the patient details of conscious level and central nervous system findings at base hospital

Exposure and radiographs—Exposure must be prevented. Keep the patient covered. Ensure documents and radiographs are sent with patient

Outcome after severe head injury

The main determinants of outcome are coma scale score at admission, age, pupillary state, raised intracranial pressure, and the presence of hypoxia or ischaemia. About 40% of patients who are in a coma after initial resuscitation and beyond 6 hours after injury will die. Prognosis should not be estimated too soon because resuscitation and stabilisation may dramatically improve the patient's conscious level.

Late sequelae

Neurological recovery after severe injuries takes about 2 years but is most rapid within the first 6 months. Mental disabilities are far more important for the patient and his or her family than physical impairment. Personality changes, poor motivation, impaired memory and concentration, and lack of emotional restraint are the most common of these. They often cause difficulty with schooling, employment, and family relationships, and patients should be advised against returning to school or employment too soon after a head injury. Psychometric testing often discloses unsuspected difficulties and allows more directed rehabilitation to be formulated.

Common physical sequelae include ataxia, hemiparesis, speech disorders, cranial nerve palsies such as anosmia, unilateral blindness, diplopia, unilateral deafness, and tinnitus. Seizures occur in 4–40% of patients, depending on the nature of the initial injury, focal injuries being more epileptogenic.

Symptoms after minor head injury

In one third of patients with minor head injury, symptoms such as headache, dizziness, irritability, poor concentration, tinnitus, poor balance, fatigue, depression, and intolerance of alcohol will persist for more than 6 months. Many of these "postconcussional" symptoms are attributable to mild diffuse axonal injury, and occur in patients who have been unconscious for only a few minutes and who may have electrophysiological and neuropsychological abnormalities. The symptoms usually subside spontaneously; depression and anxiety may lead to their persistence but malingering is rare. When the symptoms begin only after an appreciable interval psychological factors are likely to be more important.

Specific treatment for postconcussional symptoms is lacking. In the early stages reassurance that severe brain damage has not occurred is important, but patients should not resume activity too rapidly. If the patient has difficulty in coping, anxiety and depression may be provoked and lead to perpetuation of symptoms. Psychotherapeutic support is appropriate, but the value of more formal psychological rehabilitation is not proved. Analgesics are appropriate in the early stages, but the smaller their effect the greater the need for a psychological approach.

Patients who have required admission to hospital following a mild or minor head injury and have a post-traumatic amnesia greater than 1 hour are more likely to benefit from early follow-up.

References

1 Bartlett J, Kett-White R, Mendelow D, Miller JD, Pickard J, Teasdale GM. Working party, British Society of Neurosurgeons. SBNS Guidelines on management of head injury. *Br J Neurosurg* 1998; **12**: 349–52.

2 Royal College of Surgeons of England. *Report of the Working Party on the Management of Patients with Head Injuries*. BSC Print, June 1999. Available at www.rcseng.ac.uk.

Outcome at 6 months after head injury

	Dead or vegetative (%)	Moderate disability or good recovery (%)
Age		
0–29	39	50
30–59	49	34
15–60	81	11
Coma score (best number at 24 h after injury)		
3–5	84	11
6–7	56	29
8–10	28	58
11–15	16	72
Pupils (best reaction at 24 h after injury)		
Both fixed	86	6
One or both reacting	16	72

Moderate and severe deficits (%) in patients with head injuries

	Degree of overall disability	
	Moderate	Severe
Physical handicap	22	
Cognitive impairment	8	78
Personality change	18	89

Proportion (%) of patients with certain neurological symptoms after trauma

	At discharge	At 1 year
Headache	36	18
Dizziness	17	14
Depression	8	18

Suggested further reading

American College of Surgeons. *Advanced Trauma Life Support for Doctors Student Course Manual*. 6th ed. Chicago: ACS, 1997.

Bullock MR, Chesnut RM, Clifton G *et al*. Guidelines for the management of severe head injury. *J Neurotrauma* 1996; **13**: 639–734.

Maas AIR, Dearden M, Teasdale GM *et al* (for The European Brain Injury Consortium). EBIC Guidelines for Management of Severe Head Injury in Adults. *Acta Neurochir* 1997; **139**: 286–94.

Royal College of Radiologists Working Party. *Making the Best use of a Department of Clinical Radiology*, 4th ed. London: RCR, 1998.

Teasdale GM, Murray G, Anderson E *et al*. Risks of traumatic intracranial haematoma in children and adults, implications for managing head injuries. *BMJ* 1990; **300**: 363–7.

Working Party of the British Paediatric Association and British Association of Paediatric Surgeons, Joint Standing Committee in Childhood Accidents. *Guidelines on the Management of Head Injuries in Childhood*. London: British Paediatric Association, 1991.

Working Party of the Neuroanaesthesia Society and Association of Anaesthetists 1996. Recommendations for the transfer of patients with acute head injuries to neurosurgical centres. London: The Anaesthesia Society of Great Britain and the Association of Anaesthetists of Great Britain and Ireland, 1996.

7 Maxillofacial injuries

Iain Hutchison, Peter Hardee

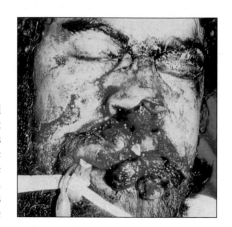

The multiply injured patient may have injuries to the face and neck that are life threatening or serious enough to need specialist advice and management. In the initial assessment such patients may present with obstruction of the airway or hypovolaemic shock as a result of profuse and continuous bleeding from the facial skeleton or its surrounding soft tissues. The resuscitation team must be aware of these problems, know which specialists to call and when, and be able to prevent the demise of the patient before their arrival.

Up to 5% of all patients attending accident and emergency departments may have an injury in the maxillofacial area.

The priority of the resuscitation team is to secure and maintain an airway. However, this action transgresses the site of maxillofacial trauma, which may be littered with broken teeth and dentures, bits of fractured bone, and macerated soft tissue.

When the airway is compromised, or there is continuous facial bleeding, call the maxillofacial team early, and simultaneously institute the measures outlined below.

Management of the airway

Six specific problems associated with maxillofacial trauma may affect the airway.

(1) A fractured maxilla may be displaced postero-inferiorly along the inclined plane of the skull base, blocking the nasal airway.
Management—Disimpact by pulling the maxilla forward, with the index and middle fingers of one hand in the mouth, behind and above the soft palate, and the palm of the other hand braced against the forehead. Advance the maxilla with gentle force initially. TAKE CARE: it is possible to avulse the maxilla totally.

(2) The tongue may lose its anterior insertion in patients with a bilateral anterior mandibular or symphyseal fracture. It may then drop back in a supine patient, blocking the oropharynx.
Management—Insert a deep traction suture (0 gauge black silk) transversely through the dorsum of the tongue and tape the suture on to the side of the face; or, if no suture is available, pull the tongue forward by using a towel clip, or pull the mandible forward manually.

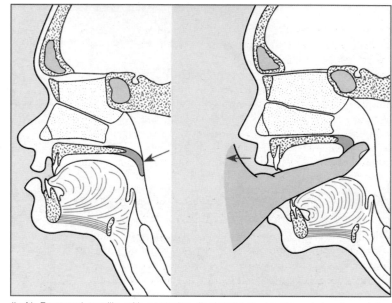

(Left) Fractured maxilla with posterior displacement, causing obstruction of the nasopharynx (arrowed). (Right) Fractured maxilla disimpacted and pulled forward to clear airway.

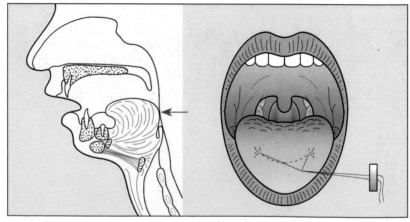

(Left) Fractured mandible with loss of anterior attachment of the tongue. The tongue drops back, blocking the airway (arrowed). (Right) Traction suture in the tongue taped to the face.

(3) Teeth, dentures, bone fragments, vomitus, haematoma, and other foreign bodies may block the airway at any site from the oral cavity through the oropharynx, larynx, and trachea down to the bronchi. The right main bronchus is particularly susceptible. *Management*—(a) Clear the oral cavity by using a gloved finger inserted laterally (just inside the cheek) to the back of the mouth, then hook the finger medially and forward to pull debris out of the mouth. (If the finger is pushed centrally, foreign bodies may be pushed further down the airway.)
(b) Repeat this manoeuvre from the opposite side of the mouth.
(c) Use a large bore sucker (plastic yankauer) and good illumination to aspirate the oral cavity.
(d) Use the laryngoscope and sucker (ignoring potential pain from mandibular fractures) to examine and clean the oropharynx and larynx.

(4) Haemorrhage may result from several causes and obstruct the airway:

(i) Distinct vessels in open wounds
Management—Insert 5 cm ribbon gauze or gauze swabs as a firm compressed pack into the open wound to achieve haemostasis and arrange for definitive treatment. Place two wide-bore cannulae in large peripheral veins and take blood for urgent cross-match and full blood count. Set up a crystalloid infusion.

(ii) The nose, as a result of damage to the anterior or posterior ethmoidal vessels or the terminal portion of the maxillary artery (see management of bleeding).
Management—see page 44 for management of bleeding and technique of nasal packing. Many patients with midface or mandibular fractures will be conscious and able to protect their own airway when upright, but lose their airway when forced to remain supine. Be aware of this and be prepared to protect the patient's airway. Patients may sit up if conscious and there are no other injuries (such as possible cervical spine fracture) that contraindicate this.

After dealing with these immediate problems consider orotracheal intubation.

(5) Soft tissue swelling and oedema. Trauma of the oral cavity causes swelling around the upper airway. This rarely presents an immediate problem, but the swelling may worsen insidiously over a few hours and cause later airway problems.

(6) Maxillofacial trauma may occasionally be associated with trauma to the larynx and trachea, which may cause obstruction of the airway by swelling or displacement of structures such as the epiglottis, arytenoid cartilages, and vocal cords.
Management—(a) Maintain a high index of suspicion if the mechanism of injury suggests trauma to the larynx and trachea: for example, in cases of blunt trauma of the neck caused by impact with a steering wheel.
(b) When there is severe oedema, high dose intravenous steroid therapy (e.g. dexamethasone 8 mg) will reduce the obstruction temporarily, allowing endotracheal intubation.
(c) Note any neck swelling, dyspnoea, voice alteration, or frothy haemorrhage.
(d) Palpate the neck for surgical emphysema (crackling), tenderness, and, before swelling progresses, laryngeal or tracheal crepitus at the site of the fracture.
(e) Arrange for lateral and anteroposterior radiographs of the soft tissues of the neck and mediastinum to be taken urgently to find out whether there is air in the soft tissue.
(f) If suspicion is maintained perform bronchoscopy to determine the site of injury.

Indications for chest radiography or bronchoscopy, or both
- A foreign body is unaccounted for
- A missing tooth or denture is unaccounted for
- Cyanosis, tachypnoea, tachycardia, and respiratory distress
- Deterioration in PaO_2

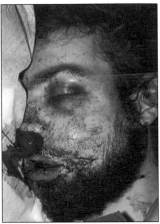
Life threatening haemorrhage from a closed bony injury of the maxilla.

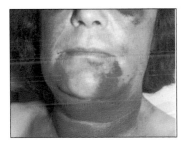
Haematoma and oedema of the neck and floor of the mouth caused by a fractured mandible.

Management of injuries to the larynx and trachea that threaten the airway
- If the injury is above the larynx
  —perform cricothyroidotomy
- If the injury is at the level of the larynx and is incomplete
  —experts may pass an endotracheal tube
  —otherwise, seek specialist opinion for tracheostomy
- If the injury is at the level of the larynx and is complete
  —seek specialist opinion for tracheostomy
- If the injury is in the trachea, below the potential tracheostomy site
  —refer urgently to a thoracic surgeon

Management of bleeding

Soft tissues

Although the scalp, face, and neck have an excellent blood supply, extensive superficial lacerations in this region are not always accompanied by blood loss of such quantity that a transfusion is required. Conversely, small puncture wounds to the skin that scarcely seem to need suturing may cause life threatening haemorrhage if they involve a moderate size artery such as the facial artery or superficial temporal artery. The danger lies in overlooking the continuous trickle of fresh blood from the puncture wound.

Management—These wounds should be dealt with by specialist maxillofacial surgeons.

Initial management comprises application of direct pressure to control haemorrhage. The facial artery can be compressed against the lower border of the mandible just anterior to the masseter muscle. The superficial temporal artery can be compressed against the cranium just anterior to the ear.

Definitive management is as follows:
(a) Assess wounds regularly for blood loss.
(b) If haemorrhage continues explore the wounds and clip or ligate bleeding vessels.
(c) Extend puncture wounds along natural skin crease lines to locate bleeding vessels.
(d) If profuse bleeding occurs from a neck wound, consider whether there is enough time for ultrasound examination or arteriography, check arm pulses, extend the wound to expose the major vessels in the neck (usually along the anterior border of the sternomastoid), control the bleeding, and assess damage.

Small vessels off the external carotid artery can be ligated. Large arteries (for example, the carotid and subclavian arteries) usually require repair. It is possible to ligate one internal jugular vein without untoward effect, and it may be possible to ligate one common carotid artery without causing a stroke.
(e) If there is a continuous trickle of fresh blood from the neck wound in a stable patient, arrange ultrasound examination or arteriography to assess major vessels before open exploration.

Bone

Significant haemorrhage also occurs occasionally in patients with closed injuries to the bony structures of the middle third of the face—that is, the maxilla, nose, and ethmoids. This presents as a steady flow of blood from the nose and oral cavity and bleeding into the soft tissues of the face, producing profound cheek swelling with a shiny, tense skin.

Two problems exist:
(i) Failure to recognise the extent of blood loss and subsequent development of a coagulopathy.
(ii) Inability to define the source of the arterial bleeding—fractures of the middle third of the face are usually bilateral, with disruption of the nasal septum, so that haemorrhage from one side manifests equally at both nostrils.

Management—(a) In the intubated patient, if possible, palpate the posterior pharyngeal wall with your index finger through the mouth, feeling for tears and fractures, which can be the site of profuse bleeding.
(b) Disimpact the maxilla, place mouth props between upper and lower molars then insert and inflate Epistats to splint the maxilla between the base of the skull and the mandible. The latter is supported by the cervical collar (which, in turn, is stabilised on the upper thorax). If Epistats are not available, use anterior and posterior nasal packs.

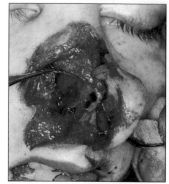

Apparently simple nasal soft tissue injury, which on exploration needed extensive repair.

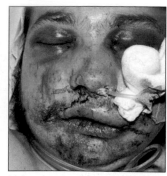

Major haemorrhage caused by closed maxillofacial trauma, treated by anterior and posterior nasal packing.

Procedure for anterior and posterior nasal packing

If the maxilla is mobile, first place mouth props between the upper and lower molars on both sides, otherwise the balloons cannot exert tamponade

A. Using Epistats

(1) Insert Epistat* into each nostril, aiming for a finger tip inserted into the mouth to the back of the soft palate, so that the posterior cuff is resting in the nasopharynx
(2) Inflate the posterior cuff (via the white colour-coded valve) with up to 10 ml of saline
(3) Withdraw the Epistat until resistance is felt at the nasopharyngeal cuff
(4) Inflate the nasal (anterior) cuff (via the green colour-coded valve) with up to 30 ml of saline
(5) Suction catheters can be inserted down the central lumen to aid in cleaning debris from the nasopharynx

B. Procedure in the absence of Epistats

(1) Insert 12/14 G Foley catheters with 20 ml balloons into the nose, aiming for a finger tip inserted into the mouth to the back of the soft palate
(2) Inflate balloons when the tip of the catheter is in the postnasal space
(3) Pull back the catheter until the balloon occludes against the choana at the back of the nose
(4) Tie the catheters together after passing behind the head, catheter from right alar to go round the left side of the head, and release periodically to prevent ischaemic necrosis
(5) Insert bismuth iodoform paraffin paste 5 cm ribbon gauze packs into the nose in front of the balloon and Foley catheter

TAKE CARE NOT TO INSERT EPISTATS OR FOLEY CATHETERS IN A CRANIAL DIRECTION.
SOME PATIENTS WILL HAVE A BASE OF SKULL FRACTURE AND THERE IS THEN A RISK OF THEM ENTERING THE CRANIAL CAVITY

Secondary survey

Once the airway has been secured and haemorrhage arrested, the definitive management of soft tissue and bone trauma of the face and neck can be deferred until life threatening neuro-surgical, thoracic, abdominal, and neurovascular limb injuries have been dealt with. It may be appropriate, however, to perform simultaneous procedures or even combined operations, particularly when cranial trauma is combined with facial trauma.

Examination

(1) Expose the affected area by cleaning all wounds and the face and scalp with Savlon (0.15% cetrimide). **Do not discard any loose bone or soft tissue fragments.**

(2) Examine the scalp for lacerations and bruises, not forgetting the back of the scalp if it is possible to move the patient—that is, if a cervical spinal injury has been excluded or the cervical spine is immobilised.

(3) Examine the eyes for:
● Visual acuity—can the patient count fingers? Can he or she read print? If possible, use a Snellen chart.
● Limitation of eye movements, diplopia, or unequal pupillary levels. If one or more of these is present suspect trauma of the orbital floor or medial wall with entrapment of periorbital tissues.
● Direct, consensual, and accommodation reflexes. Examination of these may help detect a rise in intracranial pressure, but be aware of false positive signs caused by trauma to the globe, resulting in post-traumatic mydriasis, and retrobulbar haemorrhage.
● Proptosis (or exophthalmos)—this suggests haemorrhage within the confines of the orbital walls.
● Enophthalmos—this suggests fracture of an orbital wall (usually the floor or medial wall).
● Periorbital swelling—if this is present, suspect a fracture of the zygoma or maxilla.
● Subconjunctival ecchymosis—if this is present suspect direct trauma to the globe, or a fractured zygoma.
Examine the anterior chamber and fundus for evidence of direct trauma and raised intracranial pressure.
Particularly consider the following possible diagnoses:
● Retrobulbar haemorrhage—haemorrhage within the orbit causes proptosis, pain and decreasing visual acuity. This is a surgical emergency requiring immediate specialist attention. Medical management with intravenous acetazolamide, mannitol and steroids may gain time in which to transfer the patient to the operating theatre.
● Ruptured globe—the globe must be examined in all facial trauma patients. If you are unable to do so, seek specialist advice. If the eye is painful or impossible to examine because of blepharospasm, damage to the globe is highly likely.

(4) Examine the nose for:
● Deformity, pain, mobility, and difficulty in breathing.
● Bleeding and leakage of cerebrospinal fluid. If present suspect anterior cranial fossa fracture at the cribriform plate. Do not pass a nasal endotracheal tube or nasogastric tube. Measure the intercanthal distance. If it is more than 3.5 cm suspect nasoethmoidal fracture.

(5) Examine the ears for bleeding and leakage of cerebrospinal fluid. If present, give prophylactic antibiotics.

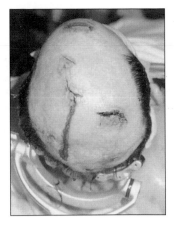
Underneath this apparently minor scalp injury was a fractured skull.

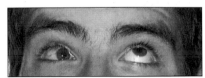
Limitation of upward gaze denoting an orbital floor fracture.

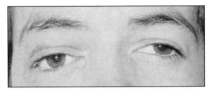
Proptosis and depression of right pupillary level caused by fractured orbital roof and intraorbital haematoma.

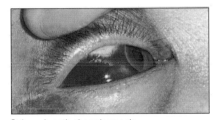
Subconjunctival ecchymosis.

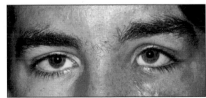
Left medial canthal damage with characteristic almond shaped palpebral fissure and increased intercanthal distance.

Causes of bleeding from the ears

Site	Indication
Anterior wall of the external auditory meatus	Fracture of the condylar neck of the mandible
Posterior wall or middle ear	Fracture of the base of the skull in the middle cranial fossa
Ecchymosis behind the ear (Battle's sign) —usually presents after 48 h	Probable middle cranial fossa fracture

(6) Examine the soft tissues for:

● Sensory (V nerve) impairment (e.g. of the upper or lower lip) and motor (VII nerve) deficit—this may have a peripheral or central cause. Consider this in relation to other injuries.

● Surgical emphysema around the eyes and on the face. This suggests continuity between sinuses and face as a result of facial fracture. To avoid emphysema instruct patients not to blow their nose. (Surgical emphysema in the face should be distinguished from that in the neck, which is caused by trauma to the larynx, trachea, or lungs.) If present, give prophylactic antibiotics (e.g. amoxycillin 250 mg three times a day for 5 days).

● Venous engorgement of the face. If present, suspect trauma to the major vessels in the thorax or neck.

● Pooling of tears and leakage from the eye. This may indicate damage to the lacrimal apparatus.

● Leakage of pink or clear fluid from a facial wound. If present suspect damage to the parotid salivary gland or duct.

(7) Examine the face for lengthening, bilateral swelling, "panda eyes", and dish face deformity.
If any of these are present suspect bilateral maxillary fracture.

(8) Palpate around the orbit for step defects, particularly at the frontozygomatic and zygomaticomaxillary sutures, and the zygomatic arch. Such defects indicate fracture to the zygoma or maxilla. Isolated zygomatic arch or body of zygoma fractures can cause a restriction in mouth opening.

(9) Palpate the mandible externally from the condyle and along the lower border for tenderness, step defects, and crepitus.

(10) Examine intraorally for haematoma (especially under the tongue—this indicates mandibular fracture), lacerations, bleeding, loose teeth, broken teeth and dentures, mobile jaw segments, abnormal alignment of the jaw and step defects, and teeth meeting prematurely. If possible, ask the patient to bite together on their back teeth. Do the teeth meet evenly? If unsure, ask the patient if it feels right. If teeth lost because of the trauma are not accounted for, a chest radiograph is mandatory.

(11) Using both hands, palpate the middle third of the face for mobility. Place the thumb and fingers of the right hand on either side of the anterior maxillary teeth (with the thumb in front and the index finger on the palatal side). Place the palmar surface of the left hand across the forehead. Pull the premaxillary segment forward gently and see whether nose or cheek bones move, indicating a maxillary fracture at the Le Fort I, II, or III level. Any combination of Le Fort fractures can be present on one or both sides.

Imaging and investigation

Good quality maxillofacial radiographs help in definitive planning and treatment. Radiologists and maxillofacial surgeons can advise on suitable investigations, but generally:

● If there are missing and unaccounted for teeth, crowns or dentures—chest radiograph (and lateral neck soft tissue exposure for dentures).

● For possible vascular damage from a penetrating neck wound —ultrasound or angiography if the clinical state allows delay.

● For possible mandibular fracture—posteroanterior view of mandible with a rotational tomogram is ideal (alternatively, right and left oblique lateral mandible if rotational tomography is not available).

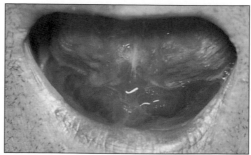
Sublingual haematoma caused by mandibular fracture.

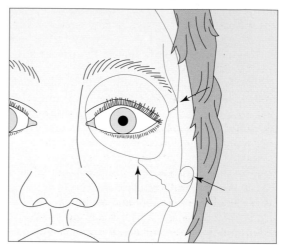
Palpate frontozygomatic and zygomaticomaxillary sutures and the zygomatic arch for tenderness and steps.

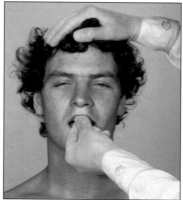
Pull on the anterior maxilla while supporting the frontal bone to show movement of the maxilla on the base of the skull, indicating maxillary fracture.

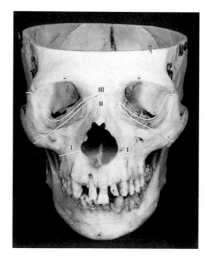
Le Fort I, II and III fracture lines marked on the skull.

- For possible midfacial fracture—occipitomental radiographs 10° and 30° after cervical spine fracture has been excluded. Lateral skull radiographs are of little additional benefit.
- If a nasoethmoidal fracture is suspected—occipitofrontal radiographs.
- For a head injury requiring computed tomography—if a rapid (spiral) scanner is available, imaging of the facial bones and mandible requires less than 1 minute of additional scanning time, and should be performed at the same session. Fine 2 mm cuts need to be requested.
- If the patient is uncooperative—consider postponing non-urgent investigations such as occipitomental and mandibular views until later. Poor quality radiographs taken in suboptimal conditions do little to help management.

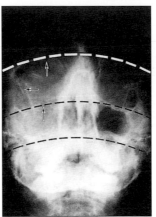

Anteroposterior occipitomental radiograph taken in the initial assessment period of a multiply injured patient. Examine along these standard arcs for evidence of fractures (arrowed).

Pain management

- Soft tissue injuries—these are rarely painful. Marked pain should therefore raise suspicion of an underlying bony injury.
- Facial or mandibular fracture—the pain here is mainly caused by the grating of bone ends. Therefore, this is more of a problem in mandibular fractures. Opiates are best avoided as it makes interpretation of eye signs in a possible coexisting head injury more difficult.

Diclofenac 100 mg followed by 50 mg three times daily is an excellent analgesic, and can be given rectally, intramuscularly or orally (but obviously avoid the oral route if the patient may need an operation). Ketorolac has the advantage that it can be used intravenously in patients aged over 16. The dose is 10 mg i.v. over 15 seconds, then 10–30 mg every 4–6 hours as required.

For patients in whom non-steroidal anti-inflammatory drugs (NSAIDs) should be avoided, such as those with asthma who are sensitive to NSAIDs, use codeine phosphate (60 mg every 4 hours in adults).

Communication with the specialist

- For all patients, mention whether there are any other injuries, particularly whether there is a head injury, and whether the patient is stable with respect to the respiratory and cardiovascular systems.
- Is there major bleeding in the maxillofacial area, or airway problems requiring immediate attendance?
- For midfacial fractures—are there any concomitant ophthalmic injuries? What is the visual acuity?
- For mandibular fractures, is there a single fracture (rare) or bilateral fractures (more common, and a greater potential risk to the airway)?

Conclusion

Major maxillofacial injuries may occur in isolation or in combination with other injuries. They pose problems because they are intimidating and obstruct access to the airway. Rarely, they may be the cause of life threatening haemorrhage, which is often overlooked. The definitive management of soft tissue and bone injuries of the face and neck can usually be deferred while life threatening thoracic, abdominal, and neurological injuries are dealt with. It may be appropriate, though, for the maxillofacial surgeon to help the anaesthetist and perform a fuller assessment, wound toilet, and preparatory procedures while the patient is anaesthetised. Combined procedures with specialists such as neurosurgeons may also be indicated.

Further reading

Banks P. *Killey's fractures of the mandible.* 4th ed. Bristol: Wright Publishing, 1991.

Banks P. *Killey's fractures of the middle third of the facial skeleton.* 4th ed. Bristol: Wright Publishing, 1991.

Hutchison IL, Magennis P, Shepherd JP, Brown AE. The BAOMS United Kingdom Survey of facial injuries. Part 1. Aetiology and the association with alcohol consumption. *Br J Oral Maxillofac Surg* 1998; **36**: 3–13.

Hutchison IL. Facio-maxillary and dental injuries. In: Skinner D, Swain A, Peyton R, Robertson C, eds. *Cambridge textbook of accident and emergency medicine.* 1st ed. Cambridge: Cambridge University Press, 1997.

Hutchison IL. Maxillofacial trauma. In: Driscoll P, Skinner D, eds. *Trauma care: beyond the resuscitation room.* 1st ed. London: BMJ Books, 1998.

Rowe NL, Williams JLl, eds. *Maxillofacial injuries* Volumes I and II. 2nd ed. London: Churchill Livingstone, 1997.

*Epistats are available from Xomed Surgical Products Inc., 6743 Southpoint Drive North, Jacksonville, FL 32215, USA.

8 The spine and spinal cord

Andrew Swain, John Dove, Harry Baker

A patient with serious multiple injuries is rarely able to provide a coherent history. Injuries that carry a risk of death or severe disability must, therefore, be suspected from the outset so that correct early management can be instituted. Any patient with trauma who is not fully conscious should be assumed to have an injury of the cervical spine until proved otherwise. The thoracolumbar spine must also be managed carefully. The most common reason for failing to detect an important spinal injury is failure to suspect one, particularly in patients with multiple trauma; but sometimes a serious injury is considered minor.

The spinal cord is most often damaged in the cervical region, but it is also particularly at risk near the thoracolumbar junction. The thoracic spine is splinted by intact ribs and sternum, but the spinal canal is narrower in this region relative to the width of the spinal cord so when vertebral displacement occurs it is more likely to damage the cord. Partial cord injuries are generally more common, and the potential for neurological improvement or deterioration is correspondingly greater.

Management at the scene of the accident

Spinal trauma may be suspected from a witness's description of an accident. It cannot, however, be excluded without a definitive examination, even in the fully conscious patient. The neck must be aligned in the neutral position without longitudinal compression or distraction. This will improve the airway and reduce spinal deformity, helping to relieve pressure on the spinal cord or arteries. If the patient is a motorcyclist the doctor should support the neck from below while an assistant carefully eases the helmet off. The neck is then splinted with a rigid collar of appropriate size to grip the chin. Collars alone are inadequate and they need to be supplemented by manual stabilisation or lateral support with bolsters and forehead tape. Be wary of swelling under the collar, which may develop from a haematoma or surgical emphysema.

In the unconscious patient the airway should be opened by chin or jaw lift and an oropharyngeal airway inserted. The supine position facilitates clinical examination, resuscitation, respiratory movements, and control of the neck, but tracheal intubation is required to prevent aspiration. Alternatively the patient can be turned into the lateral position with the trunk straight but inclined forwards by 20°, allowing secretions to discharge freely from the mouth. The three quarters prone or coma position cannot be recommended as it entails rotation of the cervical spine and splints the diaphragm, causing hypoventilation.

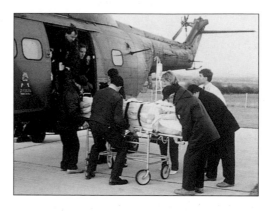

Incidence (percentage) of neurological injury in patients with fractures or dislocations of various parts of the spine

Part of spine	Incidence
Any	14
Cervical spine	40
Thoracic spine	10
Thoracolumbar junction	35
Lumbar spine	3

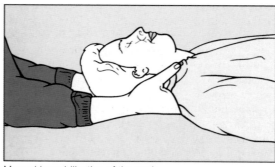

Manual immobilisation of the neck.

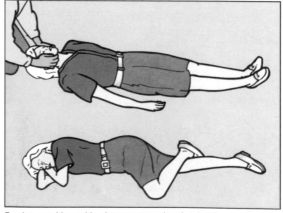

Supine position with airway protection (top); lateral recovery position (bottom).

Thoracolumbar injury must also be assumed and treated by carefully straightening the trunk and correcting rotation. The patient may be log rolled (ideally by four assistants), but it is vital that the whole spine is maintained in the neutral position.

The neck and back can be protected simultaneously in supine patients by means of a spinal board incorporating a head immobiliser. From the lateral position, the casualty is rolled back on to the board. Spine immobilisers, for example, Kendrick or Russell extrication devices, are lighter and can be applied to a sitting patient. Doctors should familiarise themselves with the splints that are available locally.

Transfer to hospital

Once the airway is protected, high-concentration oxygen has been administered and the patient positioned, one or more intravenous infusions are established. If conditions allow, the patient should be examined briefly before transportation. In the absence of life threatening injury the patient with spinal trauma should be transported steadily (not slowly) to hospital. Hard objects should be removed from anaesthetic parts of the body.

Arrival at hospital: primary survey

Safe transfer of the patient from the ambulance to a trauma trolley is best achieved with the patient strapped to a spinal board, which is not removed until spinal injury has been excluded. A scoop stretcher is less satisfactory. If the casualty is unco-operative, every effort should be made to persist with the collar although additional splintage may be resisted and counterproductive.

Airway (with protection of the cervical spine)

Patients with multiple trauma are invariably kept supine during resuscitation unless regurgitation occurs and the airway is unprotected. In such an emergency the patient may be tipped head down on the spinal board and oropharyngeal suction applied. In patients with cervical cord injury, pharyngeal stimulation by vigorous suction, manipulation of a Guedel airway or intubation may result in unopposed vagal discharge and cardiac arrest. This can be prevented by prior administration of atropine.

Many seriously injured patients require intubation, and this is not contraindicated in patients with an unstable cervical injury. The procedure should, however, be performed whenever possible by an experienced anaesthetist and spinal movement minimised by an assistant controlling the head and limiting movement. Alternative methods of intubation that do not require the neck to be moved—for example, blind tracheal intubation and use of a fibreoptic laryngoscope—should be employed only by those with the necessary experience. Whether the patient is breathing spontaneously or not, pulse oximetry is required and capnography if available. Ileus develops after spinal cord injury, and a nasogastric tube is required.

Circulation

Patients with injury to the cervical cord or high thoracic cord may have reduced sympathetic outflow between the T1 and L2 segments with associated bradycardia and hypotension. Patients must be connected to a cardiac monitor on admission. Tetraplegic patients with bradycardia should be given atropine if their pulse rate drops below 50 beats/min.

Haemorrhage is the most common cause of post-traumatic shock but bradycardia with hypotension is not a classical feature

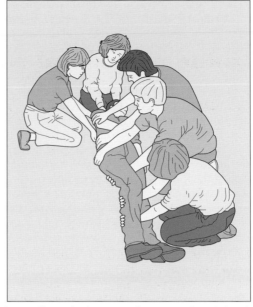

Log rolling: deployment of personnel and hand positions used when moving a patient with possible spinal injury from the supine to the lateral position.

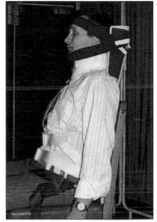

Semirigid collar and spine immobiliser.

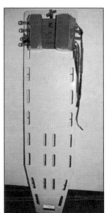

Spinal board with head immobiliser.

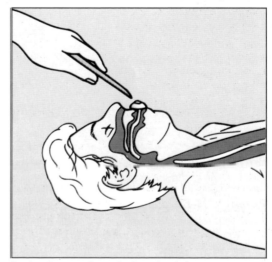

Suction: beware of vagal reflex stimulation.

of hypovolaemic shock, and in a traumatised patient it should increase suspicion of spinal cord injury. The extent of bradycardia and hypotension in neurogenic shock depends on the level and degree of neurological injury. Bradycardia may not be accompanied by hypotension, and peripheral vasodilation may be an important clue. If the systolic blood pressure falls below 80 mm Hg, inotropic support is necessary. Bradycardic shock is also seen in elderly patients and patients taking β blockers.

In recent years the importance of maintaining adequate tissue perfusion and oxygenation in patients with spinal cord trauma has been emphasised. Episodes of hypotension or hypoxia often lead to irreversible neurological deterioration. Patients with spinal trauma are likely to have hypovolaemia owing to other injuries. Circulatory volume must be restored, but aggressive fluid replacement is detrimental in patients with purely neurogenic hypotension as it precipitates pulmonary oedema. Therefore traumatised patients with bradycardia and hypotension should be subjected to a fluid challenge and the response observed and monitored by measuring central venous pressure. For this, cannulation of the subclavian vein is recommended because access to the internal jugular vein is difficult to obtain without rotating the neck.

Secondary survey

Any injury to the spinal cord carries a high risk of early and late medical complications. Important early complications include respiratory failure as a result of intercostal paralysis or partial phrenic nerve palsy, impaired ability to expectorate, and ventilation-perfusion mismatch. The patient's respiratory state may also deteriorate shortly after admission as a result of ascending oedema in the traumatised cervical cord. Opioid analgesics should be given in small doses as necessary, but care must be taken as they will further impair respiration. Cardiac arrest usually results from respiratory failure. Blood gas tensions must be checked. Pulse oximetry is important and vital capacity should exceed 1 litre.

Abdominal trauma is not easily assessed in tetraplegic patients as the abdominal wall is anaesthetic, flaccid, and areflexic and ileus results from the neurological injury. A useful positive sign is pain at the tip of the shoulder that is aggravated by abdominal palpation. Peritoneal lavage is a useful diagnostic aid in patients with cervical or thoracic cord injury although ultrasonography has gained popularity and computed tomography is recommended in stable patients.

Acute retention will develop in paraplegic and tetraplegic patients unless the sacral segments are spared. Measurement of urine output in patients with multiple trauma is important, and the bladder will usually require drainage, particularly if the patient has been drinking. In the absence of urethral trauma a narrow gauge Silastic catheter with a small (5 ml) balloon is passed under strictly aseptic conditions and taped to the anterior abdominal wall to prevent unnecessary movement of and injury to the urethra, which may lead to sepsis. Alternatively a suprapubic catheter can be inserted.

The conscious patient

Sensory loss or motor symptoms should never be disregarded, no matter how unimportant they seem. Diagnosis of spinal cord injury relies on symptoms and signs of pain in the spine with sensory loss and disturbances in motor function distal to a neurological level. The pain may radiate down the spine like an electric shock or into the limbs owing to nerve root irritation. A full neurological examination must be performed, including testing of cranial nerves, sensation to fine touch and pin prick, proprioception, power, tone, coordination, and reflexes.

Treat
- Bradycardia—pulse <50 beats/min
- Hypotension—systolic blood pressure <80 mm Hg
- Inadequate urinary excretion

Do not rotate the patient's neck during central venous cannulation unless cervical injury has been excluded by both radiographic and clinical assessment

Monitor always
- Heart rate
- Blood pressure
- Temperature
- Oxygen saturation
- Electrocardiogram
- Urine output

Monitor where practical/available
- End-tidal CO_2
- Central venous pressure
- Vital capacity

Causes of respiratory insufficiency

In tetraplegic patients
- Intercostal paralysis
- Partial phrenic nerve palsy
  —immediate
  —delayed
- Impaired ability to expectorate
- Ventilation–perfusion mismatch

In paraplegic patients
- Variable intercostal paralysis according to level of injury
- Associated chest injuries
  —rib fractures, pulmonary contusion, haemopneumothorax

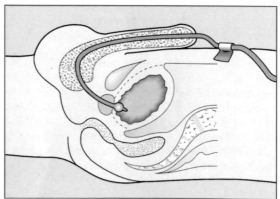

Method of catheterisation in patients with spinal cord injury.

Myotomes	Reflexes	
Muscle group	*Nerve supply*	
Diaphragm	C(3),4,(5)	
Shoulder abductors	C5	
Elbow flexors	C5,6	Biceps jerk C5,6
Supinators/pronators	C6	Supinator jerk C6
Wrist extensors	C6	
Wrist flexors	C7	
Elbow extensors	C7	Triceps jerk C7
Finger extensors	C7	
Finger flexors	C8	
Intrinsic hand muscles	T1	Abdominal reflex T8–12
Hip flexors	L1,2	
Hip adductors	L2,3	
Knee extensors	L3,4	Knee jerk L3,4
Ankle dorsiflexors	L4,5	
Toe extensors	L5	
Knee flexors	L4,5 S1	
Ankle plantar flexors	S1,2	Ankle jerk S1,2
Toe flexors	S1,2	
Anal sphincter	S2,3,4	Bulbocavernosus reflex S3,4 Anal reflex S5 Plantar reflex

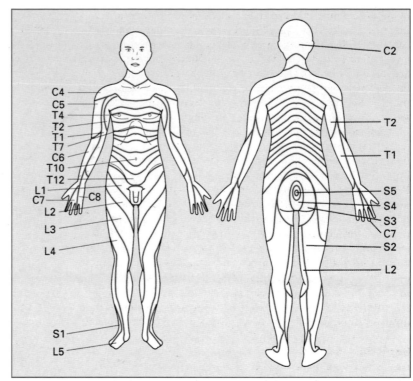

Sensory and motor neurological assessment.

Great care must be taken in managing conscious patients as the neurological symptoms and signs may be dismissed if they do not fit a classical pattern. In patients with a partial cord lesion some neurological function is preserved distal to the level of injury (for example, the sacral segments may be spared): a vascular lesion may be responsible for this.

Sometimes the zone of cord injury lies centrally, encroaching on the cervical segments of the long tracts and producing flaccid weakness in the arms (the central cord syndrome).

Anterior contusion affects the spinothalamic and corticospinal tracts and is therefore associated with weakness and impaired pain and temperature sensation (the anterior cord syndrome). Posterior cord injury causes loss of sense of vibration and proprioception (the posterior cord syndrome). Trauma may be confined to one side of the cord, producing ipsilateral weakness and impaired contralateral pain and temperature sensation (Brown-Séquard "hemisection").

The central cord syndrome is more common in patients in whom the spinal canal has been narrowed by cervical spondylosis (osteophytes, thickened ligamentum flavum, degenerate discs). Patients with this syndrome may not have an associated fracture or dislocation, whereas those with anterior cord injury usually do. Brown-Séquard lesions are more common in patients with penetrating trauma and blunt rotational injury.

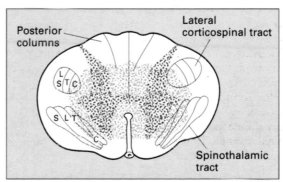

The central cord syndrome.

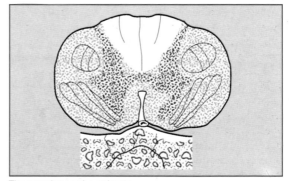

The anterior cord syndrome.

The unconscious patient

There are no truly pathognomonic features of spinal cord injury, but important signs are flaccid paralysis, diaphragmatic breathing, priapism, hypotension with bradycardia, and upward movement of the umbilicus on tensing the abdomen—this is attributable to a T10 lesion (Beevor's sign). The *whole* length of the spine *must* be examined in all unconscious patients with multiple trauma. Failure to do so has resulted in diagnoses being missed, with serious consequences.

The patient is log rolled to one side, keeping the spine in the neutral position. If performed correctly this manouevre is quite safe. Inspection may detect bruising, swelling or a kyphos;

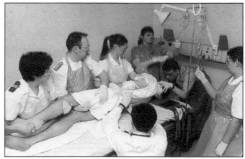

Log roll.

palpation may detect tenderness, an increased interspinous gap, or malalignment of spinous processes (rotational deformity). Suspicion of an injury to the upper cervical spine may be aroused by a retropharyngeal haematoma seen through the open mouth; the trachea may be deviated.

Neurological examination is mandatory in all unconscious patients, and baseline observations are extremely important in patients with spinal injury, not least for medicolegal reasons. Use of a Glasgow or similar coma chart will allow limb movements and strength to be charted. Some head injury charts do not include this facility. Neurological examination in unconscious patients is usually limited to completing the coma chart, funduscopy, and assessing tone and reflexes, but in patients with suspected cord injury the abdominal, anal, and bulbocavernosus reflexes should be recorded. The sensory response to pain can also be assessed in patients with depressed consciousness. Beware of flaccidity and areflexia in an arm as this may result from brachial plexus injury or spinal cord trauma, or both (particularly in motorcyclists).

By the end of the secondary survey, the history must have been gleaned from the patient, ambulance staff or witnesses. An "AMPLE" history should include details of any previous spinal problems.

Radiology

Good quality radiographs are essential for accurate diagnosis of spinal injury, and these are best obtained in the radiology department if circumstances allow. When spinal injuries are suspected radiographic examination should be supervised by a doctor to ensure that there is no unnecessary movement of the patient. Collars, bolsters, and splints are not always radiolucent, and it may be necessary to remove them once preliminary films have been obtained. Riggins found that there was no radiological evidence of trauma in 17% of adult patients with spinal cord injury.[1] When in doubt seek a radiological opinion, especially with radiographs of children, which are difficult to assess and are often normal in spinal cord injury.

Cervical spine

In a patient with multiple trauma radiographs of the cervical spine, chest, and pelvis are mandatory. If there is depression of consciousness a computed tomographic scan of the head is required.

Most radiologically detectable abnormalities of the neck are shown in a standard lateral radiograph, which must display all seven cervical vertebrae and the C7–T1 junction if injuries are not to be missed. This can usually be achieved by applying traction to both arms, but pain in the neck or exacerbation of neurological symptoms must be avoided. If the lower cervical vertebrae are still not adequately shown a "swimmer's view" and, if necessary, conventional or computed tomograms can be requested. These are helpful in excluding important lesions at the cervicothoracic junction.

The lateral radiograph will normally show fractures, subluxations, and dislocations. Unilateral facet dislocation is associated with forward vertebral displacement of less than half the diameter of the vertebral body. This produces a change in the rotational orientation of the spine at the level of injury. Displacement of more than half the vertebral width normally indicates bilateral facet dislocation.

Many patients present with more subtle signs of an unstable injury. A chip fracture of the lower and anterior margin of the vertebra ("tear drop" fracture) is commonly associated with an unstable flexion injury. This may produce widening of the interspinous gap, loss of normal cervical

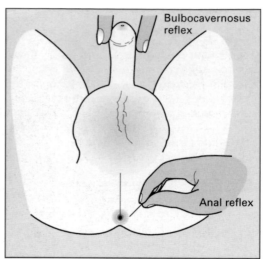
Sacral reflexes.

Assessing spinal radiographs

What to check	What to look for
Adequacy	Are all cervical, thoracic, or lumbar vertebrae shown?
Alignment	Check the line of the anterior and posterior longitudinal ligaments, the spinolaminar, and interspinous lines
Bones	Study each vertebra
	Ensure there are no separate bony fragments
	Look for fractures and cortical discontinuity
Cartilages/joints	Check disc spaces and facet joints
	Check atlanto-odontoid gap
Soft tissues	Look for prevertebral or paravertebral swelling

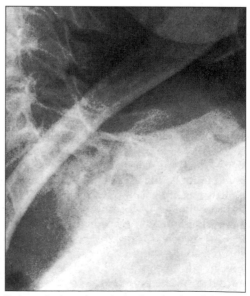
Swimmer's view of cervical spine showing dislocation of C6 on C7.

lordosis, and minor subluxation. Always look for a prevertebral haematoma, which is indicated by an increased gap between the nasopharynx or trachea and cervical spine. The retropharyngeal space (C2) should not exceed 7 mm in adults or children, whereas the retrotracheal space (C6) should not exceed 22 mm in adults or 14 mm in children. (The retropharyngeal space widens in a crying child.)

The other standard radiographs of the cervical spine are the open mouth odontoid view and the anteroposterior projection.

Abnormalities are more likely to be seen in the odontoid radiograph (for example, Jefferson fractures of the atlas as well as odontoid fractures), but the view of odontoid and atlantoaxial joints must not be obscured by overlying teeth.

In the anteroposterior radiograph look closely at the upper thoracic vertebrae and the first two ribs. Also take care to examine the alignment of spinous processes, which may be displaced laterally at sites of unilateral facet dislocation.

When standard radiographs are normal but cervical injury is suspected flexion and extension radiographs may be obtained later as long as neurological symptoms and signs are absent. Even these radiographs, however, may show no evidence of instability in children with cord injury or adults with cord compression resulting from spondylosis or acute disc prolapse. Rupture of the transverse ligament of the atlas is associated with an increased atlanto–odontoid gap, which should not normally exceed 3 mm in adults and 5 mm in children.

Supine oblique radiographs of the cervical spine help to confirm the presence of facet dislocation if standard radiographs are difficult to interpret, particularly those of the cervicothoracic junction.

Thoracolumbar spine

Anteroposterior and lateral radiographs are the standard radiographs of the thoracolumbar spine.

Unlike a cervical haematoma a paravertebral haematoma in the thoracolumbar region is best seen on an anteroposterior radiograph, in which it may be responsible for mediastinal widening that resembles aortic dissection.

In the lateral radiograph particular importance should be attached to subluxation, burst fractures, or potentially unstable injury affecting the posterior vertebral ligaments or bone (laminae and pedicles). Instability requires at least two of the three columns of the spine to be disrupted.[2]

The upper thoracic spine is usually difficult to assess in the lateral radiograph, and if symptoms or signs indicate, tomograms or computed tomograms should be considered.

Injuries of the thoracic spine can be rendered unstable by fractures of the ribs and sternum. An appreciable force is required to produce an unstable thoracic injury, which is usually evident in the standard radiographs.

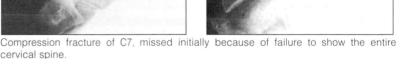

Compression fracture of C7, missed initially because of failure to show the entire cervical spine.

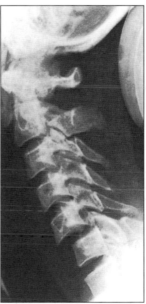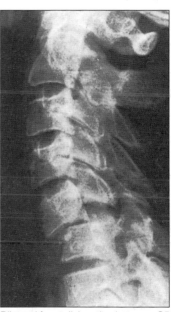

Unilateral facet dislocation between C5 and C6.

Bilateral facet dislocation between C5 and C6

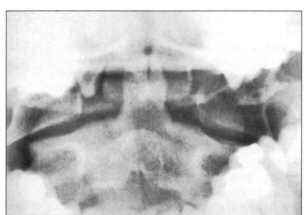

Open mouth odontoid view showing a Jefferson fracture of the atlas with outward displacement of the right lateral mass.

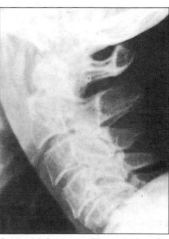

Odontoid fracture with posterior displacement of the anterior arch of the atlas.

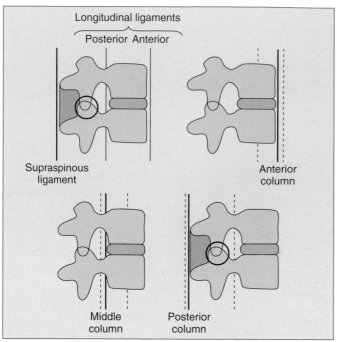

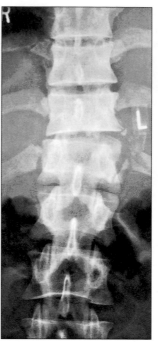

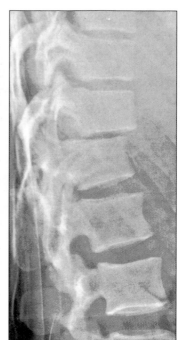

The three spinal columns. (Reproduced with permission from Denis F. *Spine* 1983; 817–31).

Fracture dislocation of T11 on T12.

Removal or replacement of spinal board

Spinal boards are unconforming and high pressures are generated at the interface between the occiput, thoracic kyphosis, scapulae, and the board. The device should therefore be removed as soon as the secondary survey has been completed and essential radiographs obtained. Removal can usually be achieved during the log-roll at the end of the secondary survey, when debris can also be cleared from the back. If further radiographs have to be taken in the radiology department, the board provides a useful means of transfer to the *x* ray table.

Patients should not be transferred to a tertiary centre on a spinal board. An effective alternative is the vacuum mattress, which contours itself to the patient and then becomes rigid when air is evacuated. It needs to be moulded around the head and neck but provides much lower interface pressures.

Referral

The basic history, physical assesment and the results of spinal, neurological, and radiological examinations need to be communicated to the orthopaedic or neurosurgeons at the receiving hospital (or spinal consultants at a tertiary centre). Details about about other injuries, as well as about the treatment initiated and the response are all extremely important pieces of information.

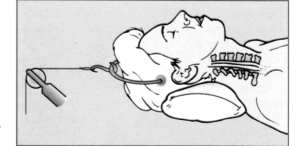

Skull traction using caliper with neck roll in position to maintain postural reduction.

Treatment

Cervical injuries

At the district hospital orthopaedic surgeons should participate in the patient's management at an early stage. Unstable cervical injuries may be immobilised by a firm collar or skeletal traction. No technique is foolproof, and treatment should be supervised by a senior member of the medical staff. Skull traction helps to correct the alignment of the injured spine, reduce fractures and dislocations, decompress the cord and nerve roots, and provide stability.

Various skull calipers are available, but spring loaded types such as the Gardner–Wells calipers are easily applied and

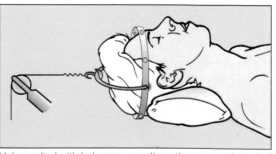

Halo applied with bale arm—an alternative approach to skull traction if early mobilisation into a halo brace is being considered.

carry a low risk of complications. In recent years halo traction has become more popular because it can be converted to a halo brace to allow the patient to mobilise. Care must be taken not to overdistract injuries of the upper cervical spine, and for some of these traction is contraindicated. For interhospital transfer, immobilisation of the head with a semirigid collar, bolsters and tape provides effective spinal protection.

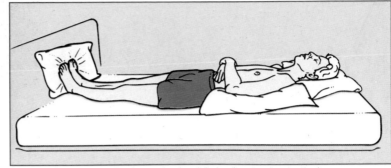

Conservative treatment for thoracolumbar injuries (postural reduction).

Thoracolumbar injuries

Thoracolumbar injuries may be treated by "postural reduction", which entails bed rest on a lumbar support to maintain the normal lordosis and help reduce the fracture or dislocation. Nowadays, treatment is often determined by the findings of computed tomography and magnetic resonance imaging. The former provide good detail of fractures or bony displacement while the latter show disc involvement and cord injury. Some surgeons commonly operate on patients with unstable injuries to enable them to be mobilised without much delay and to facilitate nursing care, though this approach is controversial.

Spinal injury associated with paraplegia or tetraplegia

Because of the medical complications associated with paraplegia or tetraplegia, early referral and transfer to a spinal centre allows the patient to receive better overall care. Many spinal centres have intensive care units, and staff are experienced in dealing with complicated cases. Referral should be the responsibility of the orthopaedic or neurosurgical team.

Routine administration of mannitol and antibiotics in these patients is of no proved benefit. However, the second national acute spinal cord injury study in the United States has shown that the degree of neurological injury may be reduced if very high doses of steroids are given during the first 24 hours after injury.[3] A policy should be agreed with the local spinal injury centre.

There is no conclusive evidence that surgery improves neurological outcome, but it is undertaken when there are signs of deteriorating neurological function and also to prevent deformity. The prognosis is always uncertain, and patients should therefore be treated actively. Magnetic resonance imaging is now the investigation of choice for visualising the spinal cord, assessing the extent of injury and the prognosis.

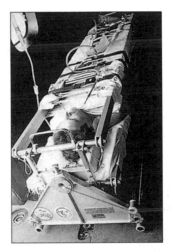

Patient immobilised in a Royal Air Force pattern turning frame for transfer to a spinal injury unit. Skull traction is maintained by means of the constant tension device.

Drug treatment in spinal cord injury
- Consult your spinal unit for advice
- Aim to give methylprednisolone at the earliest opportunity: 30 mg/kg intravenously over 15 minutes and then 5.4 mg/kg/h for 23 hours

---

Summary

Spinal injury can range in severity from insignificant to lethal. The back and the peripheral nervous system must be examined. Any neurological abnormality needs to be taken seriously, even if atypical. Radiographs may reveal no abnormality in spite of the presence of spinal cord injury. Immobilising the spine in the anatomical position will protect it without compromising emergency care and to neglect this is to risk catastrophe.

References

1 Riggins R. The risk of neurologic damage with fractures of the vertebrae. *J Trauma* 1977; **17**: 126–33.

2 Denis F. Thoracolumbar spinal injuries: classification. *Curr Orthopaed* 1988; **2**: 214–17.

3 Bracken MB, Shepard MJ, Collins WF, *et al*. A randomized, controlled trial of methylprednisolone or naloxone in the treatment of acute spinal cord injury: results of the second national acute spinal cord injury study. *N Engl J Med* 1990; **322**: 140–11.

9 The abdomen

Andrew Cope, William Stebbings

The aim of this chapter is to enable all those concerned with the management of patients with abdominal trauma to perform a thorough examination and assessment with the help of diagnostic tests and to institute safe and correct treatment.

Intra-abdominal injuries carry a high morbidity and mortality because often they are not detected or their severity is underestimated. This is particularly common in cases of blunt trauma, in which there may be few or no external signs. Always have a high index of suspicion of abdominal injury when the history suggests severe trauma. Traditionally, abdominal trauma is classified as either blunt or penetrating, but initial assessment and, if required, resuscitation are essentially the same.

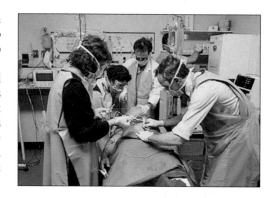

Blunt trauma

Road traffic accidents are one of the most common causes of blunt injuries. Since wearing seat belts was made compulsory the number of fatal head injuries has declined, but a pattern of blunt abdominal trauma that is specific to seat belts has emerged. This often includes avulsion injuries of the mesentery of the small bowel. The symptoms and signs of blunt abdominal trauma can be subtle, and consequently diagnosis is difficult. A high degree of suspicion of underlying intra-abdominal injury is essential when dealing with blunt trauma. Blunt abdominal trauma is usually associated with trauma to other areas, especially the head, chest, and pelvis.

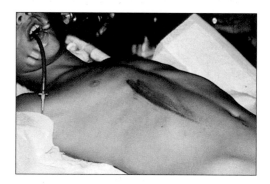

Penetrating trauma

Penetrating wounds are caused by low velocity projectiles such as knives or hand gun bullets or high velocity projectiles such as rifle bullets and shrapnel from bombs or blasts. With the increasing prevalence of civilian violence, penetrating injuries—especially those resulting from stabbing—are encountered increasingly in emergency departments. Visceral injury occurs in 80–90% of bullet wounds but only 30% of stab wounds. Penetrating wounds may seem easy to diagnose, but it is difficult to assess whether peritoneal penetration has occurred. About a third of abdominal stab wounds with serious visceral injury at operation have minimal physical signs.

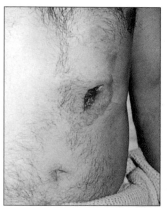

Stab wound.

Assessment

Doctors must perform the primary survey—namely, airway management with protection of the cervical spine, breathing, circulatory and initial neurological evaluation. The circulation may be compromised if there is concealed intra-abdominal

Remember the A, B, C of the primary survey

bleeding. The usual diagnostic pathway of taking the history, physical examination, and special investigations cannot always be followed as resuscitation is the highest priority. The sequence of look, feel, and listen will help in the rapid initial evaluation of the abdomen.

Procedure

Take a careful history

The patient may have limited recall of the injury owing to loss of consciousness, alcohol intoxication, or hysteria. Relatives and friends can provide information regarding medical conditions, current drugs, allergies, and alcohol or drug misuse.

In victims of road traffic accidents further information that may help clarify the type of injury, such as the speed of the vehicle, the nature of the impact, evidence of a steering wheel injury, whether seat belts were worn, and the condition of the other victims, should be sought from the police and ambulance crews.

Useful information in patients with penetrating injuries includes their position when shot or stabbed and the length of the blade or the type of gun and the number and range of shots fired.

Perform a thorough examination

Look—You cannot perform an adequate assessment without exposing the patient fully; therefore you must remove all of the patient's clothes. Look systematically at the anterior structures, including the urethral meatus in men, the flanks, and the posterior structures—the back, buttocks, and perineum—for bruises, lacerations, entry and exit wounds, and impressions of seat belts or tyres. Any abnormality should be recorded.

Feel—Palpation, both superficial and deep, should include all abdominal structures. The abdomen starts at the level of the fifth rib, and therefore penetrating wounds of the lower chest can enter the abdominal cavity.

The assessment of blunt trauma is difficult. Muscle guarding may indicate intraperitoneal injury but can also result from injury to the abdominal wall. Signs of peritoneal irritation after rupture of a hollow viscus can be slow to develop, and consequently the physical signs must be re-evaluated repeatedly. Abdominal rigidity usually indicates visceral injury; percussion and tenderness on coughing are also useful indicators of intraperitoneal injury.

Instability of the pelvic ring can be confirmed by applying direct pressure in two planes to both anterior superior iliac spines. The superior pubic rami should be palpated in addition to the symphysis. Retroperitoneal injuries are difficult to diagnose but should be considered if there is a spinal deformity or paravertebral haematoma or if the mechanism of the injury suggests possible damage to retroperitoneal structures.

Listen—The presence or absence of bowel sounds and their quality if present should be recorded. The presence of bowel sounds does not exclude major peritoneal injury.

Rectal examination—Rectal examination is essential. Loss of integrity of the rectal wall and the presence of blood indicate trauma of the large bowel; a high lying prostate indicates urethral damage.

Vaginal examination—Disruption of the pubic rami or symphysis may cause vaginal injury, therefore, vaginal examination is

To evaluate the abdomen:
- Look
- Feel
- Listen

Information required in patients with abdominal trauma

From the patient or relatives and friends
- History of allergies
- History of alcohol or drug misuse
- Medical history
- Current medication

From the police and ambulance crew when the patient has been involved in a road traffic accident
- Speed of the vehicle
- Nature and direction of impact
- Evidence of deformation of the vehicle—front, back and sides
- Evidence of steering wheel injury
- Whether a seat belt was worn
- Injuries to other victims

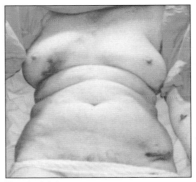

Seat belt injury.

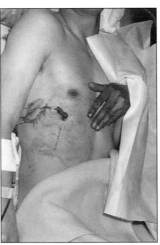

Anterior stab wound.

mandatory, not only to confirm the integrity of the vaginal wall but also to detect obvious pelvic fractures, particularly of the inferior rami.

Examination of urethral meatus—In men the meatus should be examined for evidence of urethral injury. If there is blood at the meatus a urethral catheter should not be passed, and a urologist's opinion should be requested.

The doctor must ensure that airway management with protection of the cervical spine, breathing, and circulation are adequate before proceeding to the special investigations.

Special investigations

Perform baseline tests
Determination of baseline haemoglobin concentration, white cell count, packed cell volume, and cross matching is essential in all victims of trauma. Blood for these tests may be obtained while an intravenous cannula of gauge 14 is being inserted. As a general rule it is safer to overestimate the amount of cross matched blood required. Biochemical measurements that should be made include urea and electrolyte concentrations, serum amylase activity, blood gas tensions, and a pregnancy test for female patients aged 12–50 years.

Pass a nasogastric tube
A nasogastric tube will not only empty the stomach contents but may also suggest upper gastrointestinal injury if blood is aspirated. The tube should be passed orally if there is a suggestion of a fracture of the cribriform plate.

Insert a urethral catheter
A urethral catheter is mandatory in all patients with severe trauma except those in whom urethral injury is suspected, when the suprapubic route should be used.

Perform radiography of the chest and abdomen
An erect chest radiograph is preferable to a supine abdominal film for excluding the possibility of free intraperitoneal air. Abdominal radiographs may show fractures of lower ribs, which may be the only sign of intra-abdominal damage, or fractures of the transverse processes, which may suggest ureteric injury. They can also confirm the presence of opaque foreign bodies (for example, bullets), confirm the position of the nasogastric tube, and show acute gastric dilatation.

In multisystem trauma radiography of the lateral cervical spine and pelvis must be performed.

Additional imaging
Imaging techniques such as ultrasonography and computed tomography are not usually available for routine diagnosis in an emergency department. Centres that have portable ultrasonic facilities might consider using them to assess possible subcapsular splenic haematomas or renal injuries. They should be used only after initial stabilisation and when there is no indication for immediate laparotomy. Computed tomography is valuable in diagnosing pancreatic and other retroperitoneal injuries.

The advent of spiral computed tomography has allowed more rapid aquisition of data (an abdominal scan takes about 1 minute), better picture quality and an improved ability to reconstruct organs and structures. The position of ultrasound examination and peritoneal lavage is therefore downgraded in centres that have spiral computed tomography.

Signs of urethral injury
- Blood at external meatus
- High riding prostate
- Bruised scrotum
- Bruised perineum

Baseline blood tests
- Send a blood sample for cross matching, specifying the number of units required
- Measure haemoglobin concentration, white cell count, and packed cell volume
- Measure serum urea and electrolyte concentrations, serum amylase activity, and arterial blood gas tensions

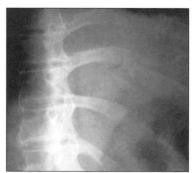
Fractures of the 10th and 11th ribs.

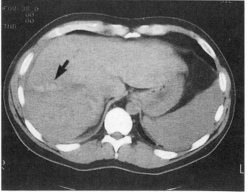
Computed tomogram showing liver laceration.

Indications for laparotomy

If laparotomy is to be performed notify immediately the most senior surgeon present and the anaesthetist, and alert the staff of the operating theatre. Urgent laparotomy is required if profound hypovolaemia caused by haemorrhage persists despite adequate replacement of fluid volume and there is no overt cause (for example, haemothorax or a pelvic fracture).

Peritoneal lavage

If there is no indication for an urgent laparotomy peritoneal lavage may help decide which patients subsequently require surgical assessment by laparotomy.

Contraindications
The only absolute contraindication for lavage is an indication for urgent laparotomy. Relative contraindications are pregnancy, coagulopathy, gross obesity, and previous lower abdominal surgery.

Procedure
(1) Explain the procedure to the patient if he or she is conscious
(2) Ensure that a urethral or suprapubic catheter and a nasogastric tube are in place
(3) Prepare the patient's abdominal skin with antiseptic, and drape sterile towels over the abdomen
(4) Infiltrate the skin with a solution of 1% lignocaine and 1 in 200 000 adrenaline
(5) Make a vertical subumbilical incision in the midline 5 cm in length centred at one third of the distance between the umbilicus and the symphysis pubis
(6) Under direct vision divide the linea alba and identify the peritoneum
(7) Make an incision into the peritoneum and insert a peritoneal dialysis catheter (without introducer) towards the pelvis
(8) Aspirate any free blood or enteric contents. If more than 5 ml of blood is aspirated an urgent laparotomy is indicated
(9) If no blood is aspirated infuse 1 litre of warm (37°C) physiological saline
(10) Allow the saline to equilibrate for 3 minutes and then place the bag and giving set on the floor with the tap open and drain as much of the original 1 litre as possible
(11) Send a 20 ml sample to the laboratory for measurement of white and red blood cell counts and microscopic examination.

Interpretation of results
If >5 ml of blood or enteric contents is aspirated laparotomy is mandatory. If fluid from peritoneal lavage is obtained from the urinary catheter or chest drain an urgent laparotomy is essential.

A positive result necessitates a laparotomy. Patients with a negative result may be managed conservatively and should be re-examined often by the surgeon responsible for the patient.

False positive results occur in about 2% of cases, particularly when the lavage is performed blind, and are caused by trauma to vessels in the abdominal wall or perforating a viscus with the trochar. False negative results also occur in about 2% of cases. Most of these are thought to result from injury to retroperitoneal structures and, occasionally, diaphragmatic injuries.

A special difficulty occurs when there is a concomitant fractured pelvis, retroperitoneal haemorrhage and intraperitoneal blood from torn pelvic vessels. The incision must then be made above the umbilicus. But in spite of this the result must be interpreted with caution because an uneccessary laparotomy with a severe pelvic fracture converts it into an open fracture, which has a greater mortality.

Indications for laparotomy
- Unexplained shock
- Rigid silent abdomen
- Evisceration
- Radiological evidence of free intraperitoneal gas
- Radiological evidence of ruptured diaphragm
- All gunshot wounds
- Positive result of peritoneal lavage

Indications for peritoneal lavage
- Equivocal clinical abdominal examination
- Difficulty in assessing the patient because of alcohol, drugs, or head injury
- Persistent unexplained hypotension despite adequate fluid replacement
- Multiple injuries, particularly if they include injuries of the chest, pelvis, or spinal cord
- Stab wounds where the peritoneum is breached

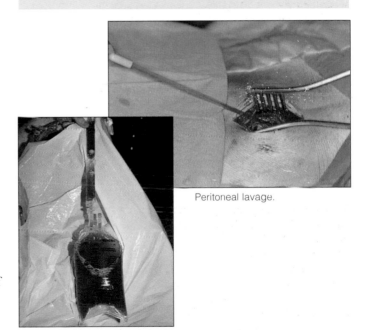

Peritoneal lavage.

Bag and giving set after drainage of saline. The result was positive.

Positive result
- Lavage leak into chest drains or urinary catheter
- Aspirate 5 ml of dark blood
- Red blood cell count more than $10^9/l$
- Presence of bile, bacteria, or faecal material

Complications of peritoneal lavage are rare but may include (particularly if the procedure is incorrectly done):
- Perforation of a viscus—for example, bladder or bowel
- Haemorrhage from mesenteric vessels
- Infection

Considerations for management

Penetrating trauma

All patients with gunshot wounds, regardless of the muzzle velocity of the gun, must have a laparotomy. The tracks of stab wounds should be explored (not probed) to show the integrity of the peritoneum. If the peritoneum is not intact a laparotomy should be considered. Lower chest wounds can be managed conservatively with careful monitoring, assuming that the results of lavage are negative. Flank and back wounds are difficult to assess even with the aid of peritoneal lavage, ultrasonography, or computed tomography, and therefore laparotomy should be considered. Evisceration of bowel necessitates laparotomy.

Blunt trauma

In all cases of blunt trauma a high index of suspicion of intra-abdominal injury is essential. Blunt trauma is more difficult to assess clinically than penetrating trauma, and therefore diagnostic peritoneal lavage is helpful in evaluating the need for laparotomy.

If laparotomy is not indicated initially

Consider admission for all patients with suspected intra-abdominal injuries so that reevaluation and observation including of vital signs can continue. Such admissions will normally be to the general surgical ward, unless the patient's other injuries require intensive care.

Conclusion

Abdominal injuries should never be underestimated. In a recent retrospective study of 1000 deaths from injury, 43% of the deaths not related to the central nervous system were judged to have been potentially preventable. Among the most common missed diagnoses were those of ruptured liver and ruptured spleen.[1] Thorough initial assessment and repeated re-evaluation with appropriate investigations are of prime importance for detecting these injuries.

Reference

1 Anderson ID, Woodford M, de Dombal T, Irving M. Retrospective study of 1000 deaths from injury in England and Wales. *Br Med J* 1988; **296**: 1305–8.

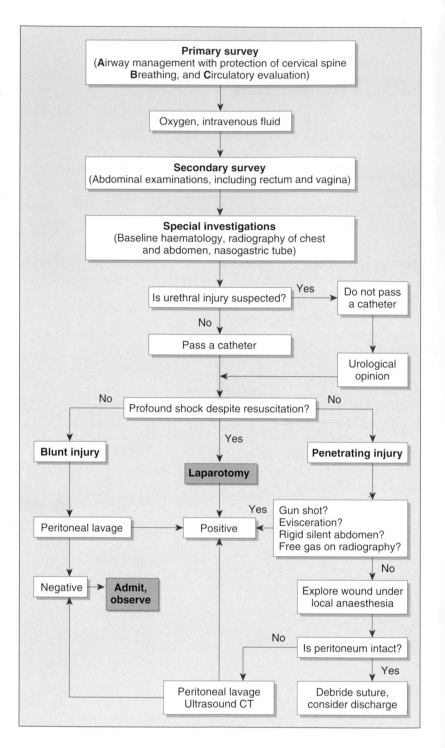

10 The urinary tract

Timothy Terry, Anthony Deane

A. Upper urinary tract

In the United Kingdom about 10% of patients who suffer abdominal trauma have injuries to the genitourinary tract. Blunt trauma is responsible for more than 90% of renal injuries. Important associated injuries occur in about 40% of patients with blunt renal trauma. A high index of suspicion of a renal lesion is required in the patient with multiple injuries, as the signs and symptoms of the renal trauma may be obscured by those of the concomitant injuries.

In children the kidney is the organ most commonly injured by blunt abdominal trauma. This may be explained by the relative lack of perinephric fat in children and the incidence (up to 20%) of pre-existing renal abnormalities (primary pelviureteric junction obstruction is the most common).

The mechanism of renal injury caused by blunt abdominal trauma may be direct or indirect. With a direct injury the kidney is crushed between the anterior end of the 12th rib and the lumbar spine—such as in sporting injuries— or between an external force applied to the abdomen anteriorly just below the rib cage and the paravertebral muscles—such as in run-over traffic accidents and injuries caused by seat belts and steering columns. Indirect injury occurs when a deceleration force is applied to the renal pedicle (as a result of falling from a height and landing on the buttocks). Such injuries can tear the major renal vessels or rupture the ureter at the pelviureteric junction.

Penetrating renal trauma occurs in about 7% of patients with abdominal stab wounds. As with blunt renal trauma associated injuries are often present (in up to 80% of cases); these affect the liver, lungs, spleen, small bowel, stomach, pancreas, duodenum, and diaphragm in descending order of frequency. Renal stab wounds are potentially serious, with the possibilities of severed major renal vessels and lacerations to the collecting system or upper ureter. Gunshot wounds that affect the kidney may be caused by a low or high velocity missile. Low velocity missiles cause injury by directly penetrating the tissue whereas high velocity missiles produce direct tissue injury plus damage to adjacent tissue because of the shock wave effect (see chapter 24).

Classification of renal trauma

Renal injuries can be classified as minor (grades 1 and 2), major (grades 3 and 4), or critical (grade 5), on the basis of clinical and radiological assessments of the patient. Minor injuries (contusions and superficial lacerations) consist of parenchymal damage without capsular tears or involvement of the

Typical victims of urinary tract trauma

- Young men while performing a sporting activity (55% of cases)
- People in road traffic accidents (25% of cases)
- Victims of domestic or industrial accidents (15% of cases)
- Victims of assault (5% of cases)

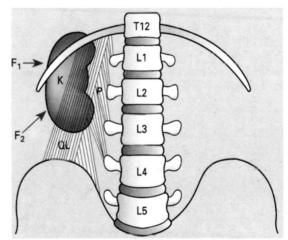

Mechanism of direct blunt renal trauma. An external force (F1) may crush the kidney (K) between the 12th rib and the vertebral column, or a force (F2) may crush the kidney against the paravertebral muscles (quadratus lumborum, QL, or psoas major in position P but deleted from diagram).

Classification of renal injuries

Grade	Nature of injury
1 and 2	- Minor (85% of cases) Contusions Superficial lacerations (capsule and pelvicaliceal system intact)
3 and 4	- Major (10% of cases) Deep lacerations (capsular tears or pelvicaliceal involvement, or both)
5	- Critical (5% of cases) Renal fragmentation Pedicle injuries (renal artery thrombosis, vessel avulsion, and pelviureteric rupture)

pelvicaliceal system. Major injuries (deep lacerations) consist of parenchymal damage with capsular tears or extension into the collecting system, or both. Critical injuries include kidney fragmentation and injuries to the pedicle (such as renal artery thrombosis, avulsion of renal vessels, and rupture of the pelviureteric junction).

Clinical presentation

Most patients (80–90%) with direct renal trauma give a history of a blow to the flank and complain of loin pain, which is followed after a variable period by gross haematuria. The haematuria may subsequently be accompanied by ureteric colic caused by the passage of blood clots. Clinical examination may show skin abrasions or bruising overlying the upper abdomen, loin, or lower thoracic area. Rigidity of the anterior abdominal wall and local loin tenderness over the affected kidney are invariably elicited. A flattening of loin contour together with a palpable loin mass indicate the presence of a perinephric haematoma with or without urinary extravasation of contrast dye. In such cases a paralytic ileus may be present. Varying degrees of hypovolaemic shock may be present, but this is usually secondary to associated injuries.

About 70% of potentially lethal injuries to the renal pedicle (indirect trauma) do not cause gross haematuria. Patients with such injuries are usually in severe shock, having been brought to hospital after a fall from a height. The same mechanism, in a milder form, usually produces intimal tearings of the renal vessels, which can lead to thrombosis.

The victim of a penetrating renal injury caused by a low velocity missile or stab wound will have an obvious entrance wound. The depth and direction of the wound track and the site of the exit wound, when present, suggest the likelihood of renal involvement.

Radiological investigations

The standard investigation for patients in whom serious renal injury is suspected is high-dose infusion intravenous urography. This includes all patients with gross haematuria or with microscopic haematuria and a systolic blood pressure below 90 mm Hg. Haemodynamically stable patients with microscopic haematuria have minor renal injuries and do not need urography. A high-dose intravenous pyelogram in the emergency room detects significant renal trauma in more than 90% of cases.

The preliminary control film shows abnormalities in about 15% of patients with blunt renal trauma. These abnormalities include pneumothorax or haemothorax; concomitant fractures of ribs and the transverse processes of lumbar vertebrae; scoliosis with concavity towards the side of injury; loss of psoas shadow or renal outline because of perirenal haematoma; a soft tissue loin mass displacing bowel shadows or raising the ipsilateral hemidiaphragm; and free intraperitoneal gas.

In 85% of patients with blunt renal trauma the postcontrast series of radiographs shows no abnormalities. The appearances in the remainder are those of distortion of caliceal pattern, extravasation of contrast dye into the perinephric tissues, or failure to visualise any part or the whole of the caliceal system. These findings suggest the presence of a major or critical renal injury, and the appearance in the intravenous urogram of a normal contralateral kidney is reassuring.

If patients with blunt trauma are clinically stable further information on the precise state of the damaged kidney (the presence of parenchymal disruption, intrarenal or subcapsular

Clinical signs of renal trauma
- Regional skin lesions (abrasions, bruising, and entry and exit wounds)
- Loin tenderness
- Loss of loin contour
- Loin mass
- Gross haematuria (up to 90% of cases)

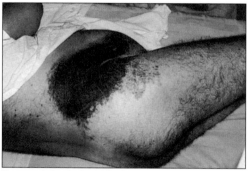

Severe abdominal and flank ecchymosis with potential urological injury (caused by a seat belt).

Findings on intravenous urography
Control film
- Fractures (of lower ribs and transverse processes of lumbar vertebrae)
- Loss of psoas shadow
- Loss of renal outline
- Loin mass (displacement of bowel or diaphragm

Postcontrast film series
- Distortion of caliceal pattern
- Contrast extravasation
- Non-visualisation of part or whole of caliceal system

haematomas, and perirenal collections) may be gained by renal ultrasonography. This technique is particularly valuable for imaging injuries to the kidneys not visualised in the urogram and following the natural course of perirenal collections.

Computed tomography with enhancement with an intravenous radiocontrast agent accurately determines the extent of the renal injury and reliably identifies renal pedicle injury. Furthermore, computed tomography also shows associated non-renal injuries. However, high-dose infusion intravenous urography complemented with ultrasonography is widely and readily available and the combined study is as sensitive and specific for renal injuries as computed tomography.

Magnetic resonance imaging may be considered in patients with renal insufficiency or contrast allergy.

Selective renal arteriography is indicated in patients with vascular pedicle injuries whose condition is stable and in patients with macroscopic haematuria persisting longer than 1 week. In the rare cases in which the mode of the accident and the findings on urography suggest the possibility of disruption of the pelviureteric junction, a retrograde ureterogram is necessary.

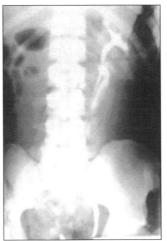

Excretory urogram showing extravasation of dye.

Management

The principle underlying the management of patients with renal trauma is conservation of the maximum number of functioning nephrons with minimal morbidity and mortality. The immediate management of any individual patient is determined, however, more by the patient's general clinical state and the presence of important associated injuries than by the mode and type of renal injury.

Fewer than 5% of all blunt renal injuries are by themselves life threatening, and hypovolaemic shock in a patient with blunt renal trauma is nearly always secondary to the presence of concomitant injuries. The initial general clinical assessment of the patient is therefore all important in deciding a plan of supportive and definitive treatment.

In patients with blunt renal trauma urgent surgical exploration for critical injuries (renal fragmentation and pedicle injuries) is mandatory. A generous midline abdominal incision allows complete assessment of the abdomen for concomitant injuries while providing access to the entire length of both ureters, the kidneys, and the vascular pedicles. If conservative renal surgery is being contemplated the ipsilateral renal vessels must be isolated and controlled before Gerota's fascia is incised. Partial nephrectomy may be possible in some patients with fragmented kidneys, but usually total nephrectomy is necessary. Retention of about 30% of one kidney is sufficient to avoid dialysis.

Lacerations to the major renal vein may be debrided and sutured. If renal artery thrombosis has been diagnosed within 6 hours of injury, thrombectomy, excision of the damaged arterial segment, and direct end to end reanastomosis may be considered. However renal salvage rates are less than 20% with open surgery and consideration should be given to endovascular repair using endoluminal stents.

Disruption of the pelviureteric junction is treated by spatulation of the ends and reanastomosis over a ureteric stent.

Minor renal injuries (contusions and superficial lacerations) and major injuries (deep lacerations), which together comprise about 95% of cases of closed renal trauma, are initially managed expectantly. Strict bed rest, appropriate analgesia, and prophylactic antibiotics (cephradine or trimethoprim) are instituted together with frequent serial clinical observations of vital signs and assessment of any loin swelling. Once the vital signs are stable ambulation is allowed only after gross

Management of renal trauma
- Treat hypovolaemic shock
- Stage renal injury radiologically
- Treat patients with stable minor and major renal injuries (up to 95% of cases) expectantly
- Operate on patients with critical and unstable major renal injuries

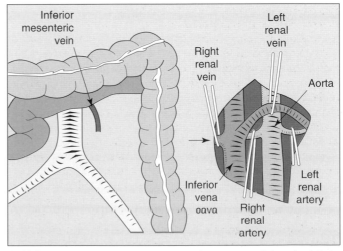

(Left) Retroperitoneal incision sited over the aorta medial to the inferior mesenteric vein to isolate the renal vessels before opening Gerota's fascia. (Right) The left renal vein crosses anterior to the aorta. With this vein retracted superiorly the left and right renal arteries may be located arising from the aorta.

haematuria has cleared (serial aliquots of urine are kept for comparison) and the perirenal swelling, if present, has clinically resolved.

Whether to perform early surgery in patients with major renal injuries is a controversial issue. It is however clearly indicated in those rare cases in which primary haemorrhage or secondary haemorrhage at 10–14 days, usually resulting from infection, endangers life. The late complications (after 6 weeks) of major renal injuries that may require surgery include hypertension, arteriovenous fistula, hydronephrosis, formation of pseudocysts or calculi, chronic pyelonephritis, and loss of renal function. Regular follow up is necessary in patients with major renal trauma during the first year after injury if these late complications, of which hypertension is the most common, are not to be missed.

Penetrating renal stab and gunshot wounds require immediate surgical exploration if the patient is clinically unstable or has critical renal injury (grade 5) or to treat associated injuries. Stable patients with grade 1–2 injuries can be observed.

Finally, an unsuspected penetrating or blunt renal injury may manifest itself at emergency laparotomy performed to control massive intra-abdominal bleeding in a patient with trauma. The clinically silent renal injury manifests itself as a retroperitoneal haematoma. In such cases on-table intravenous urography is essential to establish the presence of a normal functioning contralateral kidney and to determine the type of injury to the damaged kidney. The retroperitoneal haematoma should be explored only if a critical injury is identified in the urogram or if the haematoma is large and is seen to expand during laparotomy. In either case the renal vessels must be controlled before opening Gerota's fascia, otherwise the possible use of conservative renal surgery may be jeopardised.

B. Lower urinary tract

Injuries to the lower urinary tract cause more confusion than those of the upper urinary tract as their management is controversial. The rule in patients with suspected urethral injuries and major pelvic fractures is not to pass a urethral catheter without first seeking advice from a urologist. Even though monitoring urinary output is important in patients with major injuries, a catheter should not be passed without careful thought. Urinary extravasation is not dangerous in the short term.

External genitalia

Serious injuries to the penis and scrotum are unusual. The mobile scrotal skin can be used to cover penile defects and has good powers of recovery. Scrotal tears heal well without suturing. The erectile mechanism should always be repaired if torn with monofilament non-absorbable sutures.

The testicles can be damaged by direct trauma—usually a blow or a kick. If bleeding is confined to the scrotal skin no active treatment is required. Tense haematoceles should, however, always be explored as these usually indicate that the testis is torn and needs repair. Severe damage may require orchidectomy.

Bladder injuries

Bladder injuries may be associated with a pelvic fracture—that is, they may be caused by penetration by a bony fragment or by a direct blow to the lower abdomen, especially when the

---

Expectant management of renal injuries

- Make serial clinical observations (pulse, blood pressure, temperature, urine aliquots, abdominal palpation)
- Institute strict bed rest
- Give appropriate analgesia
- Give prophylactic antibiotics
- Perform serial renal ultrasonography

Late complications in renal trauma

- Hypertension
- Arteriovenous fistula
- Hydronephrosis
- Formation of pseudocysts or calculi
- Chronic pyelonephritis
- Loss of renal function

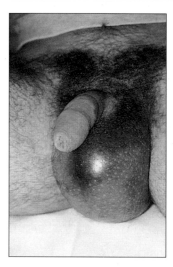

Scrotal haematoma.

Investigations in patients with lower urinary tract injuries

- Inspect the urinary meatus for blood
- Examine the abdomen for peritonism, perineal bruising, and a high riding prostate
- Perform intravenous urography to detect bladder perforation, displaced bladder, upper urinary tract injury
- Perform cystography to exclude bladder perforation if patient has a catheter in place
- Perform ascending urethrography (aqueous contrast) to exclude urethral injury (controversial)

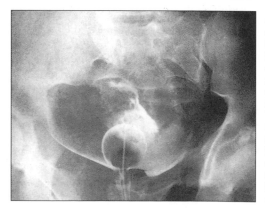

Cystogram showing a bladder full of haematoma with extravasation of contrast through a torn anterior bladder wall. The patient needed 30 units of blood before bleeding was controlled by selective internal iliac embolisation.

bladder is full. The condition may be missed in patients intoxicated with alcohol or those with a head injury. Patients with a bladder injury may have lower abdominal peritonism and not be able to pass urine. A catheter may have been passed by the receiving clinicians and the urine may contain blood.

Investigation begins by inspecting the plain radiograph to exclude pelvic fractures. Disruption of the pelvic symphysis alerts the clinician to the possibility of urethral injury and delayed rupture of the bladder as a result of stretching of the anterior bladder wall. An intravenous urogram may show an extravasation from a bladder injury. If there is no pelvic fracture and no urethral haemorrhage a urethral catheter may be passed, and cystography with 10% dilute contrast agent will show any important bladder injury. If an intraperitoneal bladder rupture is suspected then cystography should be done before diagnostic peritoneal lavage because a laparotomy will be required to repair such a lesion, making lavage unnecessary. In patients with serious pelvic fracture, especially if it affects the pubic symphysis, upward dislocation of the bladder on urography should be excluded first, although this is usually accompanied by urethral haemorrhage.

Treatment—Patients with important intraperitoneal ruptures and peritonism are best treated by laparotomy and drainage by suprapubic catheter and urethral catheter for about 7 days. Broad range antibiotics should be given. Extraperitoneal injuries are managed with drainage by a catheter without irrigation for about 10 days. A catheter of at least 20 FG is necessary, and cystography to confirm healing is advisable before withdrawal of the catheter.

Bulbar injuries

Bulbar injuries occur by direct trauma—for example, by falling on to a bicycle crossbar. Occasionally they can be caused by penetrating trauma. Patients with bulbar injuries have perineal bruising and blood at the urinary meatus. A urethral catheter must not be passed because it may aggravate the injury and introduce infection. The patient should be treated expectantly, and, if he passes urine, should be given antibiotics and followed up. Patients with urinary retention should be treated by inserting a suprapubic catheter with a small calibre percutaneously as heavy haematuria is not usually a problem. Antibiotics are given, and urethrography can be performed after about 5 days. The patient will need urological follow up to exclude the formation of a stricture.

Urethral injuries caused by pelvic fracture

The membranous urethra below the prostate is damaged in about 10% of men with pelvic fractures. Serious injuries, though rare, are devastating as impotence and stricture are common sequels. Damage usually comprises a partial tear, but, occasionally, complete disruption and upward dislocation of the bladder and prostate occurs. The prostate is fixed to the pubic symphysis by the puboprostatic ligaments, and any severe disruption of the pubic symphysis is liable to tear the prostate off the membranous urethra, which is attached to the pelvic floor.

The signs of urethral injury caused by pelvic fracture are blood at the meatus, perineal bruising, and inability to pass urine. A urethral catheter must not be passed as it may aggravate the injury, even if it passes the tear: the urethra is often traumatised and devascularised and may be eroded by the catheter or disintegrate around it; the catheter will prevent the haematoma from draining and introduce infection with

Suprapubic catheterisation: a step-by-step guide

Suprapubic catheterisation is a relatively simple procedure to perform if certain guidelines are followed. It should be used to drain a distended bladder in the patient with a torn or bleeding urethra as a result of injury, which may be iatrogenic. Repeated attempts at catheterisation can produce urethral haemorrhage and the answer is to pass a suprapubic rather than to persist. No patient with a history of a urethral stricture should be instrumented via the urethra and the suprapubic approach is the method of choice in small boys, in whom urethral strictures secondary to catheterisation are difficult to manage. Patients with large incisional hernias may not be suitable for suprapubic catheterisation and should be referred to a urologist.

Suprapubic catheterisation is safe in a patient with a distended bladder. Distention can be confirmed by suprapubic percussion or ultrasound. The bladder must always be aspirated using a narrow gauge needle—a green needle (21G), or a spinal needle (19G) in the obese.

If urine cannot be easily aspirated by suprapubic needling, percutaneous suprapubic catheterisation should be abandoned, as otherwise bowel may be perforated.

Make the initial puncture two finger breadths above the pubic symphysis and use the needle to inject local anaesthetic. For short term suprapubic catheterisation, a needle and fine catheter set can be used, such as the Bonano. Follow the instructions carefully, as otherwise the catheter may be damaged or even dislodged into the bladder. The instruments are passed into the bladder two finger breadths above the pubic symphysis, angling a little downwards in patients who have had previous surgery.

This type of temporary suprapubic catheter is not suitable in patients with significant lower urinary tract trauma as the tubes rapidly block with blood clot. In such patients, an adequate Foley suprapubic catheter (16F) can be placed via a Lawrence Add-a-Cath, which is a trocar and cannula system. In an emergency situation, this would ideally be placed by a member of the urological or surgical team.

If percutaneous catheterisation is impossible, it is safer to place a suprapubic catheter via a small suprapubic incision, opening the bladder under direct vision.

Do not perform percutaneous suprapubic catheterisation without prior needle aspiration of urine to confirm bladder distention.

Management of patients with bulbar injuries
- Do not pass a urethral catheter
- If the patient passes urine give antibiotics and follow up
- If the patient has urinary retention insert a suprapubic catheter with a small calibre and give antibiotics. Perform urethrography after about 5 days and follow up

possible fistulation on its withdrawal; and worst of all, the catheter may pass out of the tear and drain blood and urine below the prostate. Balloon inflation may convert a partial disruption into a complete one.

If there is doubt about whether a bladder is full, a small portable ultrasound machine can be used to determine bladder measurement. If an ultrasound scan shows a full bladder, it is usually safe to proceed with suprapubic catheterisation.

The safest way to treat urethral injuries caused by pelvic fracture is to pass a suprapubic catheter of adequate calibre either percutaneously or by cystotomy if the patient requires a laparotomy for other reasons or if the bladder is impalpable.

Intravenous urography should be performed to exclude total disruption with a high riding bladder above the pubic symphysis—an indication for exploration and repositioning. Some authorities advise performing ascending urethrography to delineate the extent of the injury and plan its management, but this can be difficult in the emergency room.

In general a urethral catheter can be passed in a patient with a pelvic fracture if there is no blood at the meatus or if the pubic symphysis is not severely disrupted on radiography. If any difficulties are encountered urological help should be summoned and an ascending urethrogram considered or suprapubic catheterisation performed. If there is severe disruption of the pubic symphysis orthopaedic help should be requested, as early fixation may assist in management and reduce morbidity. Later treatment of these injuries entails urethroscopy, but late strictures are common.

In women the urethra is injured only rarely, and usually a catheter can easily be passed in those with pelvic fractures and, if necessary, cystography performed to exclude the possibility of bladder injuries.

Pain management and specialist referral

Lower urinary tract injuries are painful and will usually require opiate analgesia.

Always consult a urological specialist if the patient is bleeding from the urethra or is suspected to have a ruptured bladder.

Conclusion

Injuries to the lower urinary tract may not seem important in a patient with severe multiple trauma, but these injuries often have sequelae long after other more dramatic injuries have healed. Patients with membranous injuries have a high incidence of erectile dysfunction and urethral strictures that poor management can only increase.

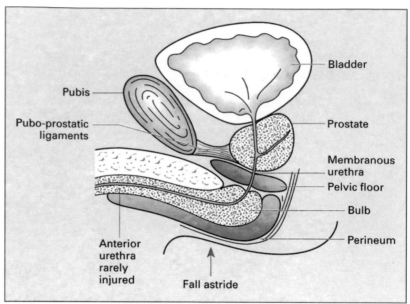

The puboprostatic ligaments carry the prostate with them in patients with pelvic fracture, tearing the urethra off the pelvic floor.

Signs of membranous urethral injury
- Pelvic fracture
- Perineal bruising
- Blood at the meatus
- Inability to pass urine
- High riding prostate

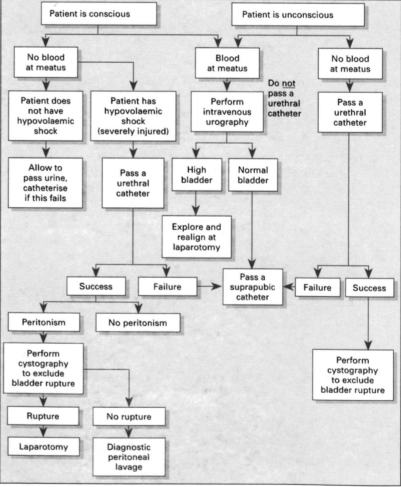

Urological management of men with serious pelvic fractures.

11 Limb injuries

Nigel D Rossiter, Keith M Willett, Raymond Ross, Hugh Dorrell, Peter Kelly

Up to 70% of multiply injured patients have injured limbs and fractures or dislocations of the appendicular skeleton. Severe limb injuries must not distract the resuscitation team from the priorities of establishing an airway, optimising ventilation, and restoring circulatory volume as limb injuries, except those that cause exsanguination, are rarely immediately life threatening.

Careful thorough examination, however, is required after resuscitation to identify injuries, particularly those threatening the overall mortality or morbidity. Apparently minor injuries, often overlooked in the face of multiple trauma and only discovered some days later, must not be neglected, because they may result in long term disability or disfigurement .

Prehospital care

Doctors attending the scene of an accident should confine themselves initially to personal safety, assessment of the scene, and management of the patient's airway, cervical spine, breathing and circulation. Attention can then be directed towards immobilisation of the injured limbs. When moving a patient with a fractured limb the pain is reduced by supporting the limb on either side of the fracture and applying gentle traction along the axis of the limb. All unnecessary handling of the injured part without splinting should be avoided. The exceptions to this rule are when severe deformity or ischaemia distal to the fracture threatens survival of the soft tissues; reduction is then indicated. This is achieved by gentle traction and restoration of the normal anatomical alignment. Perfusion of the distal limb must be checked after any manipulation, to avoid further soft tissue injury.

Splints are mandatory before the victim is evacuated. Anything rigid can be used, such as pieces of wreckage and wooden sticks. Strapping to the opposite leg is useful in solitary lower limb injuries, and "bulk" splints can be produced by bandaging blankets or pillows around the limb. External bleeding must be controlled by a compressive pad and any wounds covered with a sterile dressing. Rapid transfer to hospital is then required.

Hospital care

Haemorrhage

Blood loss from limb wounds and occult bleeding from fractures contribute to hypovolaemic shock in patients with multiple injuries. Haemorrhage from multiple fractures may result in exsanguination, particularly when the pelvis and femora are involved. Patients with hypovolaemic shock should be resuscitated immediately along the lines described in chapter 5.

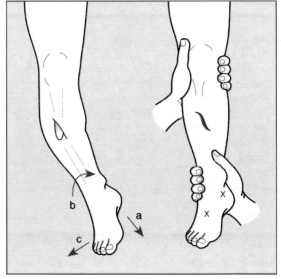

(1) Reduction of a major deformity; (a) perform gentle longitudinal traction; (b) restore the correct rotation; (c) restore the alignment.
(2) Control of the fracture; check pulses (x); maintain traction; apply a splint.

Estimated blood loss caused by fractures

Site of fracture	Blood loss (litres)
Humerus	0.5–1.5
Tibia	0.5–1.5
Femur	1.0–2.5
Pelvis	1.0–4.0

For an open fracture the loss is two or three times greater

Total blood loss can be estimated (see table), and blood for transfusion should be cross matched urgently. Blood loss from open fractures may be two or three times greater than that from closed fractures. Fractures, however, should not be assumed to be responsible for hypovolaemia, and occult bleeding into visceral cavities must be excluded. Blood loss from wounds can be reduced by a compressive bandage or hand pressure over a sterile pad. A tourniquet is indicated only for unmanageable life threatening haemorrhage or after traumatic amputation with exsanguinating haemorrhage.

Assessment

Evaluation of limb injuries is not started until life threatening conditions have been treated. Careful examination is complemented by suspicions raised by the knowledge of the mechanism of injury, information on which may only be available from the ambulance service. These witnesses should not be discharged until at least the mechanism, environment, time and immediate care of the injury have been established. For victims of road traffic accidents it is important to determine whether they were a vehicle occupant, whether they were restrained by a seat belt, the direction of impact and degree of damage to the vehicle. Ejection from a vehicle, and death and serious injury of others involved in the accident, carry a high risk of serious injury.

Certain injury patterns are common. For instance, a direct blow to the knee in a seated occupant of a car may not produce only knee injury and femoral fracture but is commonly associated with hip dislocation or fractures of the acetabulum or both. The femoral neck is injured in 10% of incidents of this type and should be carefully studied, as the injury is often initially missed, with significant morbidity resulting. A victim falling from a height and landing on his or her feet may sustain compression fractures of the calcaneum, ankle, tibial plateau and one or more vertebrae at the thoracolumbar junction or in the lower cervical spine.

The patient must be completely undressed. The assessment should begin by comparing the injured limb with the uninjured limb if possible. Observe the attitude of the limb: shortening and rotational abnormalities indicate proximal fractures or dislocations. Angular or rotational deformity may be visible or palpable.

As clinical signs are often subtle, particularly in the unconscious patient, careful inspection of the whole circumference of each limb for local swelling and bruising is necessary. Gently palpate along the axes of the bones and all the bony prominences for tenderness, fracture crepitus (grating) and abnormal interfragmentary mobility.

Carefully examine adjacent joints so that coexisting injuries are not overlooked. A co-operative patient may indicate the active ranges of joint movement. Passive ranges of motion should be assessed cautiously in a limb that is suspected to be fractured; these should not be tested if an obvious fracture exists.

Vascular state

Of prime importance to limb survival is the competence of the vasculature distal to any injury. Local contusion, penetrating injuries, fractures and, particularly, major joint dislocations may occlude or disrupt blood vessels.

In the haemodynamically stable patient examination of distal pulses is crucial in assessing distal circulation. A diminished or absent pulse strongly suggests a vascular injury and must be explained and managed promptly. Skin colour will also indicate tissue perfusion, and pallor or a blue-grey colour should arouse suspicion. It may be useful to compare pulse oximetry on the digits of the affected limb and a normal

Life threatening injuries
- Traumatic amputation
- Major vascular injury
- Pelvic fracture disruption
- Haemorrhage from open fractures
- Multiple long bone fractures
- Severe crush injury

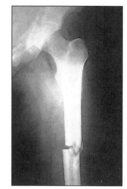

Acetabular fracture associated with a femoral shaft fracture.

Limb threatening injuries
- Vascular injury
- Major joint dislocation
- Crush injury
- Open fracture
- Compartment syndrome
- Nerve injury

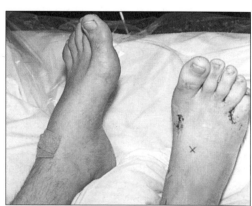

Ischaemic right foot.

limb in the same patient. Similarly, a low skin temperature indicates inadequate perfusion. A sensitive indicator is capillary return—the normal prompt pink flush of the nail bed seen after transient compression. This response will be slowed or blue if the circulation is inadequate.

Peripheral nerves are sensitive to ischaemia, and sensation is lost early. However, total insensibility in a hand or foot suggests ischaemia, because, with the exception of brachial plexus or spinal cord injury, it is unlikely that all a limb's nerve trunks would have been damaged. An inadequate distal circulation is never the result of spasm in a traumatised limb. If distal ischaemia is identified more proximal pulses should be checked and any major deformity at the fracture site corrected, the splint device checked for local compression, and an urgent surgical/vascular opinion sought.

Dislocations of major joints require urgent reduction. Doppler ultrasonography may be useful in evaluation of limb perfusion, but if a vascular injury is suspected arteriography provides the best definitive evaluation.

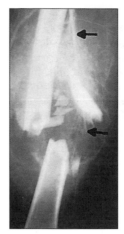

Femoral shaft fracture. Arteriogram showing occlusion of the superficial femoral artery at the level of the fracture.

Neurological state

Evidence of nerve injury may be difficult to obtain in the unconscious or multiply injured patient. There is a higher incidence of neurological damage with dislocations than with fractures. Simple tests to touch, motor function and sweating are sufficient to determine nerve integrity. When testing distal motor function the more proximal innervation of the muscle bellies must be appreciated. Injury to a peripheral nerve must be assumed if there is altered sensation in the distribution of that nerve and a wound overlying its course. Neurological function should be documented to allow later comparison.

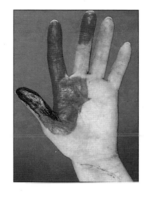

Areas of complete (black) and partial (red) sensory loss resulting from a wrist wound indicate damage to the median nerve, which was missed when the wound was sutured.

Wound management

Among patients with open fractures, 50% have multiple injuries. The extent of soft tissue damage will determine the outcome. A sterile dressing applied to an open wound at the site of an accident should not be disturbed, as repeated examinations outside the operating theatre considerably increase the risk of infection. Instant Polaroid photography of the wound has been recommended to prevent this interference.

Debridement (surgical toilet) is required within 6 hours of the injury. As an adjunct to this, prophylactic antibiotics are indicated for open wounds. A cephalosporin (for example cefuroxime 750 mg three times a day) given intravenously for at least three doses and gentamicin (3 mg/kg) as a single dose given slowly intravenously are appropriate. Tetanus prophylaxis must not be forgotten and depends on the patient's immunisation status. An immunised patient with a contaminated wound prone to tetanus requires a booster of tetanus toxoid if more than 5 years have elapsed since his or her last dose. In addition, tetanus immunoglobulin is required if no immunity exists or the immunisation state is unknown.

Pelvic injuries

Pelvic fractures must be actively sought both clinically and radiologically in all patients with multiple injuries, because they are relatively common and if missed can have catastrophic consequences. Any pelvic displacement seen on a radiograph is usually considerably less than that present at impact, because of the inherent elasticity of the pelvic structures (see chapter 13.) Considerable force is necessary to disrupt the pelvic ring and the associated extensive soft tissue and visceral damage may

---

Management of wounds

(1) Obtain samples for culture

(2) Give preventive antibiotics intravenously

(3) Administer tetanus immunisation if necessary

(4) Remove particulate contaminants by physical wound cleaning and irrigation

(5) Excise all devitalised tissue

(6) Take a split skin graft early from skin flaps of doubtful viability

(7) Anticipate swelling, decompress compartments, and leave wounds open

(8) Obtain early fracture stabilisation

result in life-threatening haemorrhage. In these cases stabilisation of the pelvis can control further blood loss and further soft tissue or visceral damage during movement of the patient. The rationale is no different from that outlined for other fractures, but action is more urgent in the case of the pelvis.

Stabilisation in the emergency department is easily and rapidly achieved with the use of a folded sheet or draw sheet. This can be placed on a trolley before the arrival of a patient, folded to about 20 cm wide and positioned to lie under the patient's buttocks. If unstable pelvic disruption is suspected, or shown radiologically, the sheet can be rapidly wrapped tightly around the front of the pelvis and secured with a sponge forceps or knotted. This will not interfere with access to the abdomen, perineum, genitalia or groins for vascular access, any further radiological investigations, or patient transfer around or between units. To avoid skin pressure necrosis, it should then be removed after 6–8 hours and replaced with another form of pelvic fixation if appropriate.

In units experienced with this type of injury the placement of an external fixator on the pelvis may be part of the initial stabilisation. This should be performed by a surgeon experienced in the rapid application of a frame and the correct positioning of pins. A poorly applied external fixator and pins may limit further management options.

Damage to pelvic organs

Damage to pelvic organs, particularly to the urinary tract, is common. If such damage is suspected (because of blood at the external meatus, perineal haematoma or displacement of the prostate on rectal examination) urethral catheterisation should not be attempted. Instead an urgent retrograde urethrogram should be done; if injury is ruled out a catheter can be passed, but if injury is confirmed an urgent urological opinion should be sought. The same algorithm applies if a single attempt at urethral catheterisation is unsuccessful (see chapter 10).

Damage to abdominal organs

Abdominal examination may be equivocal if there is a major pelvic injury. Peritoneal lavage can be performed but the result should be interpreted with caution. If the returned fluid is not frank blood the red cell count in the fluid should be measured (see chapter 9). The use of ultrasound in the emergency department by an experienced trauma surgeon is a more sensitive and specific test for free fluid in the peritoneum. This can be further refined with the use of computed tomography. Opening the abdomen without good reason can do more harm than good as the abdominal wall contributes significantly to tamponade of bleeding within the pelvis.

The problem with peritoneal lavage is that blood may enter the peritoneal cavity from the retroperitoneal haematoma associated with a pelvic fracture, so the result could be positive in the absence of damage to other organs. A negative result indicates no necessity for a laparotomy, but a positive peritoneal lavage does not necessarily mean that there is peritoneal organ damage. Continuous monitoring of the haemoglobin concentration is essential because blood loss may be immense.

Open pelvic fractures are almost always fatal unless dealt with properly. This includes diverting the bowel and washing out the distal segment. The stoma should be sited in the upper quadrants, well away from any iliac crest pin sites, to reduce pin site/pelvic infection and so increase the options for definitive pelvic fixation.

Disruption of the pelvic ring with extensive damage to the pelvic blood vessels is an important cause of death in multiple trauma. Close co-operation between orthopaedic and general surgeons is critical to avoid unnecessary deaths.

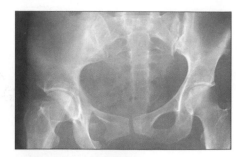

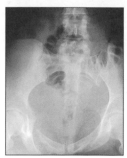

Fractured pelvis.
(Above) Anteroposterior view.
(Left) Inlet view.
(Below) Outlet view.

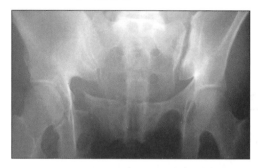

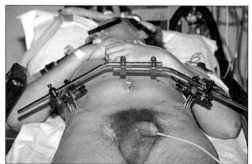

Pelvic external fixator.

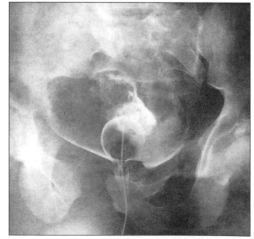

Cystogram of a bladder full of haematoma with extravasation of contrast through a torn anterior bladder wall.

Radiology

Only when the multiply injured patient is resuscitated and stable should radiographs of the limbs and additional pelvic and acetabular studies be considered. The standard two projections at right angles to one another are appropriate and must include the whole bone suspected of being fractured and the adjacent joints. Radiographs must be scrutinised for joint dislocations and subluxations that may be associated with fractures.

Two further pelvic views are indicated in pelvic fractures—the inlet and outlet views—and in acetabular fractures and hip dislocations—the Judet views (45° obliques). In suspected shoulder pathology an axial view should be performed in addition to the standard anteroposterior view.

If computed tomography is used to study head, neck, spine, chest and/or abdomen, and a pelvic or acetabular fracture is present, 5 mm cuts through the pelvis should be requested. Five mm computed tomography cuts are also useful in planning the management of tibial plateau and pilon fractures, and specialised cuts are required for os calcis fractures.

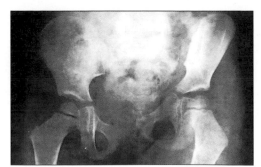
Vertical shear disruption of left hemipelvis.

Beware of requesting extensive radiographic studies if this requires the unstable patient to be moved from the resuscitation area and its monitoring facilities

Splintage

Correct use of splintage will afford considerable pain relief, avert further soft tissue damage and facilitate transport. To be effective the splint must immobilise the joint above and below the fracture and include the bone on either side of a dislocation.

The arm is best supported by a simple sling and bandaged to the body. The forearm and wrist are immobilised on padded splints or pillows. The hand should be splinted in a functional position—that is, over a bandage roll with the fingers straight. Femoral shaft fractures may be adequately controlled only by using fixed traction splints such as the Thomas splint or the modern equivalent. A traction force is applied to the leg or foot and is countered with a proximal pelvic bar.

Low pressure (30 mm Hg) inflatable double-walled polyvinyl jacket splints are commonly used to immobilise tibial, ankle and forearm fractures—they are easy to use and effective.

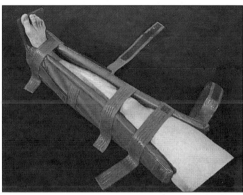
Leg splint.

Compartment syndromes

Multiply injured patients with reduced tissue perfusion and oxygenation are at high risk of developing compartment syndromes. Increasing swelling in the unyielding fascial compartments, particularly in the forearm and lower leg, as a result of tissue contusion, bleeding or ischaemia, may result in auto-infarction of the compartment muscle. The clinical symptoms and signs are increasing pain, sensory deficit in the distribution of the peripheral nerves passing through that compartment, progressive swelling and tension, and, pain on passive muscle stretching. The presence of peripheral pulses does not exclude an evolving compartment syndrome.

If signs of a compartment syndrome develop all potentially constricting dressings, casts and splints should be released. If rapid recovery is not observed then prompt fasciotomy should be performed. A high index of suspicion must be maintained in the unconscious patient and continuous instrumented compartment pressure monitoring may be indicated. A compartment perfusion pressure of less than 30 mm Hg is considered abnormal. This is calculated by subtracting the measured compartment pressure from the diastolic blood pressure. It is a fallacy that compartment syndromes do not develop in open fractures—an incidence of 15% has been reported. If the duration of a compartment syndrome has exceeded 72 hours,

Symptoms and signs of compartment syndrome
- Increasing pain—despite immobilisation of fractures
- Altered sensation in the dermatome of the nerve(s) passing through that compartment
- Palpable raised tension and tenderness of the muscle compartment
- Pain on passively stretching the muscles within the compartment

Beware:
- The pulses are often **present**
- Maintain a high index of suspicion in the unconscious or anaesthetised patient

fasciotomies should not be performed as this will expose dead muscle and increase the risk of infection. It is imperative that the orthopaedic surgeon is asked before any local anaesthetic blocks are used in severe limb injuries. This is because these may mask evolving compartment syndromes or ischaemic pain or both

> **In severe limb injuries it is imperative to ask the orthopaedic surgeon before using any anaesthetic blocks, because they may mask evolving compartment syndromes or ischaemic pain or both**

Traumatic amputations

Amputation is a catastrophic and life threatening injury. Haemorrhage must be controlled as a priority. Replantation is possible in certain instances. In these cases the amputated part should be cleaned and wrapped in a sterile cloth that has been soaked in saline. It needs to be sealed in a sterile plastic bag, which is then immersed in a container of crushed ice and water. The part must not be allowed to freeze. Rapid transfer to the definitive care centre is essential. Amputated parts that are unsuitable for grafting may be a source of bone, skin, vessel and nerve grafts and should not be discarded.

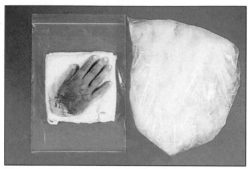
Management of an amputated hand.

Communication

Early communication with the appropriate specialties is essential. All open fractures will require early orthopaedic evaluation and management and most will also require the services of plastic surgery. Pelvic and acetabular fractures require early referral of the patient to a specialist unit, preferably accompanied by the appropriate inlet/outlet and/or Judet views plus computed tomography scans. Such patients are best managed in regional trauma units with intensive care facilities for trauma patients and should be transferred as soon as possible.

> **Polytraumatised patients are best managed in regional trauma units with intensive care facilities for trauma patients and should be transferred as soon as possible**

Definitive management of fractures

Closed fractures
In the multiply injured patient the conservative management of major fractures of long bones is not an option. The incidence, morbidity and mortality associated with adult respiratory distress syndrome, fat embolism and late systemic sepsis are significantly reduced if major long bone fractures are stabilised by internal or external fixation within 24 hours of injury. Fixation also makes nursing of the patient easier and reduces the need for narcotic analgesia.

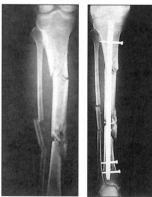
Internally fixed fractured tibia.

Open fractures
Soft tissue damage and the risk of infection are the two critical factors determining outcome in patients with serious open limb fractures. The patient's management within the first few hours can determine whether the outcome is complete recovery or lifelong disability. The infecting organisms may be the contaminating ones, and samples for culture should therefore be obtained at the outset. The priorities are to clear contamination and devitalised tissue. In so doing, the amount of potential culture medium is reduced, as is the size of an infecting inoculum.

In a multiply injured patient with reduced oxygen delivery and an anticipated rise in tissue pressure, wound hypoxia and an increased susceptibility to infection are inevitable. Closure of a wound is therefore rarely indicated.

Wound debridement is often inadequate. Debridement should be performed by the orthopaedic surgeon together with the plastic surgeon who may subsequently be required to provide tissue cover. Surrounding skin is shaved and the wound

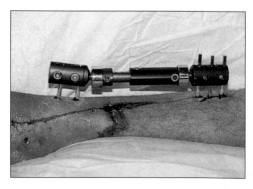
Externally fixed fractured tibia.

and surrounding area scrubbed with a brush. The wound is extended, in the long axis of the limb, as required to facilitate examination and fasciotomies performed if required. All non-viable muscle, fascia and fat are carefully but radically excised.

Large volumes of irrigation fluid should be used—in excess of 4 litres ("the solution to pollution is dilution"). The most commonly used irrigant is physiological saline, although Hartman's solution and mild antiseptics can be used. There is no evidence for the use of antibiotics in the lavage fluid. Pressurised pulsed lavage systems are advantageous, but it is the rate and volume of flow that are important rather than the pressure.

Skin flaps of dubious viability are best dealt with by taking a split skin graft from the flap surface. This will serve to delineate the margin of viability (the dead area will show no capillary bleeding). The harvested graft can be applied later if necrosis of the flap occurs. All loose fragments of bone should be removed.

Most open fractures are unstable. Stabilisation will promote tissue healing. This should be done using the most appropriate method for the fracture, the soft tissues, the unit in which the procedure is undertaken, and in appropriate cases following consultation with plastic surgeon. The debrided wound should initially be left open and covered with a dry dressing, such as fluffed gauze. Wet dressings should be avoided, except over large areas of exposed tendon or bone or both where there is no viable soft tissue that can be used to cover. The wound is ideally inspected again at 48 hours. Early closure of the soft tissue wound, when it is suitable for closure, reduces the chance of infection and non-union of the fracture.

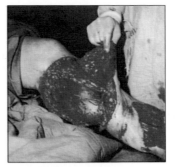
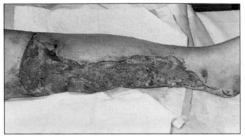

Soft tissue damage to the leg after a degloving injury (top); late flap necrosis was treated by excision and application of the split skin graft (meshed) obtained at the first operation (bottom).

Conclusions

The assessment and management of limb trauma should always be secondary to resuscitation and management of life threatening conditions.

A knowledge of the mechanism of injury and careful examination are essential if all injuries sustained by the patient are to be identified. Assessment of the peripheral circulation is crucial to allow early detection and management of potentially limb threatening injuries. Appropriate reduction of fractures and dislocations combined with correct splintage will reduce pain and can prevent serious complications.

A high level of suspicion is necessary in the multiply injured patient to identify nerve injuries and detect evolving compartment syndromes. Frequent reassessment and recordings of the circulation and neurological function of an injured limb are essential. The seriousness of open fractures should be appreciated and an aggressive approach to wound debridement adopted. As early as possible there should be consultation between orthopaedic and trauma surgeons and other teams especially the plastic surgeons for open fractures, general surgeons for open pelvic fractures and vascular surgeons for suspected vascular injuries. Operative stabilisation of major long bone fractures within the first 24 hours significantly reduces morbidity and mortality.

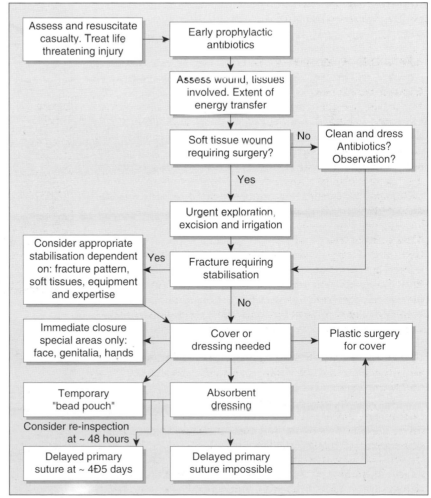

A decision-making sequence in the management of limb injuries.

12 Eye injuries

Anthony P Moriarty

The aim of this chapter is to emphasise immediate ophthalmic management and diagnosis, and to furnish the trauma team leader with the knowledge to make appropriate referral in the acute situation. This chapter will not cover long term management or definitive treatment of ophthalmic trauma.

History

An AMPLE history (see pages 10 and 82) must be taken directly from the patient if possible, and from an adult as well if a child is injured. In the unconscious patient, a history from a reliable adult is essential.

Chemical burn

Any history of alkali or acid entering the eye is an indication for immediate referral of the patient, after irrigation of the eye with a sterile fluid—preferably balanced salt or Ringer's solution—from a drip bag and stand. Use copious amounts of fluid and do not bother with pH or litmus paper. Remove particulate matter, especially lime or cement, by everting the lids and using topical anaesthetic.

Alakli injuries are devastating, and much more serious than those caused by acid. Inform the ophthalmologist immediately but continue irrigation and removal of all particulate matter.

Metal or glass foreign bodies, high velocity injuries

Any history of high velocity injuries, drilling, or entry into the eye of glass or metallic foreign bodies necessitates referral to the ophthalmologist. Radiographs are often unhelpful in locating glass and other intra-ocular foreign bodies, especially if they are not radio opaque. If genuine concern exists, the best idea is to examine the patient on the slit lamp microscope.

If an intraocular foreign body is suspected, dilatation of the pupil is necessary, followed by a retinal examination by an ophthalmologist using a binocular indirect ophthalmoscope. Often a computed tomography scan is also necessary to locate the foreign body.

If there is genuine concern about the presence of glass or an intraocular foreign body, discuss the patient with the ophthalmologist.

Is the trauma blunt or sharp?

Sharp injuries (from example, from a Stanley knife) can be devastating and transect the optic nerve or intra-orbital structures. Pad the eye if it is bleeding, refer the patient and discuss the injury with the ophthalmologist. Blunt injuries require a more measured assessment depending on the clinical findings and setting.

Eye injury: taking the history

- Chemical burn
- Metal or glass involved
- High velocity injury, or while drilling
- Trauma: blunt or sharp
- Pain
- Reduced vision/visual symptoms
- Previous eye disease

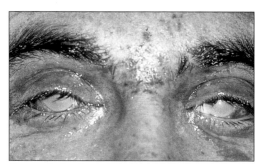
Severe alkaline burn: the corneas are already opaque.

If there is genuine concern about the presence of glass or an intraocular foreign body, discuss the patient with the ophthalmologist

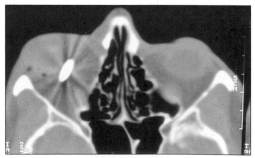
A computed tomography scan determines whether a foreign body is intraocular or intraorbital. Radiographs are often unhelpful in locating foreign bodies.

Pain

Pain may occur as a result of surface eye problems such as foreign bodies or abrasions, or deeper intraorbital causes such as a fracture or haematoma (dull ache). Assess the nature and cause. The most painful conditions are chemical burns, arc eye, abrasions, foreign bodies and orbital fractures. Pain rarely emanates from around the globe itself—a penetrating eye injury in isolation, for example, is not usually painful.

For orbital fractures simple analgesics are helpful. For surface problems, minimal use of a topical anaesthetic, such as pyroxymethocaine, is acceptable; however, do not over use in chemical burns because this further damages corneal epithelium.

Significant reduction in visual acuity

A marked reduction in visual acuity necessitates an ophthalmic opinion. Examine the vision, if possible, before discussion.

Previous eye operations or disease

The globe may be ruptured by trauma when there has been previous surgery—cataract, for example. Discuss these cases with the ophthalmologist.

Examination

Is examination possible?

A severe periorbital haematoma may make examination and any view of the globe impossible. It is then difficult to exclude serious pathology; discuss the patient with the ophthalmologist.

Visual acuity

In the acutely injured patient, gaining co-operation for long enough to check visual acuity may be impossible. Simple tests of light perception, hand movements or finger counting may be all that is feasible (check each eye separately). If the patient is more co-operative, it may be possible to check the visual acuity with a Snellen chart. Use the patient's distance glasses, if worn, for distance charts. However, if they are lost, a pinhole corrects for any error attributable to short or long sightedness. A reduced vision that fails to improve with a pinhole is indicative of pathology, reduced vision that improves to normal with a pinhole indicates simply a refractive error.

Eye movements and diplopia

Decide if double vision (diplopia) is present. Diplopia present with only one eye open is monocular; diplopia present only when both eyes are open simultaneously is binocular.

Monocular diplopia is rare in the acutely injured eye and implies corneal or lens pathology (such as a dislocated lens, which is rare in isolation).

Binocular diplopia is more common. In trauma it occurs most often in a blow out fracture, or a fracture of the maxilla in which the contents of the muscle cone are trapped in the fracture. Diplopia is then present in upward gaze, as the eye is prevented from elevation by entrapment. This must be documented, but commonly maxillofacial surgeons will be consulted at this stage and make the appropriate referral. Urgent treatment is not necessary, but documentation and referral are essential.

Binocular diplopia may also occur in the presence of palsies of the third, fourth and sixth cranial nerves. This will be obvious from abnormalities of eye movement and diplopia. All require referral and discussion, but only third nerve palsy requires urgent referral. A pupil that is dilated and unreacting in the

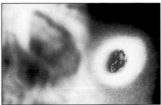
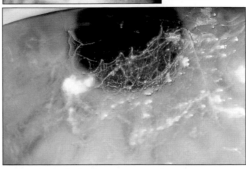
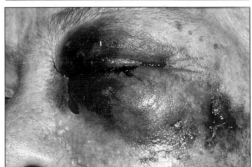

Left: corneal foreign body and surrounding rust ring. Below: corneal abrasion.

Severe periorbital haematoma.

Examination of the injured eye

- Is it possible?
- Visual acuity—use Snellen chart, and pin hole to correct refractive error
- Eye movements and diplopia
- Lids
- Sub-conjunctival haemorrhage/laceration
- **Cornea**—abrasion, foreign body
- **Pupil**—eccentric, unreacting, prolapsed, dilated, miosed
- **Soft eye/shallow chamber = perforation**
- Hyphaema
- Posterior segment complications
- **Dilation / red reflex**—in the setting of an acute injury, a reduced red reflex (the luminous red appearance on the retina during retinoscopy) implies a vitreous haemorrhage, hyphaema (blood in the anterior chamber) or traumatic cataract

Causes of reduced vision after trauma

- Hyphaema (blood in the anterior chamber)
- Corneal perforation
- Scleral perforation
- Vitreous haemorrhage
- Contusion/transected optic nerve
- Retinal detachment

All require immediate referral

ABC of Major Trauma

presence of a third nerve palsy can indicate a posterior communicating artery aneurysm or raised intracranial pressure.

An eye that is incapable of movement may be the result of a retrobulbar haematoma, with proptosis following trauma, or a combined third, fourth or sixth nerve palsy as a result of a ruptured caroticocavernous fistula (pulsatile exophthalmos). *These both require urgent referral.*

Lids

Lid margin tears require referral to the ophthalmologist, especially if the canaliculus is severed (medial to the punctum) since urgent repair is essential to prevent a permanent watering eye. Lacerations around the eye and face, not involving the lid margin, do not specifically require ophthalmic referral. This is a watershed zone between plastic surgeons, maxillofacial surgeons and ophthalmologists specifically trained in oculoplastics. Many of these can, however, be handled by the trauma team.

Subconjunctival haemorrhage/laceration

The best way to examine the globe is to get used to using the slit lamp by a microscope in your department. However, this may not be possible; in such cases some form of magnifying loupe and a bright torch, with the aid of a cobalt blue filter, are usually satisfactory. Subconjunctival haemorrhage is not a serious problem in isolation. A conjunctival laceration, however, does require referral as repair may be necessary, and exploration if there is a possibility of a penetrating eye injury.

Corneal abrasions and foreign bodies

Corneal abrasions and foreign bodies are easily visible with a loupe magnifying glass and bright torch. Use fluorescein drops and a cobalt blue filter to diagnose a corneal abrasion. To remove a corneal foreign body, use a green needle with pyroxy-methocaine anaesthetic and, preferably, a slit lamp microscope. A subtarsal foreign body requires eversion of the lid and removal with a cotton bud.

Use antibiotic ointment and a pad for comfort after removal of foreign bodies and in the treatment of corneal abrasions. A cycloplegic drop (cyclopentolate 1%) relieves spasm and can be particularly helpful. For arc eye similar ointment and padding, with a cycloplegic, often suffice. Occasionally a weak steroid drop (prednisolone 0.5% four times a day) for 3 days may also be given to minimise symptoms. These problems do not require ophthalmic referral unless complications supervene. Leave rust rings alone and simply cover with antibiotic ointment for a week.

Refer these patients if the condition fails to settle.

The pupil

Miosed pupils indicate use of narcotic drugs or pilocarpine drops.

A dilated pupil can indicate third nerve palsy (see above), a blind eye (for example, a transected optic nerve), severe visual impairment (for example, retinal detachment), or traumatic dilatation.

An irregular pupil suggests trauma or iris prolapse.

Perforating injury

Corneal perforation may be associated with iris prolapse, a shallow anterior chamber, or hyphaema (usually obvious on examination of the anterior segment)—*all require immediate referral.* In the meantime, cover the eye with a clear plastic shield and instil chloramphenicol drops.

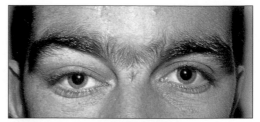

Previous right blow out fracture with sunken right globe.

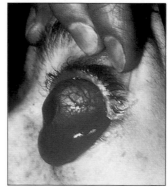

Severe retrobulbar haematoma following blunt injury.

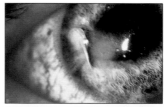

Irregular pupil: iris prolapse through corneal perforation.

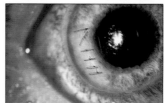

Post operative repair with normal pupil.

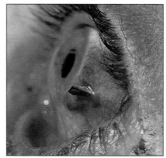

Drilling injury: scleral perforation and shallow anterior chamber.

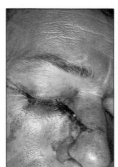
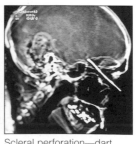

Scleral perforation—dart injury—and CT scan to show site of dart before removal.

Scleral perforation is more difficult to see and diagnose. A history of a sharp foreign body, or a high velocity injury, should arouse suspicion. Conjunctival laceration or haemorrhage may be present and the eye will be soft and may have a shallow anterior chamber. Vitreous haemorrhage may partially or completely obscure the view of the retina. The foreign body may be visible on dilated fundoscopy.

Scleral perforations are much more serious than corneal perforations because they are associated with damage to the retina. Place a clear plastic shield over the affected eye. Instil topical chloramphenicol drops and immediately refer the patient to the ophthalmologist. Do not waste time performing straightforward plain radiographs because computed tomography will almost always be necessary to locate the intra-ocular foreign body.

Hyphaema

Hyphaema—blood in the anterior chamber—from perforation or from blunt trauma *warrants immediate referral.*

Posterior segment complications

These can be difficult to diagnose.

Retinal detachment may accompany severe trauma and be associated with a reduction in visual acuity or a visual field defect. Such injuries usually require a dilated examination by an ophthalmologist with the binocular indirect ophthalmoscope.

A contused or transected optic nerve will produce a profound reduction in visual acuity and a dilated pupil.

Vitreous haemorrhage following blunt trauma or an intraocular foreign body will obscure ophthalmoscopic retinal details when the pupil is dilated. *These patients require immediate referral to the ophthalmologist.*

Should I dilate the pupil?

To diagnose posterior segment problems (retinal detachment, intraocular foreign body, vitreous haemorrhage), it is necessary to dilate the pupil and examine the posterior segment. Having said that, a dilated pupil may interfere with other observations of the acutely injured patient. Consequently if the history is suggestive of a posterior segment problem (visual acuity is reduced) an ophthalmologist will be examining the patient and dilation of the pupil is best left to him or her.

Do not dilate the pupil without prior discussion with an ophthalmologist.

Summary

Any uncertainty about the extent of injuries to the eye necessitates consultation with the ophthalmologist. There are really only two devastating eye complications that present to the trauma team: chemical injuries should be treated immediately in the emergency room; a suspected penetrating eye injury requires immediate ophthalmic referral.

Please make sure that the telephone number of the nearest ophthalmological unit, for during the daytime and at night, is clearly available in the emergency department. Remember that a telephone call at NHS expense costs you nothing, but failing to make the telephone call may cost the patient a great deal.

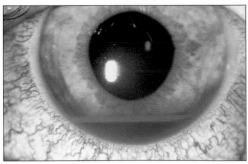
Hyphaema.

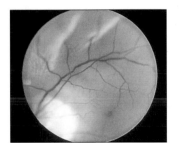
Retinal detachment—yellow folds of detached retina.

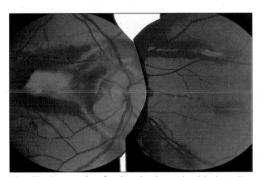
Metallic intraocular foreign body embedded in the retina

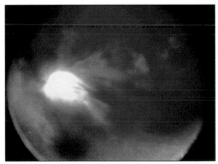
Vitreous haemorrhage following trauma.

13 Medical problems

Terry Wardle, Peter Driscoll

In this chapter we concentrate on how the trauma patient's health before injury can influence the clinical picture and the response to resuscitation. Management of coexisting medical problems during resuscitation will also be discussed.

Prevalence and effect

Only recently has attention been focused on the incidence, type, and effect of premorbid conditions on the outcome of a trauma patient. In the USA, the incidence of premorbid conditions ranges from 4.8% to 16%, whereas in the UK such conditions occur in 39% of major trauma patients. Despite geographical differences, all studies have shown that there is an increase in the mortality of trauma victims with premorbid conditions. Premorbid conditions are found in all age groups but, not surprisingly, their frequency increases with age.

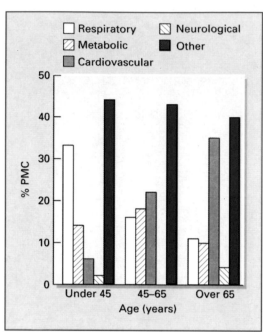

Incidence and type of premorbid condition (PMC) by age in UK trauma victims.

Assessment and management

The ABCDE approach to the trauma patient should be adhered to even if a premorbid condition is suspected.

Airway and cervical spine immobilisation

Airway—Several medical conditions may compromise the airway (see box). Although these can influence airway management with simple adjuncts, they do not usually cause problems with endotracheal intubation. In contrast, difficulties may arise if the patient has rheumatoid changes in the temporomandibular joints. These changes may be so severe that the mouth cannot be opened sufficiently to allow oral intubation. Other methods of securing the airway should be considered (see chapter 3), according to the urgency of the situation.

Immobilisation of cervical spine—Patients with rheumatoid disease or ankylosing spondylitis may have spinal involvement with instability and rigidity, and hence the potential for cervical cord injury. Minimal force can therefore cause severe injury. Care should therefore be taken when clearing and securing the airway.

Breathing

Respiratory diseases are common and many trauma victims present with coexisting pulmonary pathology. This can lead to diagnostic problems, especially when the patient has sustained a chest injury.

Several respiratory conditions may not be apparent on initial assessment but clues can be gained from the history, examination, treatment response, arterial blood gas results, and chest radiograph. Arterial blood gas results are invaluable but must be interpreted in the light of the clinical situation.

Conditions compromising the airway

- Pseudobulbar palsy
- Bulbar palsy
- Macroglossia
- Progressive systemic sclerosis

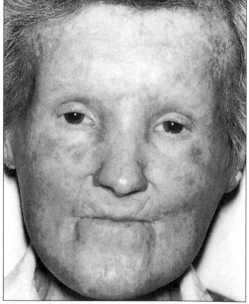

Progressive systemic sclerosis.

Assume that a cervical spine injury is present and maintain in-line immobilisation until it can be excluded clinically and radiologically

For example, hypoxia in an adequately ventilated patient indicates that there could be underlying pulmonary emboli, sepsis, or contusion. In contrast, metabolic acidosis in trauma victims, especially when associated with an increased anion gap, usually indicates hypoperfusion and lactic acidosis.

Chronic bronchitis and emphysema—These are common diseases. These patients require a fractional inspired oxygen of 0.85% because of the deleterious effect of hypoxia following trauma. Subsequently the oxygen concentration can be adjusted according to the arterial blood gas result.

Bronchospasm—An AMPLE history (see p. 82) as part of the secondary survey will help determine if this is caused by inhalation of noxious compounds or coexisting pulmonary disease. In either case, however, bronchospasm will be detected in the primary survey and bronchodilators should be given, with hydrocortisone added according to the clinical situation. It is also important to remember that patients with asthma have an increased risk of developing a pneumothorax, especially if they require positive ventilation.

Pulmonary oedema—This can result from many causes but is usually a sequel to ischaemic heart disease and, to a lesser extent, mitral/aortic valve disease. This is particularly true if pulmonary oedema is already present when the patient arrives in the accident and emergency department (providing transfer has not been delayed). These patients will benefit from early endotracheal intubation, ventilation, and measurement of right and left heart pressures. Only in this way can the correct fluid resuscitation be achieved.

Pleural effusions—Many medical conditions, including left ventricular failure, pleuropulmonary malignancy and rheumatoid disease may present with pleural effusions. A chest drain is still the management of choice and not only reduces the effect of fluid on pulmonary function but also ensures that coexisting trauma is not present.

Pulmonary emboli—Following skeletal injury, in particular multiple fractures, fat emboli may result. Although pulmonary signs predominate a variety of other clinical signs may be present. Irrespective of the many potential causes of massive pulmonary embolism, it usually presents as electromechanical dissociation. As thrombolysis would be dangerous in the presence of multiple injuries, management is symptomatic and oxygen should be given immediately.

Circulation and haemorrhage control

Hypotension—A low blood pressure after major trauma is usually due to hypovolaemia. If the patient fails to respond to an intravenous fluid challenge and there is no evidence of any occult bleeding, consider an underlying medical condition. As a minimum the clinician will require a:

● Full history and physical examination
● 12 lead ECG
● Full blood count
● Urea, glucose, and electrolyte measurement
● Arterial blood gas analysis
● Chest x-ray.

The presence of distended neck veins may indicate cardiac tamponade, pulmonary embolus, or right ventricular failure (from whatever cause). Further investigation will be required to determine the precise diagnosis.

Occult blood loss may occur from the gastrointestinal tract secondary to trauma. It can indicate pre-existent peptic ulcer disease and inflammation. That may be exacerbated by stress ulceration, particularly with burns (Curling's ulcers) or neurological injury (Cushing's ulcers).

It is unusual for trauma victims to present in *septic shock* unless there has been a prolonged delay in extrication or

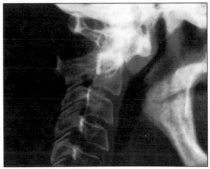

Rheumatoid cervical spine with atlantoaxial subluxation.

The presence of chronic pulmonary disease in trauma patients is an indication for early ventilation

Causes of pulmonary oedema
● Ischaemic heart disease
● Valvular disease
● Inhalation of noxious substances
● Pulmonary parenchymal injury
● Acute respiratory distress syndrome
● Neurological injury
● Myocardial trauma

Clinical features of fat emboli
● Tachypnoea
● Petechial rash
● Neurological signs

If a patient with low blood pressure after major trauma fails to respond to an intravenous fluid challenge and there is no evidence of any occult bleeding, consider an underlying medical condition

transfer. Although these patients have hypotension they also have warm, well perfused peripheries. This is a useful physical sign in the differential diagnosis of hypotension (see chapter 5).

Hypotension is an important sequel to adrenal and, rarely, pituitary insufficiency. The chances of adrenal cortical failure occurring in a trauma victim are increasing because glucocorticoids are used to treat a variety of diseases. Consequently patients may have suboptimal adrenal function even if the steroid dose has been withdrawn gradually. In such circumstances any acute stress, including trauma, can cause an addisonian crisis. This may be manifested by hypotension unresponsive to treatment, recurrent hypotension, vomiting, confusion and coma. Be aware that the classic electrolyte changes are not always present.

If an addisonian crisis is suspected, the patient should be given hydrocortisone 300 mg intravenously. This should be repeated daily until adrenal function can be assessed by a short synacthen test. A random serum sample for cortisol and ACTH concentrations should be taken before hydrocortisone is given. While these results provide useful information, they are insufficient to diagnose adrenal cortical insufficiency.

Patients with left ventricular failure, uraemia or rheumatoid disease may have a pericardial effusion before the injury. If there is clinical evidence of a pericardial effusion a pericardiocentesis is needed to improve cardiac function and exclude trauma to the pericardium or myocardium.

Hypertension—This is always a concern. The history and physical examination are important to differentiate between acute and chronic hypertension. Acute hypertension may reflect increased intracranial pressure but other circulatory signs are usually present, in particular bradycardia. Persistent or fluctuating hypertension can indicate the presence of phaeochromocytoma. While this is a rare condition it presents problems for the unwary. Patients with acute hypertension need invasive monitoring and the intravenous administration of both α and β blockers so that a careful controlled reduction of blood pressure can be achieved.

Ischaemic heart disease—This is the most prevalent disease in the Western world and will be exacerbated by hypoxia, hypovolaemia and hypotension. If the patient is unconscious, however, myocardial infarction may not be apparent. A 12 lead ECG and cardiac monitoring are essential. Hypotension is a particularly difficult problem in patients with ischaemic heart disease and haemorrhage. The most common cause is blood loss, but heart failure may coexist or be the cause. It is therefore crucial that fluid replacement is governed by accurate invasive monitoring.

Dysrhythmias—These may reflect myocardial ischaemia. However, there are other causes, for example, hypoxia, electrolyte disturbance, increased intracranial pressure, and drug therapy. Dysrhythmias may precipitate or exacerbate hypotension, cardiac failure, hypoxia, and loss of consciousness.

Tachydysrhythmias can be treated with drugs if the patient is haemodynamically stable with no evidence of cardiac failure or impaired consciousness. As all these drugs depress myocardial function, a tachydysrhythmia in the presence of cardiac failure should be treated with appropriate cardioversion.

Valvular disease—Aortic valve disease is increasingly common, especially in the elderly. The low volume pulse may be misdiagnosed as an early indicator of shock. Excessive fluid administration can cause left or biventricular failure. Cardiac decompensation may also occur because of underlying ischaemic heart disease or myocardial contusion. Patients should be given prophylactic antibiotics as soon as convenient according to British Heart Foundation guidelines. If there are no contraindications intravenous gentamycin 120 mg and

Premorbid conditions that give rise to hypotension

Pulmonary
  embolism
  tension pneumothorax
  severe bronchospasm

Hypovolaemia
  diuretic
  gastrointestinal bleed
  adrenal insufficiency

Cardiac
  left/right ventricular failure
  dysrhythmia
  cardiac tamponade
  pericardial effusion
  septicaemia
  uraemia
  opiates

Circulatory
  diuretic
  vasodilators
  septicaemia
  spinal cord injury
  anaphylaxis
  autonomic dysfunction

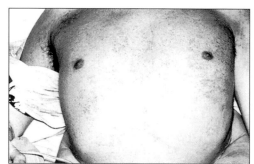

Petechial rash secondary to fat emboli.

Blind treatment of patients with diuretics or vasodilators may precipitate or exacerbate tissue hypoxia

ampicillin 1 g should be given followed by a further 500 mg of oral ampicillin 12 hours later.

Cardiac pacemakers—These can influence the clinical picture following major trauma (see box).

Chronic anaemia—This is a common condition and many patients are asymptomatic. Unfortunately information as to the presence and type of anaemia may not be available from the initial haemoglobin estimation. Therefore patients should be transfused according to symptoms and signs rather than haemoglobin concentration. Haemoglobinopathies, in particular sickle-cell disease, may precipitate or be precipitated by major trauma. Acute abdominal pain may be due to a sickle cell crisis rather than intraperitoneal injury. Tenderness is not uncommon and under these circumstances further assessment is warranted with ultrasound scan, computed tomography or diagnostic peritoneal lavage.

Coagulopathy—Whether the result of a bleeding diathesis or a procoagulant disease, coagulopathy can profoundly influence the patient's response to trauma and resuscitation. This problem may come to light only during resuscitation if a history is not available and there are no clinical features, for example of chronic liver disease. If there is any suspicion of a bleeding disorder, e.g bleeding from Venflon sites, the activated partial thromboplastin and prothrombin times should be checked. These should be corrected appropriately.

Electrolyte imbalance—This is not uncommon, especially in patients taking diuretics. Hyperkalaemia is likely to be the most important electrolyte problem in the acute situation. This should not be ascribed to a haemolysed sample because patients can have coexisting renal dysfunction, metabolic acidosis in association with shock, diabetic ketoacidosis, or even tissue (especially muscular) necrosis. This is particularly important in patients who have chronic or acute renal failure where underperfusion may exacerbate the situation and warrant early consultation with a nephrologist.

Cardiac transplants—The type of transplant will govern whether myocardium is able to respond directly to sympathetic nerve stimulation or indirectly to circulating catecholamines.

Neurological impairment

With the increasing number of elderly patients there is a corresponding increase in cerebrovascular disease. Hypoglycaemia has many manifestations and may mimic a stroke.

Many neurological problems can be identified when assessing airway, breathing, and circulation. Fits or coma are usually ascribed to intracerebral injury; however, in the presence of a normal computed tomography scan other conditions need to be considered (see box). Hyponatraemia or hypocalcaemia may be precipitated by rapid volume expansion. In contrast, hypernatraemia can be precipitated or exacerbated by dehydration and result in cerebral oedema.

Many of the chronic neurological diseases, for example stroke or demyelination, may present with lateralising signs. These can mimic or mask occult intracerebral trauma. The presence of these signs necessitates computed tomography if a history is not available.

Autonomic dysfunction may not only mask the patient's response to trauma and fluid resuscitation but can also mimic spinal cord injury. With the exception of diabetes mellitus most causes of autonomic dysfunction are rare. Ideally patients should be treated as though they have an acute spinal injury. Invasive monitoring and cautious fluid resuscitation are therefore essential and inotropic drugs should be considered.

Malignant hyperpyrexia and the neuroleptic malignant syndrome are potentially fatal disorders that may not be

Potential problems associated with pacemakers
- Damage to pacemaker/wire
- Pacemaker failure
- Inappropriate function
- Masking of myocardial damage or bradycardia
- Inappropriate response to fluid resuscitation (especially if the pacemaker has a fixed rate)

Causes of chronic anaemia
- Chronic renal failure
- Chronic liver disease
- Acute intestinal inflammation
- Chronic intestinal inflammation
- Multisystem disease
- Haemolytic anaemia
- Gastrectomy
- Ileal resection

Coagulation disorders
- Thrombocytopenia (especially if $<20\times10^9$/l)
- Congenital coagulation defects—for example, haemophilia
- Acquired coagulation defects—for example, malabsorption
- Disseminated intravascular coagulation

A serum glucose estimation is essential for all trauma patients—hypoglycaemia is easy to treat but easy to miss!

Causes of fits and coma
Drugs/chemicals:
  cocaine, solvents, tricyclic antidepressants
Infections:
  meningitis, encephalitis, toxoplamosis, malaria, intracerebral abscess
Vascular:
  thromboembolic disease, hypertension, dysrhythmia
Metabolic:
  hypoglycaemia, hyperglycaemia, uraemia, electrolyte imbalance, hypocalcaemia, anoxia, hepatic encephalopathy
Intracerebral tumours

evident during the primary survey and may only be diagnosed during or following anaesthesia. These conditions necessitate prompt treatment with dantrolene and measures to maintain an appropriate core temperature.

Exposure

Hypothermia can cause or be the result of major trauma. Appropriate means to correct the body temperature include the use of warmed intravenous fluids and overhead heating in the resuscitation room (see chapter 3).

AMPLE history

Many medical problems will be identified in trauma patients providing that an AMPLE history has been obtained. Information may have to be sought not only from the patient but also from the general practitioner, hospital records, relatives and witnesses.

Allergies—These are unlikely to influence the management of a trauma patient. However an allergic response can cause trauma and follow drug therapy. A range of clinical manifestations can occur. Anaphylactic shock, the most sinister manifestation, requires immediate adrenaline.

Medication—Many patients are who sustain trauma are prescribed drugs. The details may be unknown at the time of resuscitation. Beta blockers, calcium channel antagonists, ACE inhibitors, and, to a lesser extent, nitrates are important because they modify the cardiovascular response to trauma and resuscitation. The use of oral steroids is common and an addisonian crisis can occur if these drugs are omitted or their dose is not increased.

The use of recreational drugs may also precipitate or modify the patient's response to trauma.

Alcohol consumption influences the presentation, treatment, and outcome of major trauma. The link between alcohol and road traffic accidents is well established.

Alcohol can produce a variety of clinical manifestations, as can its withdrawal. In the presence of chronic alcohol consumption adequate thiamine should be given before glucose to prevent Wernicke's encephalopathy. Control of withdrawal is advocated.

Past medical history—This is extremely important, alerting the physician to factors that may influence the patient's clinical presentation and response to treatment.

Last meal—This information is crucial, especially if the patient needs an anaesthetic. It can also explain the cause of hypoglycaemia in the trauma patient.

Environment—Environmental details provide clues to the mechanism of injury and hypothermia. If a low core temperature cannot be attributed to exposure to the cold it should alert the physician to the presence of occult pathology, for example, pancreatitis, diabetes, hypothyroidism, and phenothiazine overdose.

AMPLE history		
A	=	Allergies
M	=	Medication
P	=	Past medical history
L	=	Last meal
E	=	Event/environment

It is better to exclude disease than to ignore it

Summary

Medical problems are common in trauma patients. They may have caused the incident or result from the injury or its subsequent treatment. Co-existing medical problems can have a tremendous impact on resuscitation after major trauma and also on the patient's survival. To overcome these problems the clinician must keep to the "ABCDE" system of trauma resuscitation and consider potential medical problems if the patient fails to respond to treatment in the expected way. An AMPLE history is invaluable, especially when supplemented by information from the hospital notes and general practitioner. Thus the physician has an important role in the management of major trauma patients.

● The illustrations were prepared by the department of medical illustration, Salford Royal Hospitals NHS trust. The photograph on p 78 is reproduced with the patient's permission.

14 Radiological assessment

James Rankine, David Nicholson, Peter Driscoll

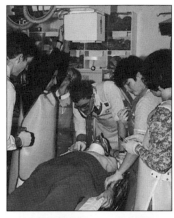

The mainstay of radiological investigation of trauma in the resuscitation room is the plain radiograph. This is also available in all emergency departments. Many immediate management decisions can be made with the aid of such radiographs, which show possible causes of cardiorespiratory compromise and detail any major bone or soft tissue injury. The development of pneumothorax, haemothorax, or early signs of aortic rupture may be clearly shown. However, radiological investigation should not interfere with the mechanics of resuscitation or be allowed to delay appropriate surgery.

The experienced radiographer is an invaluable member of the emergency team. He or she can advise on the effects of positioning and resuscitation on the images produced and give guidance as to possible delays caused by various radiographic techniques.

Unnecessary exposure of the patient and, particularly, of staff members to damaging ionising radiation must be avoided. Every radiograph should have a purpose. The quality of each image will depend on the time and effort taken to produce it. Full radiological evaluation may be deferred in patients with peripheral injuries that are not life threatening, particularly if there are other patients with trauma to be assessed.

Two important considerations in cases of major trauma are whether recognised focal injury has had hidden consequences and whether there is clinically occult damage that can be signalled early by radiography. For example, a rib or sternal fracture may be clinically quite apparent, but there may be an underlying haemopericardium; likewise a pneumothorax or pneumomediastinum may become apparent only on radiography.

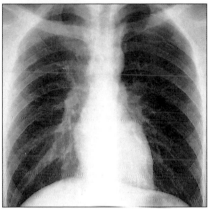

Left sided pneumothorax. The separated white line at the upper left heart border indicates pneumomediastinum.

Radiological survey

Patients with major trauma should have immediate lateral cervical spine, chest, and pelvic radiographs taken, usually at the end of the primary survey or during the secondary survey. The images should be assessed using the ABCS system as soon as they are processed and serve as a baseline for future comparison.

The patient is usually supine and immobilised by a variety of intravenous lines, airway devices and spinal stabilisers. These factors modify the quality of the radiographs. Some areas of the film may be overexposed (dark), necessitating the use of a bright light. Major trauma may affect different organ systems and parts of the body simultaneously. Once an abnormality has been identified and evaluated as far as possible attention should be turned to the possibility of an additional serious injury.

Fractures are usually represented by lucent (dark) lines, which may or may not cross the entire bone. Occasionally,

> **ABCS system of radiographic interpretation**
> A = Alignment and Adequacy
> B = Bones
> C = Cartilage/joints
> S = Soft tissues

> **General principles of radiological assessment**
> - Follow the ABCS system of interpretation
> - Plain films are most useful in the resuscitation room
> - Imaging must not interfere with resuscitation
> - All patients with major trauma should have the following radiographs taken
>   —cervical spine (lateral)
>   —chest
>   —pelvis
> - Two views are needed to exclude bone injury
> - If in doubt seek radiological advice

overlapping fragments may result in a linear density (white line) rather than lucency. Sometimes the only sign of fracture may be the alteration of the internal trabecular pattern.

Two radiographs taken from different angles are required to assess any fractured bone: a single view rarely excludes a fracture. The bone contours should be inspected for irregular steps. Abnormal angulation, particularly in children, should be regarded as suspicious. With few exceptions (one being the knee) joint surfaces should be parallel and congruent.

Injury to joints usually lead to effusions, even without fracture. Effusions may be visualised as soft tissue densities in relation to the joint capsule or by displacement of fat planes. Local haemorrhage from a skeletal fracture is also visualised as a soft tissue density with displacement or effacement of fat planes.

Soft tissue injuries may be more important than fractures, even when the two are associated. An atypical or asymmetrical soft tissue density may represent a haematoma or other fluid collection. The presence of gas in the soft tissues, visualised as dark streaks or bubbles in the tissue planes, is a sign of compound or penetrating injury involving the bowel, lungs, or neck structures.

Many accident victims have had previous trauma or disease—for example, degenerative change in the cervical spine—that will be apparent in the radiograph. Age related osteopenia predisposes patients to fractures, especially vertebral wedge compression fractures. The age of fractures may be estimated from their density, cortical thickness, and trabecular continuity. In patients with major trauma it is safest to assume that all fractures are new. Familiarity with the variety of normal appearances can develop only with experience.

Finally, if there is any doubt or mismatch of clinical and radiological appearances ask a radiologist for advice. Recent air, rail, and boating disasters have shown the advantage of experienced radiologists being present in the emergency department: they are able to provide early authoritative interpretations of radiographs, direct the taking of further films, perform any necessary further investigation, and redistribute imaging services to accommodate the volume of work.

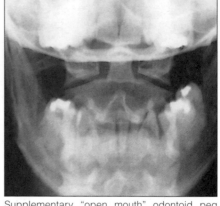

Supplementary "open mouth" odontoid peg radiograph showing symmetry of the lateral masses of C1 with regard to the peg and body of C2.

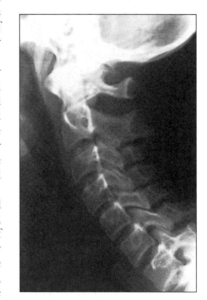

Cervical spine

Any multiply injured patient must be considered to have a cervical injury until proved otherwise. Manipulation or unguarded movement of the inadequately immobilised neck can cause cord damage, most commonly in patients with injuries below C3. A lateral radiograph shows only 70–90% of the important cervical injuries. It is therefore essential that this radiograph is supplemented by anterior, odontoid peg, and oblique views if there are clinical or radiological signs of cervical injury or any specific history. As these are best carried out in the radiology department, they cannot be performed until the patient is haemodynamically stable. Until this occurs the trauma victim's neck must remain immobilised.

Adequacy and alignment
Important cervical injury is associated with neurological damage in 40–50% of cases; instability increases this risk by 10–20%. Vital considerations are whether the radiological view supplied is adequate for assessment and whether there is evidence of injury or instability.

All seven cervical vertebrae as well as the C7–T1 junction must be visualised in the lateral radiograph. Injuries often occur at C6/7, with C1/2 next in frequency. The "swimmer's" view of the cervicothoracic junction is helpful when the lower

Interpreting radiographs of the cervical spine

What to check	What to look for
Adequacy	All seven vertebrae shown, and first thoracic vertebra
	Enough lateral projection for assessment
Alignment	Check the spinolaminar/marginal/interspinous lines
	Check the anteroposterior depth of the spinal canal
Bones	Study each individual vertebra
	Ensure there are no bony fragments
	Look for cortical continuity and obvious fracture lines
Cartilage/joints	Check disc spaces and facet joints
	Check predental space
Soft tissues	Look for local or generalised prevertebral swelling

cervical spine has not been fully visualised (see chapter 8) but is difficult to interpret and is unsafe if cervicothoracic injury is strongly suspected as it requires manipulation of the patient. Anteroposterior oblique views with tube angulation of 30° will show the lower cervical spine and also the facet joints and foraminae. The patient need not be moved for these views.

Alignment of the cervical spine radiograph is assessed by the following lines. Each line should be smooth with no angulation.

Anterior and posterior marginal lines connect the surfaces of adjacent vertical bodies and represent the sites of the longitudinal ligaments. A forward slip of one vertebral body on its neighbour may indicate dislocation. Shift of up to 25% of the antero-posterior diameter of the body is seen with subluxation and with unilateral facet dislocation. Displacement greater than 50% is a sign of probable bilateral facet joint dislocation. A forward slip of one vertebral body on its neighbour of >3.5 mm in the presence of a fracture indicates an unstable fracture dislocation

The spinolaminar line connects the white lines where laminae of each vertebra meet to form the spinous processes. C2 is often posterior to this line by up to 3 mm in normal individuals.

Spinous processes should be roughly equidistant and converge to a point behind the patient's neck. They should not diverge or "fan out".

Vertebral canal—The anteroposterior diameter of the vertebral canal, measured between the spinolaminar and posterior marginal lines, is of prime importance at the site of cervical expansion of the cord—between C3 and C6. If it is <13 mm, particularly in the presence of bone injury, the cord is at risk or already damaged. Note any pre-existing degenerative cervical spine changes with osteophytes in elderly patients; cord damage can occur in these patients without noticeable narrowing. Likewise, spinal stenosis may be a longstanding feature associated with posterior osteophytes.

Cartilage and joints

Vertebral bodies should be inspected for evidence of fracture. The height of each vertebral body should be similar anteriorly and posteriorly. A difference in height of >2 mm between the front and back is important and may indicate a crush fracture. Fractures of the spinous processes are usually shown in the lateral view; fractures of the posterior arch, however, may be apparent only in oblique projections.

The space between the anterior cortex of the odontoid peg and the posterior cortex of the anterior arch of the atlas (the predental space) should be ≤3 mm in an adult ≤5 mm in a child. Greater distances imply atlantoaxial instability.

Disc spaces should be roughly equal in height unless there are associated degenerative changes. The height of any disc space should be even throughout. Angulation greater than 10° between adjoining vertebral body end plates implies instability of traumatic origin.

Soft tissues

Above the level of the laryngeal inlet the prevertebral soft tissue should be no thicker than 7 mm. There should be no localised swelling. Below the larynx the tracheal air shadow should be separated from the anterior marginal line by no more than the equivalent of the anteroposterior diameter of a vertebral body: an upper limit of 22 mm is often quoted. Again there should be no localised swelling. Tracheal deviation in the anteroposterior view may be important providing there is no goitre present. Presphenoidal adenoidal enlargement in children and young adults may simulate a mass anterior to C1/2. Neck flexion and crying may also increase the depth of the prevertebral soft tissues substantially.

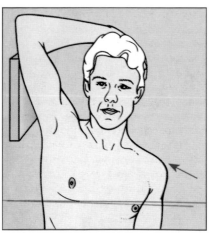

Position of patient for swimmer's view.

Important measurements on cervical *x* rays

- Overriding of vertebral bodies:
  Without fracture
    —25% indicates unifacetal dislocation
    — 50% indicates bifacetal dislocation
  With fracture
    —>3.5 mm indicates instability
- Width of spinal canal   >13 mm
- Predental space   ≤3 mm (adult); ≤5 mm (child)
- Depth of prevertebral soft tissue:
  —above larynx ≤7 mm
  —below larynx ≤22 mm (or width of vertebral body)

Radiological signs of cervical instability

- Angulation between vertebrae >10°
- Vertebral override >3.5 mm with fracture
- Complete facet override
- Facetal joint widening
- Interspinous "fanning"
- Vertebral body compression >25%

Classification of cervical injury

Stable injuries

- Hyperflexion—compression fracture (if <25%)
- Spinous process fracture
- Unifacetal dislocation
- Pure C1 arch fracture
- Pillar fracture
- Lower cervical burst fracture

Unstable injuries

- Hyperflexion "teardrop" injury
- Hyperextension "teardrop" injury
- Traumatic spondylolisthesis of C2 (hangman's fracture)
- Bilateral facet dislocation
- C2 posterior arch fracture
- Hyperextension fracture dislocation
- Jefferson fracture of C1
- Basal peg fracture

Bones

The two major mechanisms of cervical spine injury are hyperflexion and hyperextension. Hyperflexion is the more common, causing 50–80% of cervical spine injuries. There is a tendency for the posterior elements to be disrupted. Hyperextension injuries conversely tend to disrupt the anterior supports. "Teardrop" avulsion or compression fragments of the anterior aspect of a vertebral body may be the only residual features of major disruption and ensuing instability.

Compression fractures are generally stable. The Jefferson burst fracture of C1, however, is not, and the lateral radiograph may well show only soft tissue swelling. An open mouth view is essential to judge the integrity of C1 and the symmetry of its position on either side of the odontoid peg (see chapter 8). C2 fractures may be associated. Neurological damage is rare as the canal is wide at this level. Conversely, neurological damage caused by stable lower cervical compression fractures is fairly common because of posterior displacement of fragments into a relatively narrow canal. A wedge fracture in an elderly patient with osteopenia should be differentiated if possible as it is unlikely to be important.

Fractures of the odontoid peg are most common at its base. They are unstable, though neurological damage is uncommon. There is variable displacement, and soft tissue swelling is often seen only in the lateral radiograph. Ideally, a fractured peg should be excluded before intubation is attempted. An experienced anaesthetist may, however, be willing to proceed without radiological proof if the clinical situation dictates.

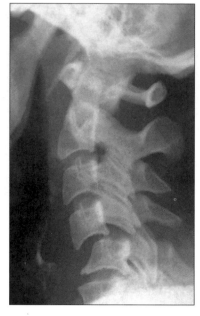

Forward slip of C4 on C5 of >50%. No fracture is present and the facets are overriding, indicating a bilateral facet dislocation.

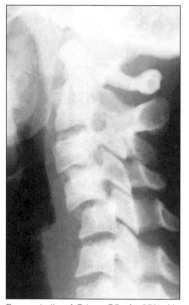

Forward slip of C4 on C5 of <25%. No fracture is visible. The disc space is slightly narrowed.

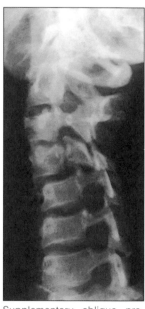

Supplementary oblique projection shows malalignment of the facet joints, indicating a unilateral facet dislocation.

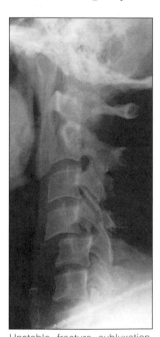

Unstable fracture subluxation. C4 has slipped forward on C5, the disc space is narrowed, and there is a fracture of the posterior elements and a fracture of the spinous process of C6.

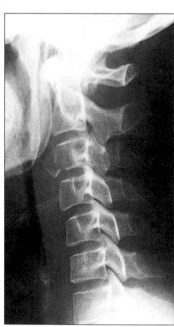

Hyperextension "teardrop" fracture of C3 showing avulsed anteroinferior fragment from the body of C3 and some localised prevertebral soft tissue swelling. This injury was unstable.

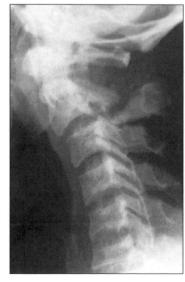

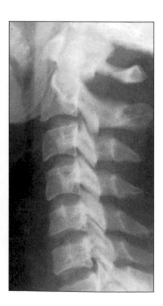

(Far right) "Hangman's" traumatic spondylolisthesis of C2. C2 is subluxed forward on C3 and the posterior elements are clearly separated. The posterior arch of C1 is also fractured. (Right) Pure C1 arch fracture. There is an undisplaced fracture line passing vertically through the posterior arch of C1. This injury was stable.

Chest injuries

About 25% of deaths caused by major trauma result from thoracic damage. The most useful radiograph in patients with thoracic trauma is the erect posteroanterior view. In the resuscitation room, however, the standard radiograph is often the supine anteroposterior view. This has the disadvantage of causing apparent enlargement of heart and mediastinal shadows, distending the upper lobe vessels, and making inspiration less efficient.

With a patient in the supine position, large amounts of free pleural air can collect in the anterior part of the chest without a characteristic lung edge being visible. This causes the costophrenic angle to extend more inferiorly than usual. If the patient does not have a bilateral pneumothorax it can be helpful to compare this with the normal side. On a normal chest radiograph the area of the liver is relatively opaque as the exposure is set to optimise visualisation of the low density lungs. When air collects in the costophrenic angle anteriorly, the liver will appear more radiolucent than usual. On the left, air will outline the medial aspect of the hemidiaphragm under the heart.

The characteristic appearance of a pleural fluid collection in an erect radiograph, with fluid tracking up the lateral aspect of the chest, is not seen with the patient lying supine. In this position the fluid lies posteriorly within the chest giving rise to a general opacification of the hemithorax. Even with the patient lying supine most of the fluid collects in the lower half of the chest. This obliterates the outline of the hemidiaphragm, with a gradual change in density from opacification to lucency going up the radiograph.

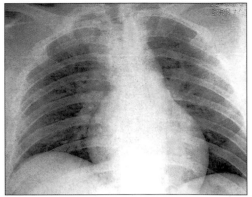

Anteroposterior supine chest radiograph showing poor inspiration and prominent upper lobe vasculature.

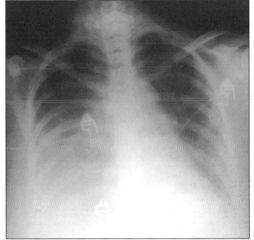

A supine chest radiograph showing a right sided pleural fluid collection. Note the basal opacification with a gradual shift towards lucency going up the radiograph. Lung markings can still be seen superimposed over the area of opacification.

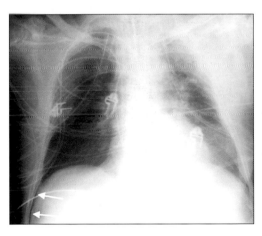

A supine chest radiograph showing a pneumothorax. The deep sulcus sign (arrows). Compare with the costophrenic angle on the other side.

Adequacy and alignment

Poor inspiration and rotation of the patient in relation to the radiographic beam may result in artefactually abnormal appearances. Ideally, five anterior ribs and ten posterior ribs should be counted above the level of the hemidiaphragm. The medial ends of the clavicles should be equidistant from the vertebral spinous processes.

The basic rules for assessment of the chest radiograph are that the transverse diameter of the heart should not be greater than half the transverse diameter of the thorax and that two thirds of the heart should lie to the left of the midline. Vascular distribution should be symmetrical on each side, and each hemithorax should have equal translucency. The hilar shadows should be clearly defined, with the left hilum being about 1–2 cm higher than the right. Cardiac, mediastinal, and diaphragmatic contours should be clearly outlined.

The position and consequence of resuscitation procedures (e.g. endotracheal intubation) need to be assessed.

Interpreting chest radiographs

What to check	What to look for
Adequacy	Check for adequacy of inspiration, penetration of film, and artefacts of resuscitation
Alignment	Check natural curve of ribs and thoracic cage
	Check position of spinous processes with respect to medial ends of clavicles
Bones	Look for fracture lines and cortical continuity
	Rib fractures: How many ribs fractured? How many fractures per rib?
Cartilage/joints	Look particularly at the sternoclavicular joint
Soft tissues	Ensure density of each hemithorax is equal and mediastinum central
	Localised opacities may be pulmonary, pleural, artefactual, or chest wall
	Check smooth contour of diaphragm
	Observe the mediastinal outline and width
	Check aortic knuckle for contour and definition
	Look for abnormal gas in pleural, mediastinal, subcutaneous, and subphrenic spaces

Bones

All the bones visible on the chest radiograph must be assessed for breaks in the cortical margin or disruption of the trabecular pattern.

Injuries to the chest wall frequently accompany pelvic trauma. The fifth to ninth ribs are most commonly injured. Lower rib fractures may be associated with splenic, hepatic, or renal damage, while fractures of the first two ribs imply that the patient has sustained a considerable force and is likely to have associated cranial, cervical, or intrathoracic injury. A fracture of the first rib with displaced fragments carries a 60% risk of underlying major vascular damage. The presence of surgical emphysema in the neck or mediastinum highlights the severity of the injury.

Flail chest occurs when multiple and adjacent rib fractures allow an area of the chest wall to move paradoxically with respiration. Sternal fractures are best shown in the lateral radiograph and may be associated with underlying pulmonary or cardiac injury. Complications caused by rib fractures include pneumothorax, haemothorax, and pulmonary contusion or laceration. Beware also of scapular fractures, whose presence indicates a high kinetic energy injury.

Cartilage and joints

All joints visible on the radiograph must be checked for congruity of the articular surfaces. Posterior sternoclavicular joint dislocation can be identified by obvious asymmetry at the manubrium. The condition is associated with risk of brachiocephalic vein disruption.

Soft tissue

Pulmonary and pleural features of injury—Sequelae of thoracic trauma include segmental, lobar, or pulmonary collapse. Features of opacification and alteration of hilar and fissure positions must be sought.

Fluid aspiration causes patchy air space consolidation, typically in the upper lobes or apices of the lower lobe. Acute pulmonary oedema may appear solely as "bat's wing shadowing" extending from the hila resulting from fluid exudation into the alveolar spaces. Interstitial oedema is hallmarked by peribronchial thickening, the septal lines of interlobular fluid, and, indeed, pleural fluid.

A pleural effusion may also indicate an abdominal injury such as splenic or hepatic laceration, and signs of subdiaphragmatic air from a visceral perforation should be sought in the upright chest radiograph.

Diaphragmatic injury—Rupture of the diaphragm is more common on the left side and can be caused by either blunt or penetrating trauma.

Haemothorax, pulmonary collapse caused by compression, rib fractures, and hepatic or splenic injuries may coexist. Ruptures resulting from blunt trauma are usually larger and more immediately apparent. The appearances are easily misinterpreted as a subpulmonic effusion, loculated haemopneumothorax, or just a high hemidiaphragm of unknown cause.

A contrast examination may be necessary to show bowel loops within the thorax.

Mediastinal injuries—Penetrating injuries may result in mediastinal or pericardial emphysema. The former is apparent in the radiograph as a white line that parallels the mediastinal border, particularly on the left side. Free mediastinal air may extend to the neck, where streaky air lucencies are readily visible in the soft tissue planes.

The tracheobronchial tree and oesophagus may be injured in patients with blunt, penetrating, or deceleration

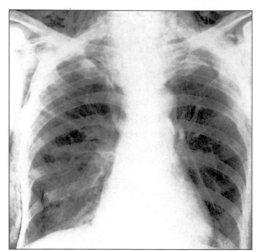

Extreme surgical emphysema and pneumomediastinum caused by multiple rib fractures. There is outlining of the pectoral muscle fibres on the right side.

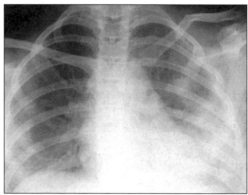

Left sided pulmonary contusion, with ill defined opacification over the left mid-zone and base. The left clavicle is fractured, but no obvious rib fracture is shown.

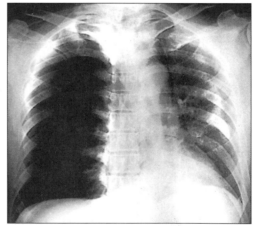

Right sided tension pneumothorax. The right hemithorax is very translucent with absent lung markings. There is flattening of the right dome of the diaphragm and considerable shift of the heart and mediastinum to the left.

Signs of major thoracic trauma

- Mediastinal widening or shift
- Mediastinal emphysema
- Multiple rib fractures
- Fractured first or second ribs
- Pleural fluid
- Loss of aortic definition

trauma. Oesophageal rupture typically causes mediastinal emphysema with an accompanying left sided pleural effusion. Bronchial fracture may cause segmental or lobar collapse but can be very subtle radiologically.

Major vascular and cardiac injuries—Major vascular and cardiac injuries may be found in association with sternal or first rib fractures and in patients with injuries caused by deceleration forces. Patients with aortic rupture may well survive to reach the resuscitation room. Vital features include mediastinal widening, loss of definition of the aortic knuckle, deviation to the right of the trachea, and thickening of the apical pleura on the left side (see chapter 4).

Cardiac and pericardial trauma may cause haemopericardium with the risk of tamponade. The heart size will be increased, but the classically described features of a globular appearance and notable clarity of cardiac outline because of reduced motion are unreliable.

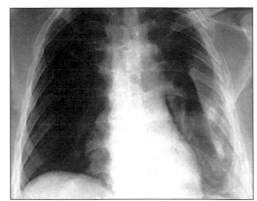
Flail chest caused by at least six fractured ribs both in the posterior axillary line and anteriorly.

Pelvic injuries

In 94% of cases a correct diagnosis can be made from just an anteroposterior radiograph of the pelvis. In the remaining 6% of cases, this radiograph needs to be supplemented by inlet, outlet and Judet (ie acetabular view at 45°) views. In addition, many patients with pelvic fractures require contrast examinations because of the high association of soft tissue damage. Computed tomography is also an essential element in the preoperative work up of haemodynamically stable patients with pelvic trauma. Arteriography may be used diagnostically or for therapeutic embolisation of bleeding vessels.

As with the other radiographs described in this chapter, the antereoposterior view of the pelvis should be assessed using the ABCS system.

Adequacy and alignment
All the pelvis must be seen, including the iliac crests, hips and femurs distal to the lesser trochanters. Pelvic rotation is determined by lining up the symphysis pubis with the midline of the sacrum.

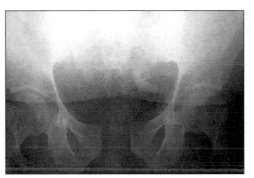
"Open book" pelvic fracture showing wide separation of the pubic symphysis and diastasis (widening) of the right sacroiliac joint.

Bones
The pelvic brim and the two obturator foramina should trace out smooth, uninterrupted circles. The superior aspect of the obturator fossa continues laterally along the inferior aspect of the femoral neck to form Shenton's line.

Disruption of these circles cannot occur at a single point. Therefore once one break is found a search must be made for a second fracture or joint diastasis. Significant opening of the sacroiliac joints is associated with tearing of the major blood vessels which overlie this joint. This radiological feature is therefore a sign of vascular damage and a potential source of major blood loss.

Fractures of the pelvic brim are caused by different types of forces. Lateral compression may result from inward rotation of the hemipelvis with disruption of the sacroiliac joint. The pubic rami are usually fractured and occasionally the sacrum as well. In contrast anteroposterior forces tend to drive the iliac wings apart and disrupt the symphysis (the "open book" fracture).

Pubic ramus fractures may also be present and, when bilateral (the "straddle" injury), are associated with urethral damage. Vertical shear forces have the highest risk of producing vascular damage because they tend to displace the hemipelvis upwards in relation to the sacrum. Additional pelvic fractures will usually be present.

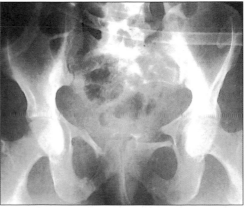
Bilateral pubic ramus fractures with separation (the "straddle" injury). Catheterisation for cystography has been performed. There is also an undisplaced left iliac wing fracture.

Individual fractures may also occur. Consequently the outer edges of the pelvis, as well as its internal trabecular pattern, should be assessed. The sacral foramina must also be assessed for symmetry. A break in their smooth border may be the only indicator of a lateral compression fracture.

Open fractures are important to detect because they are associated with a significant increase in mortality.

With every pelvic fracture consider the mechanism of injury and the high kinetic force needed; remember that during the injury the bones may have been much more separated than their final position on the radiograph, with consequent major soft tissue damage.

Cartilage and joints

All the joints must be assessed for congruity, disruption of the articular surfaces and widening.

The most common type of acetabular fracture occurs in the posterior wall. It is accompanied by a posterior dislocation and is found in people who have sustained a strong anterior force to the femur while in the sitting position. A lateral force may result in a central dislocation with associated acetabular fracture. Nevertheless relocation, spontaneously or by manipulation, may leave only subtle soft tissue changes. Anterior dislocation is rare.

Soft tissues

Intra and extrapelvic soft tissue planes must be assessed. Displacement by large haematomas may be the only indicator of fractures or vascular damage. Major pelvic trauma is associated with bladder rupture in 10–15% of cases.

Interpreting radiographs of the pelvis

What to check	What to look for
Adequacy	Check that whole pelvis is visible and not too rotated
	Should include hips and necks of femurs
Alignment	Check smooth contours of the pelvic and obturator rings and Shenton's line
Bones	Look for cortical and trabecular interruption
	Ensure that there are no fragments or overlap
	Don't ignore the sacrum
Cartilage/joints	Check symmetry of hips and sacroiliac joints
	Check width of pubic symphysis
Soft tissues	Check fat and soft tissue planes inside and outside the pelvis
	Look for abnormal gas shadows

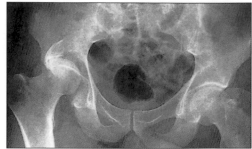

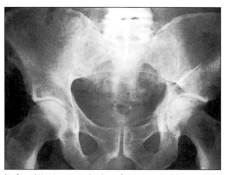

Acetabular fracture with posterior dislocation of the right femoral head. The acetabular fragment shows as a white line above the hip joint. The hip joint space is considerably widened medially and inferiorly.

Left sided acetabular fracture with central dislocation of the femoral head. There is narrowing of the medial aspect of the hip joint space and medial displacement of the femoral head. Note the thick white line of overlapping bone fragments.

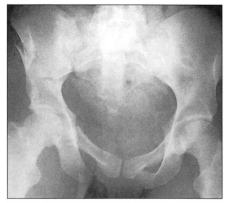

Vertical shear fracture involving both right sided pubic rami and iliac wing with a small amount of superior displacement. A sacral fracture is also visible.

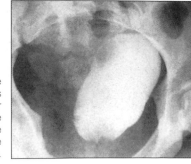

Contrast material within the bladder from an intravenous urogram shows bladder displacement by a large haematoma. The transverse sacral fracture can be clearly seen.

Skull injuries

Unnecessary importance is sometimes given to radiography of the skull. Criteria for its use have been proposed that essentially require that a neurological deficit of intracranial origin is present or that assessment of such a deficit is not possible. Once taken, this radiograph should be assessed using the ABCS system. Some features to aid differentiation of fractures from other lucencies appearing in the skull radiograph are given in the table.

Interpreting skull radiographs

What to check	What to look for
Adequacy	Ensure a good lateral view showing the vault, mandible and C1/2
Alignment	Check the contour of the skull tables and the relationship of the facial bones to the skull
Bones	Check for linear lucencies of fractures
	Do not ignore overlapping fragments causing white lines
Cartilage/joints	Look for obvious sutural diastasis and temporomandibular joint disruption
Soft tissues	Check for intracranial air
	Check for air or fluid levels in the sinuses
	Remember that the film may be "brow up"

Differentiation of lucencies in the skull

Feature	Artery	Vein	Suture	Fracture
Shape	Regular and roughly straight	Wandering	Tortuous but inner junction straight	Usually straight
Calibre	Even	Uneven	Even	Variable
Cortical margin	Present	Present	Present	Absent
Branching	Common, even	Common, irregular	Rare (eg, lambdoid suture)	May be stellate if depressed
Anatomical site	Fairly constant	Very variable	Constant	Anywhere

Other imaging techniques

The use of further imaging modalities will depend on the clinical problem and how stable the patient is. Delaying life saving surgery by inappropriate imaging must be guarded against. Ultrasound (US) is therefore very useful because it can be performed in the emergency department with minimal disruption to the resuscitation process. Modern US machines are small, highly portable and produce high quality images. Obesity and gaseous distension of bowel are the main factors limiting the examination, as US waves do not pass well through fat and air.

Ultrasound has many of the benefits of diagnostic peritoneal lavage in being a quick, economical, bedside test but is non invasive with no complications. Furthermore US does not compromise future investigation by CT and can be repeated if the clinical condition changes. The primary role of US is in the detection of free peritoneal fluid (which is usually blood), which requires prompt surgical intervention. In some centres members of the emergency department use US in this role as an almost routine extension of the clinical examination. The diagnostic value of US, however, extends beyond the demonstration of intraperitoneal blood. Even in the absence of peritoneal blood close scrutiny of the spleen is required as delayed splenic rupture is well recognised, with extensive splenic lacerations and haematoma occurring with an initially intact splenic capsule.

The retroperitoneal space can be examined, with the primary concern being the integrity of the kidneys. This examination is often performed when haematuria is detected in the setting of blunt abdominal trauma. In suspected diaphragmatic rupture US, after a chest radiograph, is the imaging modality of choice.

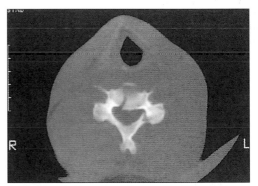

Axial computed tomogram through the C6 level shows not only the extent of the fracture through its body with some posterior fragment displacement but also a fracture through the arch (not apparent in the plain radiograph).

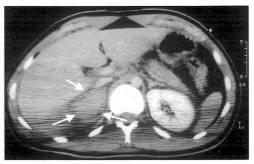

Abdominal computed tomography. The upper aspect of the right kidney (arrows) shows no contrast enhancement because of vascular disruption (compare with the normal left kidney).

Computed tomography (CT) is confined to imaging in the axial plane, which is the least favourable for imaging the diaphragms. Pleural fluid, which can be difficult to appreciate on a chest radiograph performed in a supine patient, is easily seen on US. CT is more sensitive than US in the detection of hollow viscus damage, and can be performed after the US examination in stable patients. Water soluble oral contrast is administered, which can be given via a nasogastric tube, and aids in the detection of upper bowel perforation. Intravenous contrast is used routinely to assess vascular integrity of the solid organs, particularly the kidneys, and better demonstrates solid organ lacerations.

Conventional CT scanners can take 10 min or more to image the abdomen with 1520 slices acquired individually. Multiple injections of intravenous contrast may be required to ensure vascular and organ enhancement. In contrast, spiral CT scanners allow the chest and abdomen to be imaged in a matter of seconds. Instead of acquiring the images in a stepwise manner, these machines scan continuously as the patient moves through the scanner. Speeding up the scanning process enables one injection of intravenous contrast to be adequate and ensures that images are acquired with good vascular and organ enhancement.

CT is used in the chest to diagnose aortic disruption and damage to the great vessels by demonstrating blood in the mediastinum. Angiography localises the exact site of the injury more accurately, but is less often used because of the non-invasive nature of CT. Nevertheless it has a role in some cases of pelvic haemorrhage associated with pelvic fracture where therapeutic embolisation can be performed.

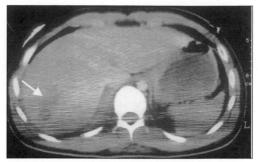

Computed tomogram showing a liver laceration. Intravenous contrast enhances the normal liver, making organ damage easier to diagnose.

Summary

There are three crucial radiographs that are needed during the resuscitation of trauma victims: those of the cervical spine (lateral), chest and pelvis. These need to be systematically assessed using the ABCS system so that all necessary information can be obtained. Subsequently, other plain radiographs, and specialist investigations, can be carried out depending upon the patient's clinical state.

Acknowledgment

The authors acknowledge Drs NM Perry and MD Lewars for their help in the earlier versions of this text.

15 Role of the trauma nurse

Lisa Hadfield-Law, Andrew Kent, Lorna McInulty

Good trauma care relies heavily on a multidisciplinary approach. Many individuals make a contribution, whether as part of an informal group of staff or a more formal resuscitation team.[1] In addition to nursing and medical staff—the more obvious members of the team—there are numerous others who have less direct though also important roles. These include clerical, portering and domestic staff, pharmacists, laboratory technicians, radiographers and the hospital chaplain. From all of these perspectives, the patient and his or her family must remain the focus of the team.

Many of those attending a trauma resuscitation are there to provide a service of one type or another. Others are there to learn. It can be tempting to send some of the learners away. However, this may discourage collaboration at a later date, and will prevent students from experiencing irreplaceable learning opportunities, thus jeopardising optimal patient care in the future.

Groups of people who are unsure of their roles can cause confusion and chaos. To work well, teams need organisation and training, a coordinated approach, and mutual trust and respect. An effective way of achieving this is to devise shared learning programmes, based on the same principles, where everyone can learn and develop an understanding of each other's roles.

Roles in trauma care must be clearly defined and tasks delegated. Nurses, whether based in the emergency department, operating theatres, the intensive care department or wards, can assume pivotal roles in the care of trauma patients. Such roles should be defined locally.

> **Role of the nurse in trauma care**
> - Preparation
> - Assessment
> - Resuscitation
> - Monitoring and evaluation
> - Transfer to definitive care

The role of the trauma nurse

The role of the nurse in trauma care has five main elements. These are preparation, assessment, resuscitation, monitoring and evaluation, and transfer to definitive care.

Preparation

Hospital staff will usually have been alerted to the impending arrival of a trauma patient. There is therefore an opportunity to prepare resources, to ensure that resuscitation can begin immediately. It is essential that all team members appreciate the importance of this preparation period so that when the patient arrives, valuable time is not lost trying to locate a general surgeon, a radiographer or the keys to the drug cupboard. Adequate preparation prevents unnecessary pressure on the team.

Throughout the resuscitation, if the nurse can stay one step ahead of the rest of the team, more time can be saved. For example, anticipating that the patient will need a CT scan allows arrangements to be put into place to locate portable equipment and alert appropriate staff.

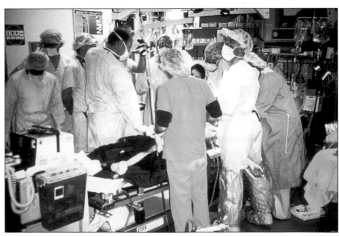

Nurses can assume pivotal roles in trauma care.

Assessment

The nurse is often the team member who receives the patient at the ambulance doors. Skills in effective and rapid initial assessment are, therefore, crucial. The principles underpinning these assessment skills must be integrated with those adhered to by colleagues in the trauma care team. Mistakes are more likely if team members do not "speak the same language".

Resuscitation

The training of nurses to perform the invasive procedures required by trauma patients during resuscitation is controversial. However, it is essential that nurses are fully cognisant with resuscitation procedures and equipment, and the best way to support patients and relatives. As team members, nurses are generally more familiar with moving and handling patients and able to approach procedures such as log rolling with skill and confidence.

Monitoring and evaluation

A nurse who remains with the patient throughout resuscitation and transfer will be in an excellent position to pick up any subtle changes in the patient's condition. This provides an essential and early indicator of the response to injury and treatment. Observations of respiration, pulse and blood pressure are basic but vital noninvasive procedures. They should be recorded as often as every 3 minutes in the early stages of resuscitation, and the frequency re-evaluated according to the patient's condition.

Transfer to definitive care

Many patients are transported to theatre for urgent surgery and may not be in a stable condition when moved to the operating theatre. Before transfer, the nurse must consider the geography of the hospital and ensure that all appropriate personnel have been informed. Portering staff should be made aware of any potential problems associated with the transfer and, if necessary, should arrange clearance along the corridors and hold lifts.

A telephone "hand over" from the primary nurse in the emergency department to the nurse who will receive the patient will allow colleagues to plan ahead; if the receiving team are aware of the patient's condition they can be ready with compatible monitoring equipment or interventions.

Resuscitation equipment must be readily available during transfer—oxygen, suction apparatus and airway devices in particular. Oxygen cylinders must contain sufficient oxygen for the transfer and airway devices must be compatible with the skills of the person transferring the patient.

Cardiac monitoring and noninvasive measurement of blood pressure and oxygen saturation provide adequate monitoring during transfer. However, the nurse must be in a position to observe the *patient* during transfer, rather than the monitors.

After transferring the patient to a bed or theatre trolley, a detailed, undisturbed hand-over, involving the receiving primary nurse, is crucial. It is useful to exchange direct telephone numbers so that further information can be passed between nurses.

Specific roles of the nursing team

The specific responsibilities of the trauma nursing team include leadership, management of the patient's airway, documentation of the patient's condition, and keeping the patient's family and friends informed.

Leadership

The nursing team leader should be appropriately trained and have a working knowledge of the location. Pending the patient's arrival, he or she should liaise with other team members.

Important nursing tasks in the early phase of trauma care

- Time can be saved during resuscitation if the nurse anticipates and prepares for procedures, such as a CT scan
- Detection by the trauma nurse of subtle changes in the patient's condition provides an essential and early indicator of the response to injury and treatment
- Transfer of the trauma patient to definitive care can be hazardous. The primary nurse in the emergency department must ensure that appropriate individuals are informed about the transfer; a telephone "hand over" to the receiving nurse facilitates appropriate preparations
- During the transfer of a trauma patient, the nurse should always be in a position to observe the *patient* rather than the monitors

---

Observations of respiration, pulse and blood pressure are basic but vital noninvasive procedures

---

Before transfer of the patient, the nurse must consider the geography of the hospital and ensure that all appropriate personnel have been informed

---

Specific responsibilities of the trauma nursing team

- Leadership
- Maintenance of the patient's airway
- Documentation of the patient's condition
- Care of the patient's family and friends

Awareness of colleagues' abilities and limitations is important, as are the skills required to recognise signs of stress. A "hands off" approach allows an overview of the team's progress. The team leader is responsible for the safety aspects of the resuscitation, and must make sure that all team members are taking appropriate protective measures. The key to success in this role is to maintain open channels of communication.

Airway

The nurse who assumes responsibility for the patient's airway can assume the role of team leader if the team is under resourced. This team member should have a working knowledge of the other roles within the team structure and the necessary skills to confidently maintain an airway in a trauma victim.

During preparation for the patient's arrival, the airway nurse must ensure that all appropriate equipment required to assess and monitor the patient's airway is available and in good working order. He or she is also responsible for ensuring the co-ordinated movement of the patient on to the hospital trolley.

Being positioned at the patient's head, the airway nurse is responsible for talking to the patient, whether he or she is conscious or unconscious.

Documentation

Documenting the patient's condition is one of the most important roles of the trauma nursing team. One nurse should avoid becoming involved in any clinical activity during the early stages of resuscitation, and be available to note and record all information. The nurse should be familiar with the hospital's system of documentation, as trauma charts can be initially confusing.

Black pens should be available, so that records made will be suitable for photocopying later. A clock should be visible so that important events can be accurately logged. All data gathered and recorded are crucial for clinical audit. Audit is important, to check the team is working safely and effectively. Without information from audit, necessary improvements to the team's structure or operation cannot be identified and acted upon.

The patient should be identified as soon as possible to allow correct labelling of blood samples and test results. However, precious minutes must not be wasted seeking identification when the patient needs urgent cross matching for blood transfusion. If the patient's identity is in doubt, use a "non-name" system; be cautious about using names such as "Mr Smith" or "Unknown male/female". If there are two or more unknown trauma patients in the hospital this sort of "labelling" is confusing.

All observations made, and any drugs or intravenous fluids given, should be noted. For intravenous fluids, record the start time, the site of administration and the finish time.

Any property taken from the patient can be handed to the recorder nurse, who can document the items and store them safely for later collection.

Family and friends

The patient's family and friends should be kept informed of progress with resuscitation (see box). If staff who are likely to be caring for the patient later are available, they can begin a valuable and supportive relationship in the emergency department, with the patient or family or both.

Those who know the patient best can be an invaluable source of information. Their input into the resuscitation effort will be beneficial to the patient and themselves. In the event of a patient's death, there is good evidence that witnessing the resuscitation effort eases the grieving process for the partner or relatives. Relatives should therefore be offered the opportunity to witness resuscitation if staff training has prepared the trauma team to accommodate the presence of relatives.[2]

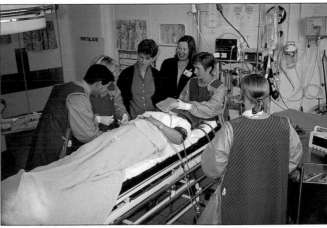

An organised, team approach to the care of the trauma patient makes for a more co-ordinated resuscitation phase. Shared learning programmes enhance team members' understanding of each other's roles.

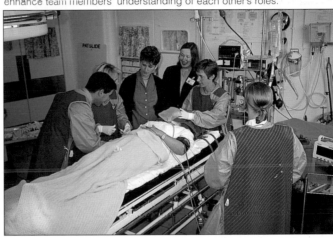

Precious minutes must not be wasted seeking identification when the patient needs urgent cross matching for blood transfusion

If nursing staff with trauma care skills are required in the resuscitation room, other members of the team, a chaplain, or a social worker, can be drafted in to assist with the care of family and friends

Trauma care in under-resourced units

Many emergency departments lack the equipment and number of skilled staff available at larger hospitals. However, underpinning the Advanced Trauma Life Support® course is the principal of one doctor using a systematic approach to resuscitation. If staffing levels are minimal, the principles remain the same. When the number of medical staff is limited, nurses may enhance their roles under the Scope of Professional Practice. This allows them, after appropriate training, to perform such skills as intravenous cannulation.

Communication

Communication entails both the transfer of information and the sharing of meaning. Under severe stress communication diminishes markedly in quantity and quality—verbal interchange becomes short and incomplete. It is important therefore to practise concise speech patterns until effective communication becomes a habit.

Each emergency department requires a well developed system by which staff can share administrative plans, changes and concerns; methods adopted may include newsletters, bulletin boards, suggestion boxes and committee meetings.

Successful resuscitation of the trauma patient depends on effective communication surrounding and supporting the efforts of the trauma team. The chance of incomplete or misinterpreted communication is increased in high pressure situations, as is a lack of coordination between departments and individuals, and this can put vulnerable patients at risk.

The transfer of information and the sharing of meaning are vital components of clinical judgment and decision making. Team members who can communicate—share information and acknowledge and respond to what others say—are safer, and less prone to errors of judgment. The main factor contributing to human error during trauma resuscitation is attitude; a good attitude demands a basic understanding of human behaviour.

Pain relief

Pain can be defined as "An unpleasant sensory and emotional experience associated with actual or potential tissue damage". "It is whatever the experiencing person says it is, existing whenever he says it does."[3]

Several factors influence pain perception in the trauma patient (see box). Pain relief can be forgotten during the activity of resuscitation, but it is an essential part of good patient care. Intravenous opiates are usually most effective, in doses titrated to control pain. Avoid giving opiates by intramuscular injection or orally, because of poor absorption following trauma. Giving an antiemetic will help avoid nausea and vomiting. Entonox can be useful in the initial stages of resuscitation. In skilled hands regional nerve blocks can be most effective, particularly before insertion of chest drains and after fractured shaft of femur.

Pain assessment

The aim of pain management is to reduce pain to a level acceptable to the patient. The first part of this process must be to assess the initial level of pain; the second part—often forgotten—is to reassess pain after providing analgesia. Several pain assessment tools are available. Visual analog scales use a numerical "1 to 10" scale, a "ladder" or descriptive

---

Trauma care with limited resources
- When staffing levels are low, remember the underlying principle of one doctor using a systematic approach to resuscitation

Effective communication is vital
- Lack of coordination between departments and individuals can put vulnerable patients at risk.
- Each emergency department requires a well developed system by which staff can share administrative plans, changes and concerns.
- Under severe stress, communication diminishes markedly. It is important to practise concise speech patterns until effective communication becomes a habit.
- Team members who can communicate effectively are safer, and less prone to errors of judgement.

Factors influencing pain perception
- Extent of tissue injury
- Culture and racial background
- Prior pain experience
- Anxiety
- Perception of control over pain and situation

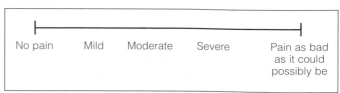

Visual analog scale for the assessment of pain.[3]

words to help patients quantify their pain. The Wong–Baker Faces Rating Scale can be used for children as young as 3 years. Information to record is listed opposite. Providing patients with a sense of control over their situation can help to reduce pain. An example of this would be in the use of a patient-controlled analgesia system.

Non-drug pain management

There are alternatives to pharmacological pain management. Muscle spasm, strain, fatigue and coincidental pain can often be reduced by positioning the patient and immobilising body parts. Psychological techniques can also have a marked effect. Information about what to expect, including sensations, will help the patient relax. Relaxation reduces anxiety and muscle tension. Rhythmic breathing, extremity relaxation, massage and a quiet environment will also help. Distraction—guiding the patient to focus on stimuli other than the pain sensation—can substantially reduce non-severe pain. Family visitors and other such diversions can enhance the effect. Guided imagery and hypnosis have produced interesting results in some centres.[4]

On-going trauma care

An organised, team approach to the care of the trauma patient makes for a more co-ordinated resuscitation phase. Ideally, this co-ordination should continue when the patient leaves the resuscitation room. Often it does not and patient care becomes increasingly fragmented. The problem intensifies when several specialties and disciplines are involved.

Whether they have single system or multisystem injury, trauma patients are vulnerable to many potential hazards as they move through the hospital system (see box). Given these potential difficulties, it is advantageous if a designated person acts as a co-ordinator or "lynch-pin" throughout the patient's admission. One approach is to appoint a trauma nurse co-ordinator (TNC)[5] charged with ensuring optimal care for the trauma patient from admission to discharge (see box).

The appointment of TNCs has been successful in the USA, and is being investigated in the UK. Evidence suggests that establishing links between the emergency department and staff caring for trauma patients later in their progress through the system leads to more co-ordinated care, reduced complication rates, shorter hospital stays and greater satisfaction for patients and their families.

Summary

Trauma teams are only effective if individual members have clear responsibilities and are trained to fulfill them. When staffing levels are low and the number of trauma admissions potentially high, as at night, some roles in the trauma team, such as airway nurse and team leader, may have to be merged.

Roles assumed by trauma nurses depend on the unit itself, its available resources and the types of patient attending. There is a growing trend for trauma nurses to expand their role, for example into the medical and radiographic spheres. However, fulfilment of traditional nursing roles, such as the psychological aspects of patient care, care of family and friends, documentation of the patient's condition and assessment of pain, should be carefully reviewed, to ensure evidence-based practice.

Attitude is the greatest contributor to human error during trauma resuscitation, and a good attitude demands a basic understanding of human behaviour. It is essential to maintain open channels of communication to support the complex networks that underpin excellent trauma care.

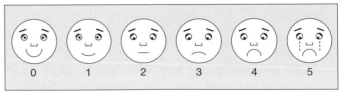

Wong–Baker faces rating scale for the assessment of pain.[3]

Pain assessment: information to record
- The site of the pain
- The intensity of the pain
- The nature of the pain — "What does it feel like?"
- What makes the pain worse or provides relief
- What the patient thinks is causing the pain

Factors that may compromise care beyond the emergency room
- Delays in investigation and definitive treatment
- Poorly executed transfers within the hospital or to a different hospital
- Lack of a systematic method of exchanging information when a patient moves to a new area
- Suboptimal care for a patient on a "nonspecialist" ward
- Delayed recognition of a patient's deterioration because of lack of knowledge of the pathophysiology of trauma
- General lack of trauma care skills
- Inadequate pain management
- Communication difficulties between different specialties and disciplines

A trauma nurse co-ordinator ensures optimal care through:
- Clinical activities and co-ordination of care
- Educational activities
- Quality assurance activities
- Promotion of evidence-based practice

References

1. Driscoll PA, Vincent CA. Organising an efficient trauma team. *Injury* 1992; 23:107–10.

2. Barratt F, Wallis DN. Relatives in the resuscitation room: their point of view. *J Accident Emerg Med* 1998; 15. 109–11.

3. Bayley EW, Turcke SA. *A comprehensive curriculum for trauma nursing*, 2nd edn. Park Ridge, Illinois: Roadrunner Press, 1998.

4. Patterson DR. Non-opioid based approaches to burn pain. *J Burn Care Rehab* 1995; 16 (Suppl Pt 2): 372–6.

5. Emergency Nurses Association. *Trauma co-ordinators resource manual*. Chicago, Illinois: ENA, 1994.

16 Scoring systems for trauma

Maralyn Woodford

Trauma care systems deal with patients who have an almost infinite variety of injuries requiring complex treatment. The assessment of such systems is a major challenge in clinical measurement and audit . Which changes are most effective in improving patient care? Do some changes produce unexpected delays or complications? Implementing recommendations for improved procedures will often incur additional costs—will the expense be worthwhile? Clearly, statistical analysis must replace anecdote and dogma, but the complexity of the task should not be underestimated.

The effects of injury can be defined in terms of input—an anatomical component and the physiological response—and outcome—mortality and morbidity. These must be coded numerically before we can comment with confidence on treatment or process of care. Elderly people and young children survive trauma less well than others, so age must be taken into account. The mechanism of injury is also important: the effect of a blunt impact from a fall or a car crash is quite different from that of a stab or gunshot wound. Most recent work has been concerned with measurement of injury severity and its relation to mortality. Assessment of morbidity has been largely neglected, yet for every person who dies as a result of trauma there are two seriously disabled survivors.

Input measures

Injury is assessed through the anatomical component and the physiological response. These two elements are separately scored.

Anatomical scoring system

The *abbreviated injury scale* (AIS), first published in 1969, is anatomically based. There is a single AIS score for each injury a patient may sustain. Scores range from 1 (minor) to 6 (incompatible with life). There are more than 1200 injuries listed in the dictionary, which is in its fourth edition. Intervals between the scores are not always consistent—for example, the difference between AIS3 and AIS4 is not necessarily the same as that between AIS1 and AIS2. (Copies of the booklet are available from the UK Trauma Audit & Research Network; see p.102).

Patients with multiple injuries are scored by adding together the squares of the three highest AIS scores in three predetermined regions of the body (see box). This is the *injury severity score* (ISS). Scores of 7 and 15 are unattainable because these figures cannot be obtained from summing squares. The maximum score is 75 ($5^2+5^2+5^2$). By convention, a patient with an AIS6 in one body region is given an ISS of 75. The injury severity score is non-linear and there is pronounced variation in the frequency of different scores; 9 and 16 are common, 14 and 22 unusual.

Analysis of trauma care

Input
Anatomical injury
Physiological derangement

Process
Variations in the system of care
Variations in patient care

Outcome
Survival: alive or dead?
Disability
  —temporary or permanent?
  —neurological?
  —musculoskeletal?
  —visceral?

Examples of injuries scored by the *Abbreviated injury scale* (**AIS90**)

Injury	Score
Shoulder pain (no injury specified)	0
Wrist sprain	1 (Minor)
Closed undisplaced tibial fracture	2 (Moderate)
Head injury—unconscious on admission but for less than 1 h thereafter, no neurological deficit	3 (Serious)
Incomplete transection of the thoracic aorta	4 (Severe)
Complex liver laceration	5 (Critical)
Laceration of the brain stem	6 (Incompatible with life)

Injury severity score (ISS)

To obtain this:

- Use the AIS90 dictionary to score every injury
- Identify the highest AIS score in each of the following six areas of the body:
  (1) head and neck
  (2) face
  (3) chest and thoracic spine
  (4) abdomen, lumbar spine and pelvic contents
  (5) bony pelvis and limbs
  (6) body surface
- Add together the squares of the highest scores in three body areas

Case study

A man is injured in a fall at work. He complains of pain in his neck, jaw, and left wrist and has difficulty breathing. There are abrasions around the left shoulder, left side of the chest, and left knee.

Examination of the cervical spine (with radiography) suggests no abnormality. There is a displaced fracture of the body of the mandible. There are also fractures of the left wrist, and left ribs (5–9), with a flail segment.

Injury	AIS score
Fracture of body of mandible	2
Fracture of lower end of radius (not further specified*)	2
Fracture of ribs 5–9 with flail segment	4
Abrasions (all sites)	1
Neck pain†	0

AIS, *Abbreviated injury scale*
*If fracture of radius was known to be displaced or open the AIS would be 3. If not specified the lower score is used.
†Symptoms are not scored if there is no demonstrable anatomical injury.

$$ISS = 2^2 + 2^2 + 4^2 = 24$$

For the purpose of the analysis described here, the ISS should be calculated only from operative findings, appropriate investigations, or necropsy reports. The overall injury severity score of a group of patients should be identified by the median value and the range, not the mean value. Non-parametric statistics should be used for analysis.

Physiological scoring systems

The physiological responses of an injured patient are assessed by the *revised trauma score* (RTS). After injury the patient's physiological response is constantly changing but for the purposes of injury scoring, and by convention, the RTS is measured when the patient arrives at hospital. If the patient is intubated before arrival an RTS cannot be measured. The physiological parameters that make up the RTS are respiratory rate, systolic blood pressure and Glasgow coma scale score.

The Glasgow coma scale (GCS) is the accepted international standard for measuring neurological state. The score may be represented as a single figure (for example, GCS = 15) or as the response in each of the three sections of the scale (for example, eyes = 4, verbal response = 5 and motor response = 6). Coma is defined as a Glasgow coma scale score of <8. Various modifications of the scale have been suggested for use in small children. Some doctors reduce the maximum score to that which is consistent with neurological maturation. A more useful clinical device, which ensures more accurate communication and simplifies epidemiological research, is to retain the maximum score of 15 but redefine the descriptions.

The RTS combines coded measurements of respiratory rate, systolic blood pressure, and Glasgow coma scale to provide a general assessment of physiological derangement. This scoring system was developed following statistical analysis of a large North American database to determine the most predictive independent outcome variables. The combination of these three variables is independently related to outcome. Selection of variables was also influenced by their ease of measurement and clinical opinion.

In practice the RTS is a complex calculation combining coded measurements of the three physiological values. To calculate the RTS, the coded value for each variable is

Glasgow coma scale

	Score
Eyes open:	
—spontaneously	4
—to speech	3
—to pain	2
—never	1
Best verbal response:	
—orientated	5
—confused	4
—inappropriate words	3
—incomprehensible sounds	2
—silent	1
Best motor response:	
—obeys commands	6
—localises pain	5
—flexion withdrawal	4
—decerebrate flexion	3
—decerebrate extension	2
—no response	1

Modification of Glasgow coma scale for children

	Score
Best verbal response:	
appropriate words or social smiles, fixes on and follows objects	5
cries but is consolable	4
persistently irritable	3
—restless, agitated	2
—silent	1
Eye and motor responses	
—scored as in scale for adults	

Revised trauma score (RTS)

	Coded value	×	Weighting factor	= Score
Respiratory rate (breaths/min):				
10–29	4			
>29	3			
6–9	2		0.2908	———
1–5	1			
0	0			
Systolic blood pressure (mm Hg):				
>89	4			
76–89	3			
50–75	2		0.7326	———
1–49	1			
0	0			
Glasgow coma scale:				
13–15	4			
9–12	3			
6–8	2		0.9368	———
4–5	1			
3	0			

Total = revised trauma score: _____

multiplied by a weighting factor derived from regression analysis of the database. This correction reflects the relative value of the variable in determining survival.

TRISS methodology

The degree of physiological derangement and the extent of anatomical injury are measures of the threat to life. Mortality will also be affected by the age of the patient and by the method of wounding. A blunt assault produces different injury characteristics and physiological abnormalities than does a penetrating object.

The "TRISS methodology" combines four elements—the revised trauma score (RTS), the injury severity score (ISS), the patient's age, and whether the injury is blunt or penetrating—to provide a measure of the probability of survival (Ps). (The acronym is tortuously developed from **TR**auma score and **I**njury **S**everity **S**core).

It is important to realise that Ps is merely a mathematical calculation (see box); it is not an absolute measure of mortality but only an indication of the probability of survival. If a patient with a Ps of 80% dies the outcome is unexpected because four out of five patients with such a Ps would be expected to survive. However, the fifth would be expected to die—and this could be the patient under study. The Ps is used as a filter for highlighting patients for study in multi-disciplinary trauma audit.

Comparing systems of care

Comparison of the probabilities of survival of all patients seen at a particular hospital with the observed outcome can be used as an index of overall performance. Probabilities of survival are combined in the "standardised W statistic" (Ws) to assess a group of patients.

Standardised W statistic

The Ws provides a measure of the number of additional survivors, or deaths, for every 100 patients treated at each hospital accounting for different mixes of injury severity. The "standardised Z statistic" (Zs) provides a measure of its statistical significance.

A high positive Ws is desirable as this indicates that more patients are surviving than would be predicted from the TRISS methodology. Conversely a negative Ws signifies that the system of trauma care has fewer survivors than expected from the TRISS predictions.

Comparisons have become more relevant to clinicians after extensive work was undertaken to base the regression analysis on statistics derived from the *Trauma Network* database. The Ws can be shown graphically with their 95% confidence intervals to illustrate clinical differences between hospitals (see graph).

UK Trauma Audit & Research Network

First developed in North America, the method used in the *UK Trauma Audit & Research Network* (developed from the major trauma outcome study) is now also used in the UK and throughout Europe and Australia to audit the effectiveness of systems of trauma care and the management of individual patients.

The TRISS methodology is applied in all patients with trauma who are admitted to hospital for more than 3 days, managed in an intensive care area or referred for specialist care, or who die in hospital. Additional information is sought

---

TRISS methodology

Probability of survival of individual patient $(P_S) = 1/1 + e^{-b}$

$b = b_0 + b_1 (RTS) + b_2 (ISS) + b_3 \times A$

The constant $e = 2.718282$, the base of Napierian logarithms.

$b_0 \ldots b_3$ are coefficients derived from regression analysis applied to data from the Trauma Network. They differ for blunt and penetrating injuries.

RTS = revised trauma score
ISS = injury severity score
A = 0 if age <55 years
 −1.1655 if age = 55–64 years
 −1.8339 if age = 65–74 years
 −2.8182 if age = 75–84 year
 −3.4448 if age >84 years

Case study

A 65 year old pedestrian is knocked down, sustaining head, abdominal, and leg injuries. On arrival in the emergency department he has a Glasgow coma score of 9, respiratory rate of 35 beats/min, and systolic blood pressure of 80 mm Hg. Computed tomography shows a small subdural haematoma with swelling of the left parietal lobe. There is a major laceration of the liver but no other intra-abdominal injury. Radiographs of the lower limbs show displaced fractures through both upper tibias.

Revised trauma score (RTS):
Glasgow coma score = 9;
 coded value 3 × weighting 0.9368 = 2.8104
Respiratory rate = 35;
 coded value 3 × weighting 0.2908 = 0.8724
Blood pressure = 80;
 coded value 3 × weighting 0.7326 = 2.1978

RTS = 5.8806

Injury severity score (ISS):

	AIS score
Subdural haematoma (small)	4
[Parietal lobe swelling]	[3]
Liver laceration (major)	4
Upper tibial fracture (displaced)	3

ISS = $4^2 + 4^2 + 3^2 = 41$

Probability of survival
Coefficients for blunt injury from the *Trauma Network* database:

$b_0 = 0.5600$ $b_2 = -0.1132$
$b_1 = 0.7281$ $b_3 = -1.8339$

$b = 0.56 + (0.7281)(5.8806) + (-0.1132)(41) + (-1.8339)(1)$

$P_S = 1/1 + e^{-b} = 0.1634$

Probability of survival = 16%

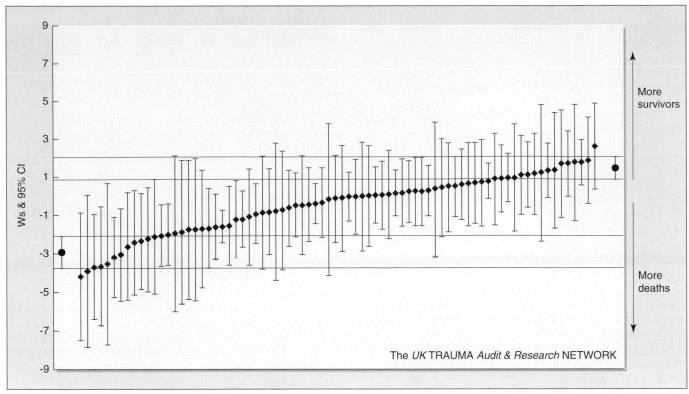

Outcomes at different hospitals for patients with blunt injuries, excluding referrals and burns, 1994–98: summary Ws statistic (see text for definition) and 95% confidence intervals. Each dot represents one hospital's performance over 5 years.

about the process of care, for example prehospital interventions, the seniority of doctors attending the patient on arrival at hospital, the initial management, and the timing of consultations and operations.

Outcome measures

Measurement of the change in mortality that may occur in patients with a given combination of anatomical injury and physiological derangement is only one method of assessing the effects of modifications in a system of care. The quality of life of survivors may vary considerably, but there is at present no adequate system of measuring this.

The Glasgow Outcome Score is a recognised method for measuring severity of permanent neurological impairment. In North America and in some areas of the UK, the Functional Independence Measure (FIM) has been developed for assessing original disability after all types of trauma, and can be used for monitoring progress, but this is only one of several methodologies. There is no universally accepted system for measuring disability following injury to the musculoskeletal system. Most research has concentrated on quantifying disability in the elderly and chronically infirm and has not addressed the issue of temporary disability that may result from injury to the locomotor system and incapacitate a young person for many months.

Future developments in emergency care services

Provision of emergency medical services varies widely throughout the world, and the optimal system for the UK is still under debate.

The UK Trauma Audit & Research Network

- Supports multidisciplinary clinical audit by analysis of individual case management
- Provides confidential comparative statistics to clinicians about institutional performance
- Provides summative information to local health commissioners about trauma workload and its management
- Provides population-based statistics on the epidemiology of trauma
- Collaborates with the Cochrane Centre to identify areas of potential research interest
- Refines methods of measuring injury severity

The *Trauma Network* provides an invaluable method of comparing patterns of care in different parts of the country. It is reliant on careful collection of data in a consistent format to allow collation and comparison of results. Deaths caused by trauma are too varied, too complicated, and too important to be discussed in isolation in individual hospitals, however sophisticated their computer software.

The wider perspective of the *Trauma Network* is increasingly recognised as the only valid approach to trauma audit and is being taken up by regional and national bodies for this purpose. Identification of deficiencies is valuable only if a mechanism exists to correct them. Local audit meetings and national comparisons must be used to stimulate appropriate changes in systems of trauma care.

The development of TRISS methodology has been a major advance in the measurement of injury severity. The detailed structure of the scales and the method of developing a single number to represent threat to life are, however, under constant review.

An alternative method of measuring anatomical injury has been described. The method uses the root sum squares of the AIS scores for the head and trunk (anatomic profile). It has been incorporated into a system for the characterisation of trauma (ASCOT), using different weightings for the RTS and age. Other recent methods have combined the AIS scores of a patient's most severe injuries regardless of body region.

These developments can be expected to lead to more accurate scoring systems, but for the present the TRISS methodology has a worldwide reputation for consistency and reasonable prediction of outcome. Immediate improvement in its usefulness could be made if, as is happening in most areas, ambulance crews measured the RTS at the scene of the accident. This would allow more scientific appraisal of the value of prehospital care. The accuracy of anatomical information could also be improved, particularly in necropsy reports; these are often inadequate for coding purposes and spinal cord injuries are rarely described in detail.

Measurement of outcome in terms of survival or death is, however, a crude yardstick. Further progress is required in measuring disability after noncerebral injury. Most life threatening visceral injuries leave the patient with little disability. In contrast the many more patients who sustain musculoskeletal sequelae are largely ignored in the statistics. Much effort will be required to develop outcome measures based on disability; these are essential if the treatment of the multiply injured patient is to be based on sound scientific principles.

● The latest edition of the *Abbreviated Injury Scale* booklet (AIS90) and information about the *UK Trauma Audit & Research Network* are available from the author at the Clinical Sciences Building, Hope Hospital, Salford M6 8HD.

Definitions of impairment, disability, and handicap

Impairment has an anatomical or physiological basis and is usually a consequence of musculoskeletal or cerebral injury (e.g. an amputated finger). It is easy to measure but variably related to the patient's activity

Disability is a functional consequence of an impairment that affects the patient's ability to perform the activities of daily life. Its measurement is relevant to the patient's needs but it is influenced by the environment

Handicap refers to disability within an individual's social and professional role. It may reflect a change in lifestyle, which is influenced by society. Handicap is difficult to relate to specific injury and difficult to measure.

17 Handling distressed relatives and breaking bad news

C A J McLauchlan

Coping with major trauma is stressful for both staff and relatives. Handling distressed relatives is an underemphasised part of the work, and medical staff may have had little training or experience of it. It is a time that the relative will always remember and, if handled badly, will leave lasting scars. Alternatively, skilled early handling of the bereaved will enable them to make a smoother journey through grief and improve the long term outlook.

Giving bad news is never easy, but it can be especially difficult in cases of major trauma when there is physical damage to the loved one. The nature of the patient's problem and the bad news can be varied. The management of the relatives may begin before they arrive at hospital and carry on until well after death or discharge of the patient. The principles of management apply to the emergency department as well as the intensive treatment unit or admitting ward. Providing genuine care and support for relatives is the key to their management.

Initial contact

When a victim of major trauma arrives in the emergency room the priority is immediate resuscitation. Once identified, the closest relatives or friends should be notified.

Communication with the emergency services can provide important information that is useful when handling the relatives. The ambulance crew and police, as well as giving details about the incident, may have already seen the relatives or know their whereabouts. It is usually better for a sympathetic police officer to make the initial contact in person rather than for a telephone call to be made from the hospital, but local knowledge may be important. The police may also be able to help with transport.

If the telephone is used, information should be given by an experienced nurse or doctor and a lone relative advised strongly against driving to hospital alone. Mentioning that the victim is unconscious often helps to impart a certain severity to the lay person, although the full severity or death is usually best explained in person at the hospital. If relatives are not told of the victim's death, however, they may blame themselves for not arriving at the hospital in time to be with their loved one at death. It is important to dispel any self recrimination by giving the relatives the exact information, including the time of death, when they attend.

If the relatives have to travel great distances or from overseas the full details, including death, may have to be explained over the telephone. Find out if the relative is alone and, if so, suggest that he or she seeks support locally. Offer to telephone for support.

Arrival of relatives at the hospital

Anxious relatives should be met by a named link nurse and not be kept waiting around at reception. It is important that the nursing sister coordinates the information so that the staff, in particular those at reception, know that potentially distressed relatives are expected. They should be welcomed and not made to feel in the way. Staff should remember that it is not only the victim's relatives who may be distressed: in some instances close friends or partners of either sex may be severely distressed and should be handled in the same way as the relatives.

There should be a private room or office where relatives and friends can wait and be seen. Ideally this room should be solely for relatives and friends, have a homely decor, yet be nearby and not isolated. An outside view is desirable, or at least a controlled view of a corridor. It is a myth that such details are not remembered by distressed relatives.

Breaking the news

Remember to ask relatives for the medical history of the patient. This history may be vital if the patient is receiving certain drugs such as steroids or anticoagulants, and an idea of the quality of life may be useful in elderly victims or those with disease. Providing a history can also make relatives feel that they are doing something useful.

During attempted resuscitation relatives should at least be given early warning if the patient's condition is critical. Regular updates by the same person (usually the link nurse) are also appreciated and may help to break the bad news in stages. It also allows relationships to form, which will help in providing the support that may be needed later.

The link nurse should introduce a doctor, preferably a senior one, to the relatives as soon as possible to provide further information. There are no firm rules as to who should break the news, but ideally it should be someone senior with the time, warmth, and communication skills. Relatives will expect to see a doctor for medical information and an idea of the prognosis: "Will he be all right, doctor?"

Advice for the doctor (or other breaker of news)

Breaking bad news has to be tailored to the situation and the particular relatives, but the following principles generally apply:

● On leaving the resuscitation area or operating theatre you may be stressed, so take a moment to compose yourself and think about what you are going to say while you take a few deep breaths. Also remove evidence of blood stains, etc, so that you are physically and mentally prepared.
● Take an experienced nurse with you. The link nurse can be a great support and can carry on where you leave off.
● Confirm that you are speaking to the correct relatives. Briefly ascertain what information they already have.
● Enter the relatives' room, introduce yourself, and sit down near the patient's closest relative at eye level. Do not stand holding the door handle like a bus conductor ready to jump out. Giving the impression that you have time to talk and listen is important.
● In general look at the person you are talking to, be honest and direct, and keep it simple. Be prepared to emphasise the main points. Avoid too much technical information at this stage (although if a patient has multiple injuries there may be much going on). If death is probable say so; do not beat about the bush.

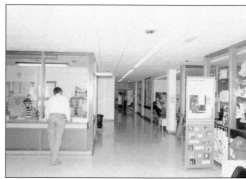

Distressed relatives should be given privacy and not kept waiting in reception areas, which may be impersonal and busy.

Essential features of a relatives' room
● Privacy
● Telephone, preferably direct dial
● Hand basin
● Mirror
● Appropriate decor and furniture
● Advice and information leaflets (out of sight)
● Tea cups and drink facilities
● Toys for children

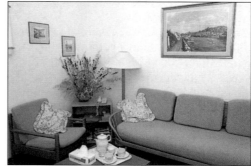

Relatives' room.

Some immediate grief reactions
● Numbness—that is, acceptance but no feeling
● Disbelief
● Acute distress
● Anger—including that against the medical care; blaming themselves or others
● Guilt
● Acceptance

- After breaking bad news allow time and silence while the facts sink in.
- If the seriousness of the situation does not seem to have been accepted, re-emphasise the facts and consider showing them the patient or deceased person immediately.
- Be prepared for a variety of emotional responses or reactions. Some people stick at one reaction, whereas others go through several reactions. These reactions are not your fault—rather they imply that you have got the message over.
- Allow and encourage reactions such as crying. Provide tissues and facilities for relatives to make themselves presentable to the world again.
- Although it is upsetting, close relatives appreciate the truth and your honest empathy.
- At this stage there is no substitute for genuine care and support. A sensitive nurse is a great asset.
- Tea usually appears, and this is another sign that the relatives' distress is appreciated.
- During the interview it is a helpful and natural comfort for staff to touch or hold the hand of the relative. Various social and cultural factors may influence the appropriateness of touching, but generally if it feels right then it is probably right.
- Likewise, during the interview it may be natural for the staff to have sad feelings, and these need not be completely hidden. Some sign of emotion may help distressed or bereaved people to realise that the staff do have some understanding and it is not just another case.
- Avoid platitudes—for example, after a death comments such as "You've still got your other son" are not helpful, as it is the dead person whom the relatives want back. Also avoid false sympathy, as in "I know what it's like," but rather empathise, as in: "It must be hard for you . . ." or "It must feel very unreal and a shock for you . . .," etc, reflecting back their emotions.

Encourage and be prepared for questions to be asked during the interview. These may disclose any misunderstandings and present a chance to re-emphasise the message. The question of pain and suffering is common and should be discussed routinely, with reassurance as appropriate. The prognosis may be unknown initially, and you should say so. If death or serious disability is possible, however, then it is only fair to be honest and warn the relatives. It will be a worse shock later if they have been protected from this knowledge.

Do not be afraid to answer that you do not know the answers to medical or philosophical questions such as "Why me?" Other difficult questions may arise from feelings of guilt or when a relative was involved in but not injured in the same accident. Special problems may arise if the relative feels responsible directly—for example, as the driver in an accident. Other complications may include a recent squabble before the accident, with subsequent self recrimination. The "If only . . ." rumination can be a type of guilt response that is fruitless and should be understood but discouraged at the outset. Just listening may be all that is needed.

If death has already occurred the same principles as discussed above apply. It is important to use the word "death" or "dead" early and avoid euphemisms such as "passed on" or "lost", which can be misinterpreted. The news is usually hard to accept and so it must be as clear as possible, abrupt as it may seem. People usually need an explanation as to the cause of death of a loved one. It may be helpful to explain the inevitability in the light of known injuries and that "everything possible was done". Worries about their own first aid at the scene of the accident may need talking through.

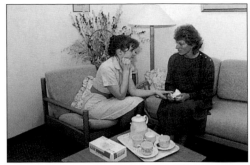

A sensitive nurse is a great asset after bad news has been broken.

Staff actions during the interview with the bereaved

Allow
- Time
- The bereaved to react
- Silence
- Touching
- Questions

Avoid
- Rushing
- "Protecting" from the truth
- Platitudes
- False sympathy
- Euphemisms
- Talking instead of listening

Whenever possible relatives should be given a clear explanation of the cause of death

Children should not be excluded from the proceedings in the mistaken belief that they need protection. They will be afraid and may have fantasies and feelings of guilt, and need more information and listening to rather than less. Parents and carers may need support and explanation about a child's or teenager's reaction.

> **Children should not be excluded from procedings—they need more information and listening to, rather than less**

Management of relatives

Seeing the patient

Depending on the urgency of further treatment it should be possible, as well as beneficial, for close relatives to see the patient briefly before he or she is rushed off to theatre, the intensive treatment unit, or even another hospital. Although distressing, reality is usually preferable to fantasy. Also, sometimes this may be the last time that they will see their loved one alive and this contact may be beneficial to the conscious patient. Relatives may ask to enter or remain in the resuscitation area during emergency treatment, especially of infants and children.

> **Reality is preferable to fantasy, so allow relatives to see even critically ill patients, albeit briefly**

Should relatives enter the resuscitation room? It is becoming more accepted practice for relatives to be offered this opportunity, and evidence suggests that it can be beneficial if certain safeguards are in place.[1,2] These include constant support and explanation from an experienced member of staff and a free choice to stay or leave—although, of course, if their presence in any way impedes the resuscitation effort, the team leader must be aware that they can be taken out. By being present, even briefly, a relative may better appreciate the seriousness of the situatuion and the vigour of resuscitation efforts.[3] In major trauma, particularly, the level of invasive procedures can increase rapidly, and careful explanation and the opportunity (or encouragement) for the relatives to leave must be provided by the support nurse.

Initially hospital staff are apprehensive about the presence of relatives but the concept should be gently introduced, with reminders of the benefits to relatives. Staff should respond promptly to relatives' requests to see a dying or dead loved one.

Seeing the body after death

The opportunity to see the dead person should always be offered and gently encouraged if there is any doubt. Well meaning friends may try and discourage this act, which is an important part of accepting reality, and relatives may also like to see the place of death.

The imagination is usually far worse than reality, and cruel fantasies about the victim being disfigured or squashed flat can be dispelled. The actions and words of staff when relatives are with the body should give "permission" for relatives to touch, hold, kiss, or say goodbye to their loved one. Staff will often carefully prepare a body before viewing in the clinical area or chapel. Ideally there should be a private cubicle near the resuscitation area, made as non-clinical as possible, to allow relatives time with the deceased person. There should also be a non-religious "chapel of rest" for later opportunities for visiting. Religious insignia can be added as appropriate. The relative may also like to be left alone with the body and must be given permission to stay as long as they wish or is practically possible.

Other actions

Although they are stunned by events, it is often the small touches of care that relatives appreciate and remember, such as being given a lock of hair from their dead child (or adult relative) by a thoughtful nurse.

Seeing the patient

- Offering relatives the opportunity to be present during resuscitation is becoming more accepted practice
- By being present, even briefly, a relative may better appreciate the seriousness of the situation and the vigour of resuscitation efforts
- Staff should respond promptly to relatives' requests to see a dying or dead loved one.
- Seeing the dead person is an important part of accepting reality, and relatives may also like to see the place of death
- If a relative wishes to be left alone with the body, he or she must be given permission to stay as long as they wish or is practically possible.

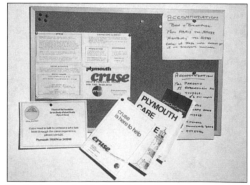
Useful information in the relatives' room.

Always ask if there is anyone else whom the relatives would like to be contacted—for example, a close friend or a minister. The relatives or appropriate minister should be consulted about any religious or ethnic issues and the correct procedures. Staff should be aware of the main minority ethnic groups in their area. The hospital chaplains can be a source of great support to both relatives and busy staff.

The patient's wishes regarding organ donation can be raised sensitively, particularly if a donor card is found. Corneas and heart valves can be donated up to 24 hours after death.

If a mechanism of counselling and follow up exists locally consider borrowing their expertise in appropriate cases of trauma.

Sedation may be requested for relatives, usually by a third party, but is generally inappropriate as it dulls reality and may delay acceptance. Grieving cannot be avoided so easily.

Information and follow up

Long term management and bereavement counselling is not within the scope of this chapter, but arrangements for follow up may need initiating at the outset. If the nurse or doctor concerned in the emergency department feels able, he or she can offer to be available for any questions later. Some departments have a social worker who can provide practical help and coordinate follow up. If death occurs it is helpful to have a routine checklist, which includes notifying the general practitioner. An open invitation can be posted to the relatives, offering an interview with a consultant so that questions on the events or necropsy findings can be answered. Many take up this offer, sometimes months later, to fill in gaps in their information which helps them to make some sense of it.

An up to date leaflet explaining official procedures slipped into a relative's pocket is useful for later perusal (for example, leaflet D49, *What to do after a death*, published by the Department of Health). Participation by the coroner's officer, who may be a policeman, should be explained. Warning relatives of the possibility of them developing symptoms of post-traumatic stress disorder is appropriate in certain cases. Such symptoms include depression, anxiety, and flash backs, with a wide range of severity. Also, a necessary part of follow up may be to warn them about the possibility of avoiding or unhelpful actions by neighbours. A local leaflet explaining possible reactions, and local information on the coroner, registration of a death and arranging the funeral, should also be provided. Details of any support organisations such as CRUSE, RoadPeace or any local groups should be included.

Staff support

Lastly, do not forget the carers. Staff do not recognise their own needs, and encouragement and "permission" are needed for them to express their feelings. Senior staff should be responsible for facilitating this, and for recognising that some staff may need further support or even professional counselling. There are many different reactions, the most common of which are sadness, anger, and guilt.[4] Staff, including the ambulance crew, may identify with particular people or situations. For example, the death of a child will be particularly upsetting, especially for staff with children of the same age. Part of the debriefing on major trauma must include an opportunity for members of staff to express their feelings. After a major trauma (or any emotive incident) staff should be allowed a short break to recover and perhaps discuss the incident before returning to more mundane duties.

After a critical incident (that is, any incident causing an unusually strong emotional reaction) staff should be given an opportunity to defuse. This is done by compulsorily calling

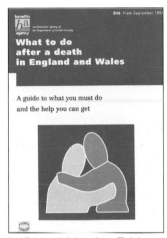
Leaflet explaining the official procedures after a death.

together all staff involved and providing key facts; then, with the leader keeping a low profile, the group should be allowed to freely discuss the incident and their roles. The beginning of nurse report or handover may also be an opportunity to defuse. The meeting is best terminated, once all is said, by the leader expressing thanks and noting the team's strengths, and that distress is normal after such events; for example, "It was the event that was abnormal, not you...".

After a large-scale or major incident staff should be demobilised at the end of the incident or shift. As with defusing, everyone who took part should attend; however, demobilisation has a time limit (10–15 min), and is characterised by clear leadership and limited participation by staff. The leader provides a factual overview of the incident, the casualties and their progress, and reassures the staff that they did a good job. The meeting should finish in the same way as a defusing session, with the additional offer of further support if necessary.

Occasionally, staff may request or need critical incident stress debriefing. This is a more formal procedure, where the staff member sees a trained counsellor over several sessions. There is probably no advantage in providing such debriefing routinely, but staff should have access to a local facility.

The purpose of informal or formal support is to allow staff to return to normal function, acknowledge distress, and show them that someone cares. Senior staff must not be forgotten, and should support one another. Facilitating such support presents a challenge in busy, often understaffed, departments, but meeting the challenge is rewarded by a reduction in staff stress and related problems.

Conclusion

The suddenness and severity of major trauma makes it especially difficult to cope with, for relatives and staff. However bad the news is, relatives need direct, honest information and genuine care and support. Many doctors find this important part of their work difficult. Reasons have been suggested for this.[5] Awareness may help the situation, and lead to more emphasis during training on acquiring the appropriate skills.

The principles of dealing with distressed relatives can be summarised as follows:

- Empathise; sit, listen, and reflect back relatives' reactions rather than making assumptions or categorising them.
- Enable relatives to accept the reality and pain by being honest and allowing them easy access to their loved one
- Encourage them, as in "You will be able to cope" (with help if needed).
- Encounter your own feelings and express them later, perhaps as part of a debriefing or defusing meeting.

Acknowledgment

I thank Sister Susan Judge, Reverend Bob Irving, Dr Sheila Cassidy, and the staff of the accident and emergency department, Derriford Hospital, Plymouth, for ideas and advice; Jackie Eccleson for typing the manuscript; and the photographic department. I also thank the relatives, whose reactions, comments, and questions have formed the basis of this chapter.

National contact addresses

- **CRUSE** (bereavement care)
  Cruse House, 126 Sheen Road, Richmond, Surrey TW9 1UR. Tel. 0207 940 4818 Helpline 0208 332 7227, Mon-Fri, 9.30-5.00
- **Compassionate Friends** (for bereaved parents)
  6 Denmark Street, Bristol BS1 5DQ.
  Tel. 0117 929 2778
- **Foundation for the Study of Infant Deaths**
  14 Halkin Street, London SW1X 7DPPS.
  Tel. 0207 235 0965
- **RoadPeace** (information and support after deaths on the road) PO Box 2579, London NW10 3PW.
  Tel. 0208 964 1021
- **Samaritans** (for the despairing)
  17 Uxbridge Road, Slough SL1 1SN. Tel. 01753 32713
- **Sudden Death Support Association** (support for families after accidental or traumatic deaths)
  Chapel Green House, Chapel Green, Wokingham, Berkshire RG11 3ER. Tel. 0118 979 0790
- **TACT: Trauma After Care Trust** (support for bereaved people experiencing post-traumatic stress disorder) Buttfields, The Farthings, Withington, Gloucestershire GL54 4DF. Tel. 01242 890306

References

1 Doyle C, Post H, Burney R, Maino J, Keefe M, Rhea K. Family participation during resuscitation: an option. *Ann Emerg Med* 1987; **16**: 673–5.

2 Robinson S, MacKenzie-Ross S, Campbell Hewson G, Egleston C, Prevost A. Psychological effect of witnessed resuscitation on bereaved relatives. *Lancet* 1998; **352**: 614–7.

3 Resuscitation Council (UK). *Should relatives witness resuscitation?* London: Resuscitation Council (UK), 1996.

4 Wright B. Sudden death: aspects which incapacitate the carer. *Nursing* 1988; **3**: 12–5.

5 Buckman R. Breaking bad news: Why is it still so difficult? *BMJ* 1984; **288**: 1597–9.

Further reading

Kuebler-Ross E. *On death and dying.* New York: MacMillan, 1969.

Wright B. *Sudden death* 2nd edn. Edinburgh: Churchill Livingstone, 1996.

18 Trauma in pregnancy

Pamela Nash, Peter Driscoll

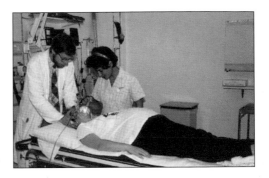

When a pregnant woman is seriously injured, two lives are at risk. Survival of the fetus depends on maternal survival. Treatment priorities are the same as in patients who are not pregnant, although resuscitation and stabilisation should be modified to account for the anatomical and physiological changes of pregnancy. Early participation of an obstetrician and a surgeon is advocated. A conscious patient will be anxious about herself and her baby. It is important to establish rapport with her quickly. Allocation of an experienced nurse to this task will facilitate communication and allow other members of the trauma team to complete the primary and secondary surveys.

Anatomical changes

In the first trimester of pregnancy the fetus is protected within the thick walled uterus by the mother's pelvis. As the uterus enlarges to become an intra-abdominal organ, it is increasingly vulnerable to injury. The fetus is cushioned by a large volume of amniotic fluid in the second trimester but by full term there is little protection for the fetus from the relatively small volume of amniotic fluid and the thin walled uterus. Unlike the uterine wall, the placenta is devoid of elastic tissue; consequently shearing forces to the abdomen—for example, those caused by blunt trauma—may cause placental abruption.

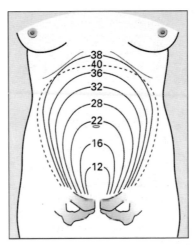

Size of the uterus at various stages of pregnancy

Physiological changes

Airway
The airway may be compromised because of the increased risk of regurgitation and aspiration during pregnancy.

Breathing
The "physiological hyperventilation" of pregnancy results in respiratory alkalosis with $PaCO_2$ at full term falling to 4.0 Kpa. A $PaCO_2$ of 5.3 Kpa at this stage of pregnancy indicates maternal and fetal acidosis.

Circulation
Interpretation of maternal pulse and blood pressure readings can be difficult as blood is shunted away from the uteroplacental circulation to maintain maternal vital signs. The fetus may be shocked before the mother develops tachycardia, tachypnoea, or hypotension. In the supine position the enlarged uterus compresses the great vessels, impairing venous return and causing a fall in cardiac output. This may be sufficient to produce a fall in maternal blood pressure (the aortocaval compression syndrome). During pregnancy, blood volume increases by up to 50% and cardiac output by 1.0–1.5 litres.

Physiological changes in pregnancy

Respiratory
- Tidal volume is increased by 40%
- Respiratory rate is unchanged
- Respiratory alkalosis

Cardiovascular
- Pulse rate is increased to 85–90 beats/minute
- Blood pressure falls by 5–15 mm Hg in second trimester
- Plasma volume is increased
- The aortocaval compression syndrome

Other changes
- Gastric emptying is delayed
- Risk of eclampsia

Compared with patients who are not pregnant, pregnant women have to lose more blood before signs of hypovolaemia develop.

Primary survey

During the primary survey, life-threatening injuries to the mother are detected and treated. Control the airway, stabilise the neck, assess ventilation, and give high flow oxygen through a mask-bag-reservoir system.

The patient should be positioned to prevent aortocaval compression. If she is immobilised on a long spine board, this can be tilted to the left and held in position by a Cardiff wedge. Alternatively, if the patient is supine the uterus can be manually displaced to the left. Once spinal injury is excluded, nurse the patient in the left lateral position.

Establish venous access with two large bore cannulae (14 gauge) in the antecubital fossas. Take blood for grouping and cross-matching and measurement of full blood count, and urea and electrolyte concentrations. Start vigorous fluid replacement with crystalloid or colloid. Haemacel has a product licence for use in pregnant patients and can be used before group-specific or cross-matched blood is available. Occasionally O negative blood is required for immediate, life saving transfusion.

If a pneumatic antishock suit is used, only the leg compartments should be inflated.

Following assessment and treatment of life threatening airway, breathing and circulatory problems, a rapid neurological assessment should be made and all the patients clothes removed.

Secondary survey

Assessment of the mother
During the secondary survey the mother is examined from head to toe. Urgent radiography should not be withheld as the priority is to detect life threatening maternal injuries. The radiation dose to the fetus can be reduced by keeping repeat abdmoinal or pelvic radiograohy to a minimum and using lead abdominal shields when taking peripheral x-ray films. This is a sensible precaution for injured, unconscious women who may be in the early stages of pregnancy. The presence of a pelvic fracture should alert the clinician to the possibility of damage to the dilated pelvic veins and subsequent massive retroperitoneal haemorrhage.

Injuries should be treated in the same way as in those patients who are not pregnant. Peritoneal lavage can be done if indicated through a supraumbilical minilaparotomy after placement of a urinary catheter and nasogastric tube. Pregnancy should not delay abdominal surgery.

Assessment of the fetus

Assessment of the fetus is part of the secondary survey of the mother and should be made by an obstetrician. Clinical examination assesses fundal height, uterine tenderness or contractions, and fetal position. Vaginal examination detects vaginal or amniotic fluid loss, cervical dilatation, and effacement.

Monitoring of fetal heart rate and pelvic ultrasonography are the most useful investigations to assess fetal wellbeing. Doppler ultrasonography can be used to auscultate the fetal heart rate from 12–14 weeks' gestation. Fetal bradycardia (<110 beats/minute) and loss of beat-to-beat variation are signs of fetal distress. Beyond 20 weeks' gestation the fetus may be monitored by cardiotocography, which compares fetal heart rate with uterine contractions. Signs of fetal distress include inadequate acceleration in fetal heart rate in response to uterine contractions and late decelerations in response to contractions.

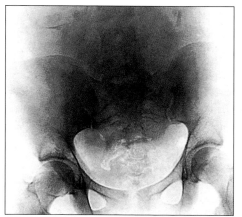

Radiograph taken after a fall excludes pelvic fracture.

In early pregnancy, fetal gestation and viability can be confirmed by transvaginal ultrasound, the fetal heart beat being visible from 5–6 weeks' gestation. Transabdominal ultrasound may show a fetal heartbeat from 7 weeks. Ultrasonography is also useful in late pregnancy to assess placental position, volume of liquor, intra-amniotic haemorrhage and placental abruption.

All Rhesus negative women should be given anti-D at the time of injury to protect against rhesus isoimmunisation as a result of fetomaternal haemorrhage.

Blunt trauma

Road traffic accidents are the most common cause of blunt trauma during pregnancy. Other causes are assaults and falls. Obstetric complications of blunt trauma include uterine contractions, placental abruption, abortion or fetal death.

Maternal hypovolaemic shock is the most common cause of fetal death. Placental abruption often leads to fetal death after blunt trauma. Clinical signs are usually obvious but fetal distress may be the only indicator of placental abruption.

Major placental separation with or without amniotic fluid embolus can lead to disseminated intravascular coagulation.

Late in pregnancy the uterus is susceptible to traumatic rupture, which has a wide range of presentations from massive haemorrhage and shock to minimal symptoms and signs. A separately palpable uterus and fetus is pathgnomonic.

Penetrating trauma

As pregnancy progresses the uterus becomes vulnerable to penetrating trauma, with the uterus and fetus acting as shields for the maternal abdominal organs. After gunshot or stab wounds to the abdomen, fetal injury and death are common but maternal survival is good because the uterus is not a vital organ.

Burns

In the late stages of pregnancy a significant percentage of the cardiac output is taken up by the utero/placental circulation. Aggravating factors that put further demand on the cardiac output can therefore lead to maternal death. An example of this is the woman in the second or third trimester of pregnancy who has high percentage surface area burns. In such cases there is high maternal and fetal mortality unless the fetus is delivered urgently. Fetal prognosis is not improved by waiting.

Indications for admission

Admission to a hospital with obstetric and surgical facilities is indicated when there is vaginal bleeding or amniotic fluid loss, uterine irritability, abdominal tenderness, pain or cramps, evidence of hypovolaemia, or abnormality of fetal heart sounds. Cardiotocographic monitoring is advocated during the first 4 hours of admission to detect signs of fetal distress if there is no immediate indication for surgery.

Conclusion

The priorities in the management of pregnant women with trauma are the same as for patients who are not pregnant. The aims are to resuscitate and stabilise the mother, and then assess the fetus with the help of an obstetrician.

Obstetric complications of blunt trauma
- Uterine contractions
- Premature labour
- Preterm delivery
- Placental abruption
- Abortion/fetal death
- Fetal decelerations
- Vaginal bleeding

Signs of placental abruption
- Vaginal bleeding
- Uterine irritability
- Abdominal tenderness
- Increasing fundal height
- Maternal hypovolaemic shock
- Fetal distress

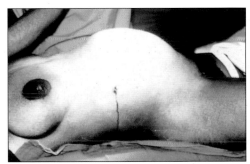
Penetrating abdominal trauma.

Immediate delivery is indicated when maternal burns exceed 50% of body surface area in the second or third trimester

Indications for surgical or obstetric intervention
- Need for treatment of maternal injuries
- Penetrating abdominal trauma
- Uterine rupture
- Placental abruption
- Fetal distress at >26 weeks' gestation
- Burns affecting >50% of body surface area in second or third trimester
- Need for caesarean section after maternal death

19 Paediatric trauma

J J M Black, A R Lloyd Thomas, I Anderson

Trauma is the most common cause of death in childhood; road traffic accidents and falls account for more than 80% of significant injuries.

The response of children to injury is quite different from that of adults—physically, physiologically and emotionally. The more frightened the child, the less will he or she be able to contribute to management. All symptoms may be denied.

Because children are small, blunt mechanisms of injury often result in multisystem injury. An injured child must therefore be assumed to have multiple injuries until proven otherwise. Life-threatening injuries found in the primary survey must be treated as soon as they are identified—treatment must not be delayed while evaluation of the child is completed.

Although injured children present several specific problems, the protocol for their initial management is similar to that adopted for adults. They must be assessed and treated simultaneously by a well directed, experienced clinical team. A structured approach is essential to ensure correct identification and prioritisation of injuries.

Primary survey and resuscitation

During the primary survey a limited history must be obtained from personnel who have attended the scene of the accident. If relatives of the child have accompanied him or her to hospital, a team member should obtain an "AMPLE" history.

With an estimate of the weight of the child, it is possible to predict appropriate volume replacement and drug doses. An approximate weight can be derived from nomograms based on head-to-toe length (Broselowe tape, or the Oakley Paediatric Resuscitation Chart; see opposite). Alternatively, for children aged 1–10 years the following formula can be used:

$$\text{Body wt (kg)} = \{\text{Age (years)} + 4\} \times 2.$$

Airway management with cervical spine control

Maintenance of airway patency is the most critical part of initial assessment and management of the injured child. Children under 6 months of age are obligate nasal breathers.

Children have specific anatomical differences from adults that can hinder maintenance of a clear airway and tracheal intubation. These include:
- Relatively large occiput, which causes flexion of the head on the neck when the child lies on a firm surface, e.g. a spinal board; this may cause complete upper airway obstruction.
- Small oral cavity with a relatively large tongue
- A compressible floor of the mouth
- Hypertrophy of the tonsils and adenoids (common in preschool children)—more likely to bleed if traumatised

- A large, horseshoe-shaped, floppy epiglottis which, with its more acute angle with the laryngeal opening, makes access to the relatively cephaled and anterior larynx difficult
- Short (in infants, non-existent) cricothyroid membrane makes needle cricothyroidotomy difficult; surgical cricothyroidotomy is impossible in infants.
- Cricoid ring is the narrowest part of the upper airway
- Short trachea; this increases the risk of mainstem bronchus intubation
- Symmetry of the carina in the infant, which may result in inadvertent intubation of either main bronchus.

All injured children must receive supplemental oxygen via a Hudson (non-rebreathing) reservoir mask, which will deliver an inspired oxygen concentration of about 85%. Fogging of the inside of the mask will confirm airway patency and spontaneous ventilation. If the child appears to be apnoeic, the head should be placed in the neutral position. If this alone is not adequate to open the airway, a jaw thrust will passively bring the tongue anteriorly and thus potentially relieve airway obstruction at the oropharynx. A jaw thrust is less likely than a chin lift to exacerbate an unstable cervical spine injury. Take care to place the fingers accurately under the mandible to avoid precipitating airway obstruction (see figure).

Gurgling when the child starts to breathe may indicate blood or secretions in the upper airway, which should be cleared by judicious suction under direct vision. Grunting or snoring indicates upper airway obstruction by the tongue. If a jaw thrust relieves this, an oropharyngeal airway of appropriate size is likely to be needed to maintain airway patency. If there is no clinical suspicion of a cribriform plate fracture, a nasopharyngeal airway may be better tolerated in a child with a score above 12 on the Glasgow Coma Scale. Stridor in an injured child implies upper airway obstruction at the level of the larynx and the need for a definitive airway at the earliest opportunity.

In any child with significant injury above the level of the clavicles, an unstable cervical spine injury must be assumed until excluded. Restore the child's head and neck to the neutral position and hold manually with in-line mobilisation in the first instance. Hold the head thus until a suitable semi-rigid collar or sand bags and tape have been applied. The child will usually have been log-rolled onto a spinal board by pre-hospital personnel to immobilise completely the thoracolumbar spine and to facilitate transfer to hospital.

Breathing

If opening and clearance of the child's airway does not result in spontaneous ventilation, then assisted ventilation via a bag valve mask (BVM) with a reservoir attached will be required to deliver 100% oxygen. Placing an oropharyngeal airway before starting assisted ventilation will improve airway patency and also reduce gastric distension and thus the risk of aspiration. The BVM must have a blow-off valve set at 30–40 cm of water to reduce the risk of causing barotrauma and life-threatening gastric dilatation. It may be necessary to obstruct (with caution) the BVM blow-off valve in the face of low pulmonary compliance to achieve satisfactory ventilation. Presence or absence of a gag reflex is a poor predictor of a patient's ability to protect the airway—inability to swallow is a much better predictor of the need for a definitive airway.

Tracheal intubation—Indications for tracheal intubation in an injured child are summarised below:
- Failure to maintain or to protect the airway
- Failure of ventilation or oxygenation
- The anticipated clinical course.

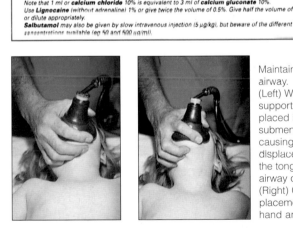

Endotracheal tube		Paediatric resuscitation chart
Oral length (cm)	Internal diameter (mm)	
18–21	7.5–8.0 cuffed	
18	7.0 uncuffed	
17	6.5	
16	6.0	
15	5.5	
14	5.0	
13	4.5	
12	4.0	
	3.5	
10	3.0–3.5	

	Weight (kg)					
	5	10	20	30	40	50
Adrenaline (ml of 1 in 10000) *initial* intravenous or intraosseous	0.5	1	2	3	4	5
Adrenaline (ml of 1 in 1000) *subsequent* intravenous or intraosseous (or *initial* endotracheal)	0.5	1	2	3	4	5
Atropine (ml of 1 in 100 µg/ml) intravenous or intraosseous (or double if endotracheal)	1	2	4	6	6	6
Atropine (ml of 600 µg/ml)	–	0.3	0.7	1	1	1
Bicarbonate (ml of 8.4%) intravenous or intraosseous (dilute to 4.2% in infants)	5	10	20	30	40	50
Calcium chloride (ml of 10%) intravenous or intraosseous	0.5	1	2	3	4	5
Diazepam (ml of 5 mg/ml) emulsion) intravenous or intraosseous	0.4	0.8	1.6	2	2	2
Diazepam (mg rectal tube solution) rectal	2.5 mg	5 mg	10 mg	10 mg	10 mg	10 mg
Glucose (ml of 50%) intravenous or intraosseous (dilute to 25% in infants)	5	10	20	30	40	50
Lignocaine (ml of 1%) intravenous or intraosseous	0.5	1	2	3	4	5
Naloxone *neonatal* (ml of 20 µg/ml) intravenous or intraosseous	2.5	5	–	–	–	–
Naloxone *adult* (ml of 400 µg/ml)	–	0.25	0.5	0.75	1	1.25
Salbutamol (mg nebuliser solution) via nebuliser (dilute to 2.5–5.0 ml in normal saline)	–	2.5 mg	5 mg	5 mg	5 mg	5 mg
Initial DC defibrillation (J) for VF or VT with no pulse	10	20	40	60	80	100
Initial DC cardioversion (J) for SVT with shock (synchronous) or VT with shock (non-synchronous)	5	5	10	15	20	25
Initial fluid bolus in shock (ml) crystalloid or colloid	100	200	400	600	800	1000

CAUTION! Non-standard drug concentrations may be available:
Use **Atropine** 100 µg/ml or prepare by diluting 1 mg to 10 ml or 600 µg to 6 ml in normal saline.
Note that 1 ml or **calcium chloride** 10% is equivalent to 3 ml of **calcium gluconate** 10%.
Use **Lignocaine** (without adrenaline) 1% or give twice the volume of 0.5%. Give half the volume of 2% or dilute appropriately.
Salbutamol may also be given by slow intravenous injection (5 µg/kg), but beware of the different concentrations available (eg 50 and 500 µg/ml).

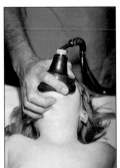

Maintaining a clear airway.
(Left) WRONG—supporting fingers placed in the submental triangle causing posterior displacement of the tongue and airway obstruction.
(Right) CORRECT placement of the hand and jaw lift.

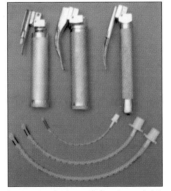

Laryngoscopes—left to right, Wisconsin, Sewerd, MacIntosh—with endotracheal tubes of various sizes for 0–10 years.

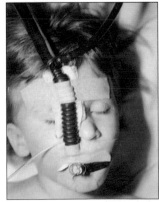

Correct fixation of Rees modified Ayres's "T" piece, endotracheal tube, and oral airway.

Failure to anticipate upper airway obstruction after an inhalation burn or penetrating wound to the anterior neck may be catastrophic, because distortion of the upper airway anatomy may make later intubation extremely difficult. Injured children with a GCS score of 9 or less require immediate rapid sequence intubation. Children who will require early surgery or transfer to a tertiary centre should be intubated before leaving the emergency department. The hazards of transfer, even to nearby intrahospital imaging facilities, cannot be over-stated.

Laryngoscopes with straight blades are widely used in infants. Traditionally curved blades have been used in older children, and the "adult method" adopted for laryngoscopy (blade inserted into the vallecula). However, with airway trauma and a distorted upper anatomy, the straight Miller blade can be extremely valuable if inserted into the proximal oesophagus and then slowly withdrawn; the tip is used to control the epiglottis directly, thus providing optimal exposure of the glottis. This is particularly helpful when in-line mobilisation has left the glottis in an unfavourable position. Any semi-rigid collar must be undone before laryngoscopy, to prevent needless restriction of mandibular movement.

Immediate management of critically ill children is greatly enhanced by storing airway, breathing and circulation equipment in colour-coded resuscitation cart drawers using the Broselow system. For those who may be required to manage seriously injured children at the scene of an accident, the prepackaged roll-up towel Broslow–Hincke Resuscitation Systems (Armstrong Medical Industries Inc., Lincolnshire, IL, USA) are invaluable.

Endotracheal tubes must be well secured; they are easily displaced, especially in small children.

Cricothryoidotomy—the indication to perform a needle cricothyroidotomy is the "cannot oxygenate, cannot ventilate" scenario. Surgical cricothyroidotomy should be avoided in children under 12 years old, because of the high risk of damage and late stenosis to the narrowest part of the paediatric airway—the cricoid ring. If a surgical airway is needed formal tracheostomy should be undertaken.

Gastric intubation—An orogastric tube must be passed as soon as the airway has been secured, to prevent gastric distension, diaphragmatic splinting and compression of inferior vena cava, which has the potential to seriously compromise oxygenation and cardiac output.

Circulation and haemorrhage control

Major external haemorrhage must be controlled by direct pressure. Then record the pulse rate and blood pressure, estimate the capillary refill time, and note the peripheral skin temperature and colour. Capillary refill time is the best indicator of the adequacy of peripheral perfusion.

Normal values for vital signs vary with age. A child's normal systolic blood pressure can be estimated by using the formula:

$$\text{Systolic BP (mm Hg)} = 80 + (2 \times \text{age in years}).$$

The physiological reserve of a child's circulation is greater than that of an adult, so vital signs may be only slightly abnormal despite considerable blood loss. Therefore the early diagnosis of impending shock in children is based on the

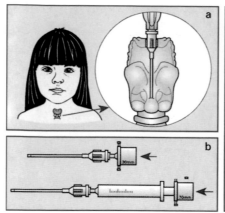
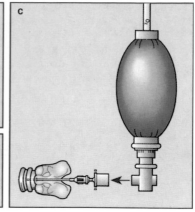

Technique for needle cricothyroidotomy.
(a) The cricothyroid membrane is pierced at an angle of 45° by a 14 G cannula. Free aspiration of air confirms correct placement, and the cannula is advanced over the needle, which is then withdrawn;
(b) a 3.0 mm endotracheal tube connector fits into the female end of the intravenous cannula or a 7.0 mm connector into the barrel of a 2 ml syringe;
(c) the connector is attached to the oxygen circuit.

Uncuffed endotracheal (ET) tubes should be used until puberty

The correct size can be derived from the formulae:

ET tube length (cm) = {age (years) / 2} + 12

ET tube diameter (mm) = {age (years) / 4} + 4

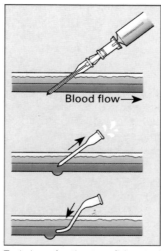

Transfix the vessel.

Withdraw the needle then the cannula until blood flows freely.

Advance the cannula into the vessel.

Technique for the transfixion and cannulation of a peripheral artery.

Appropriate sizes and indications for use of paediatric equipment according to the age (approximate weight) of the child

Equipment	0–6 months (1–6 kg)	6–12 months (4–9 kg)	1–3 years (10–15 kg)	4–7 years (16–20 kg)	8–11 years (22–33 kg)
Airway/breathing:					
Oxygen facepiece	0	0/1	1	1/2	2/3 (Adult)
Oral airways	000/00	0/1	0/1	1/2	2
Resuscitator	Baby	Baby	Baby/adult	Adult	Adult
Breathing system	"T" piece	"T" piece	"T" piece	"T" piece	Coaxial
Tracheal tubes (uncuffed; mm diameter)	2.5–3.5	3.5–4.0	4.0–5.0	5.0–6.0	5.5–7.0
Stylet	Small	Small	Small/medium	Medium	Medium
Suction catheter (FG)	6	8	10–12	14	14
Circulation:					
Intravenous cannula (G)	24/22	22	22/18	20/16	18/14
Central venous pressure cannula (G)	20	20	18	18	16
Arterial cannula (G)	24/22	22	22	22	20
Ancillary equipment:					
Nasogastric tube (FG)	8	10	10–12	12	12–14
Chest drain (FG)	10–4	12–18	14–20	14–24	16–30
Urinary catheter (FG)	5 Feeding tube	5 Feeding tube/ Foley (8)	Foley (8)	Foley (10)	Foley (10–12)

Exact measurements in children are extremely important. Endotracheal tubes are measured in mm outside diameter (OD). Catheters, naogastric tubes and chest drains are measured in French Gauge (FG) or Charrière (CH) (the same) which is the circumference in mm. ΠD is the formula for a circumference, so divide by Π (roughly 3) for the diameter in mm. G is short for SWG (standard wire gauge), which is an entirely different method of measuring needles.

appearance of the skin, the temperature of the extremities, the capillary refill time (normal less than 2 seconds), and altered sensorium. The degree of shock, and hence blood loss, can be estimated from the classification of shock (see table). A resting tachycardia may be the result of fright, pain or hypovolaemia. Hypotension is a late, preterminal sign of hypovolaemic shock. Fluid resuscitation should therefore not be withheld until vital signs are abnormal.

Circulatory access—Venous access in hypovolaemic children with collapsed veins is difficult, especially in those under 6 years of age. All seriously injured children require a minimum of two large peripheral intravenous cannulae.

If there is any difficulty in gaining peripheral access, immediate intraosseous access should be established. The usual sites are the medial upper tibia, distal to the proximal epiphysis, or the distal third of the femur, proximal to the lateral femoral condyle. It is important that there is not an ipsilateral proximal femoral fracture.

Intraosseous access enables vascular access to be established in less than a minute and improves the prospect of gaining further peripheral venous access by allowing aggressive volume replacement. All intravenous fluids (crystalloid or blood) must be actively injected into the marrow, usually with a 50 ml syringe.

Alternative sites of venous access include the femoral and external jugular veins. Internal jugular access is hazardous to attempt in a child with a potential cervical spinal injury. Subclavian access should be attempted only by those with considerable experience of this technique in children, but may be the central access of choice. The widespread adoption of early

Normal values for paediatric vital signs in patients not crying

Age	Heart rate (beats/min)	Blood pressure (systolic) (mm Hg)	Respiratory rate (breaths/min)	Blood volume (ml/kg)
<1 year	120–140	70 90	30–40	90
2 5 years	100–120	80–90	20–30	80
5–12 years	80–100	90–110	15–20	80

Advanced Trauma Life Support classification of shock in children

	Class I <15%	Class II 15–25%	Class III 25–40%	Class IV >40%
Cardiovascular system (heart rate in beats/min)	Heart rate ↑ 10–20% Blood pressure normal	Tachycardia (>150) Systolic blood pressure ↓ Pulse pressure ↓	Tachycardia (>150) Systolic blood pressure ↓↓ Pulse pressure ↓↓	Tachycardia/ bradycardia Severe hypotension Peripheral pulses absent
Respiratory rate (breaths/min)	Normal	Tachypnoea (35–40)	Tachypnoea	Respiratory rate falls
Skin	Normal	Cool, peripheries cool and clammy	Cold, clammy, cyanotic	Pale, cold
Central nervous system	Normal	Irritable, confused, aggressive	Lethargic	Comatose
Capillary refill time	Normal	Prolonged	Very prolonged	

intraosseous access has made venous cut down a rarely performed procedure in children.

Cellulitis, osteomyelitis or extravasation of intravenous fluids fluids producing a compartment syndrome are potential but rare complications; the intraosseous needle should be removed as soon as adequate venous access has been obtained.

As soon as there is venous access, blood must be drawn for group and cross-matching and blood glucose estimation, and also for a full blood count and baseline biochemistry assay. A full cross-match will take about 45 minutes if the child has not been previously transfused. Type-specific blood can usually be obtained in 15 minutes and O rhesus negative blood should be stored in every resuscitation room.

Arterial access should be obtained. Attempts to achieve it should not delay transfer of the child to an operating theatre or tertiary centre, but it will facilitate close monitoring of the child's gas exchange and response to therapy. A transfixion technique as illustrated is easiest in infants, and should initially be attempted in peripheral arteries.

Fluid administration—The use of colloids and human albumin in critically ill hypovolaemic patients has been questioned by the Cochrane investigators; until we have more clinical data from much needed randomised trials it would seem wise to use crystalloid (either Hartmann's solution or physiological saline) in the initial resuscitation of children.

All intravenous fluids should be warmed. An initial bolus of crystalloid 20 ml/kg should be given rapidly and the cardio-vascular response must be dynamically determined. Unless cardiovascular stability is achieved, a second bolus of crystalloid should be given. If stability is still not obtained, blood should be given and surgical advice promptly obtained. If patients present with the features of class III or IV shock, blood should be transfused immediately and surgical advice sought.

Whole blood, especially fresh whole blood, is rarely available. Red blood cells with a packed cell volume of 65–75% are often supplied. Administration of blood with a high packed cell volume is difficult through the small (22 G or 24 G) cannulae used in infants.

The earlier that life-threatening haemorrhage is identified and controlled ("switching off the taps"), the better will be the child's outcome.

Neurological dysfunction

The major determinants for survival following a severe head injury are oxygenation and cerebral perfusion. There is there-fore little to be gained by focusing on assessment of the head and possible spinal injury until the airway and breathing has been secured and cardiovascular stability obtained. In practice, an initial brief minineurological examination is performed; this incorporates a rapid assessment to calculate a score on the (modified) Glasgow Coma Scale, and determination of pupil-lary sizes and response to light.

Exposure

Removal of all clothing is essential to allow a complete physical examination and facilitate practical procedures. However, children, especially infants, lose heat rapidly as a result of their high ratio of surface area to weight, thin skin, and lack of subcu-taneous tissue. Considerable heat loss may have occurred at the site of injury and during transportation. Monitoring tem-perature is a vital component of initial assessment. A fall in body temperature causes a rise in oxygen consumption as endogenous processes begin to increase heat production, with peripheral vasoconstriction, and consequent metabolic acidosis. The ambient temperature of the resuscitation room should be raised

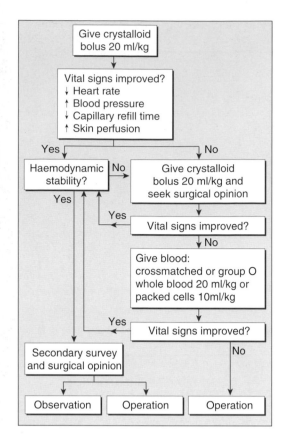

Glasgow coma scale

	Score
Eyes open	
—spontaneously	4
—to speech	3
—to pain	2
—never	1
Best motor response	
—obeys commands	6
—localises pain	5
—flexion withdrawal	4
—decerebrate flexion	3
—decerebrate extension	2
—no response	1
Best verbal response	
—orientated	5
—confused	4
—inappropriate words	3
—incomprehensible sounds	2
—silent	1

Modification of Glasgow coma scale for children

	Score
Best verbal response:	
—appropriate words or social smiles, fixes on and follows objects	5
—cries but is consolable	4
—persistently irritable	3
—restless, agitated	2
—silent	1
Eye and motor responses	
—scored as in scale for adults	

and overhead heaters and warming blankets used. Plastic sheets can be used to cover exposed body parts. Children do not respond well to being exposed in unfamiliar environments and covering the child will also help preserve his or her dignity.

Trauma x ray series

Radiographs of the chest and then the pelvis must be taken at the earliest opportunity towards the end of the primary survey —that is, within the first 15 minutes of admission when there is an experienced and well co-ordinated trauma team. Cervical spine radiographs are not an immediate priority, as injured children should always be treated and handled as if they had an unstable injury of the cervical spine. They should be delayed until cardiorespiratory stability has been obtained. Better quality films will be obtained in the radiology department, where they can be combined with computed tomography if necessary.

Computed tomogram showing right subdural haematoma.

Secondary survey

Head and neck

Fully examine the head for lacerations, the skull for fractures, the eyes for injury (also remember penetrating injury) and pupillary function, the ears and nose for leakage of cerebrospinal fluid, the face for fractures and lacerations, the mouth for loose teeth, and, finally, the neck for cervical vertebral displacement. Frequent assessment of the Glasgow coma score is essential. In the infant, palpation of the open fontanelle may give a direct assessment of intracranial pressure.

Primary brain damage that occurs at the time of the injury cannot be reversed. Secondary brain damage occurs as a result of cerebral hypoxia or ischaemia and can be minimised by maintaining oxygenation and an adequate cerebral perfusion pressure.

A child's brain is vulnerable to accelerative, decelerative, and shear forces that result in focal intracranial mass lesions (cerebral contusions, lacerations and haemorrhages) and cerebral oedema. Raised intracranial pressure secondary to diffuse cerebral swelling is the most common cause of death in children with head injuries.

Acute subdural haematomas are often bilateral; there is a high incidence of an associated primary brain injury and seizures, and a low incidence of skull fractures.

If there is no history of appreciable trauma, consider the possibility of non-accidental injury.

Extradural haematomas are most often unilateral and associated with a high incidence of skull fractures and a low incidence of seizures. The biphasic presentation of extradural haematomas ("lucid interval") is less common in children.

About 75% of skull fractures are linear, but they may be depressed, compound, or basal, and in children younger than 3 years, the cranial sutures can undergo traumatic separation (diasteal fractures).

The clinical manifestations of raised intracranial pressure or skull fractures are the same in children as in adults. Infants with open fontanelles and mobile sutures, however, are more tolerant to an expanding intracranial mass, although when decompensation does occur it is rapid and often irrecoverable. A bulging fontanelle or suture diastases in an infant implies serious cerebral trauma.

The indications for establishing a definitive airway in children with head injury are coma (GCS < 9, i.e. not obeying, speaking or opening eyes), loss of protective laryngeal reflexes, ventilatory insufficiency (PaO_2 < 9 kPa on air or < 13 kPa on oxygen; $PaCO_2$ > 6 kPa), spontaneous hyperventilation ($PaCO_2$ < 3.5 kPa), or respiratory arrythmia. The aim should be to

Principles for the secondary survey

- Assess the child systematically, from head to toe, front and back
- Finding an injury should not stop the remainder of the evaluation
- Log roll the child to prevent secondary injury to the spinal cord
- Be gentle and explain clearly to the child any procedure to be performed
- Record vital signs repeatedly and assess response to therapy

Causes of secondary brain damage

- Hypoxia
- Hypercarbia
- Cerebral ischaemia
  - —systemic hypotension
  - —fall in cerebral perfusion pressure secondary to raised intracranial pressure from cerebral oedema or an intracranial mass lesion

Initial management of severe head injury

- Adequate oxygenation (PaO_2 > 15 kPa on oxygen)
- Tracheal intubation
- Hyperventilation ($PaCO_2$, 4.0–4.5 kPa)
- Restoration of mean arterial pressure (> 70 mm Hg) and haemorrhage control
- Prompt neurosurgical referral
- Administration of mannitol 0.5–1.0 g/kg (following neurosurgical advice)
- Timely and safe transfer to a neurosurgical or intensive care unit

achieve a $PaO_2 > 15$ kPa on supplemental oxygen and a $PaCO_2$ of 4.0–4.5 kPa.

Restoration of systemic blood pressure by judicious volume replacement is vital and should not be limited by concerns about the potential for aggravating cerebral oedema. For serious head injuries, a neurosurgical opinion should be sought early and a brain CT scan performed as soon as the patient is haemodynamically stable. There is good evidence that therapy directed at lowering intracranial pressure (ICP), guided by direct ICP monitoring, improves neurological outcome.

In children, head injury alone does not usually produce shock and hypotension as a result of hypovolaemia; most bleeding usually occurs elsewhere in the body. Extensive scalp lacerations, however, may bleed sufficiently to cause hypovolaemic shock in young children. In small infants intracranial haemorrhage alone may be sufficient to cause hypovolaemia.

After head injury vomiting and seizures are more common in children than in adults. Both symptoms tend to be self limiting, but if either persists a serious head injury should be suspected. Repeated seizures cause an increase in intracranial pressure by increasing cerebral blood flow, and anticonvulsants should be given. Intravenous diazepam 0.15–0.25 mg/kg is the drug of first choice; this may cause respiratory depression, and may precipitate the need for ventilation. Phenytoin 15–20 mg/kg by slow intravenous injection (1–2 mg/kg/min) may subsequently be necessary with continuous electrocardiogram monitoring.

Minor head injury is extremely common in children. Plain radiography of the skull should be reserved for children who are well enough to be discharged from hospital (full level of consciousness, no neurological symptoms and no neurological signs) but are known to have been unconscious at the scene. The identification of a skull fracture by x-ray increases the likelihood of intracranial haemorrhage 10-fold. Such children must be admitted. Most children with such injury do not develop intracranial pathology.

Spinal cord injury

Spinal cord injuries are rare in children, constituting only 5% of all spinal cord trauma. Nevertheless, there should be a high index of suspicion in any child with major trauma, especially if he or she has an appreciable head injury and a reduced level of consciousness.

Careful clinical and radiological examination should be undertaken (see chapter 8). Assessing paralysis and altered sensation, however, can be very difficult, especially in infants. Mass flexion withdrawal in response to stimulation may be indistinguishable from normal withdrawal in this age group. Furthermore, 50% of children with serious spinal injuries have normal radiographs, and radiological normality should not deter a clinical diagnosis of spinal injury. Conversely, there are several peculiarities in radiographs of the immature spine that may lead to over-diagnosis of spinal injury. The thoraco-lumbar spine can be cleared radiologically.

Clearing the cervical spine in unconscious children is difficult and spinal cord injury may occur in the absence of a spinal fracture. The cervical spine may be unstable because of ligamentous injury alone, especially in children. Recent clinical experience with the use of fluoroscopy (in theatre or the intensive care unit) to achieve dynamic imaging of the cervical spine has shown it to be highly sensitive and specific for identifying unstable injuries. Safe removal of cervical collars within 48 hours of admission has important nursing implications and may also be helpful in lowering raised intracranial pressure.

Relative indications for skull radiography after head injury in children

- Age less than 1 year
- History of loss of consciousness
- Fall from significant height onto solid surface
- Clinical signs of possible vault fracture, depressed fracture or vault penetration

---

Indications for brain CT following head injury in a child presenting to the emergency department

- Deteriorating GCS or developing focal neurological signs
- Skull fracture with
  —GCS < 15
  —focal neurological signs
  —seizures
  —any other neurological symptoms or signs
- Persistent coma following resuscitation

Confusing radiological features of the cervical spine in children

Growth centres resemble fractures

- Cartilaginous plate at the base of the odontoid (closes at 3–5 years)
- Secondary ossification centre at apex of odontoid (present from 2–12 years)
- Secondary ossification centre at tip of spinous processes

Pseudosubluxation

- Anterior displacement of C2 on C3 (30% of children under 7 years). Much less commonly C3 on C4

Hypermobility

- Increased distance between dens and anterior arch of C1 (15% of children under 5 years)

It is essential that all children are transferred from spinal boards at the earliest opportunity in the emergency department to prevent decubitus ulceration and unnecessary discomfort. A common misconception is that emergency department trolleys do not provide adequate thoracolumbar support.

Thorax

Blunt chest trauma is common in children, whereas penetrating injury is rare. The approach to diagnosis and management is the same as in adults. About 15–20% of children with major injuries have chest trauma that requires immediate management. Early diagnosis is essential: of the children who die of chest injury more than 90% die in the first few hours after the accident. Most thoracic injuries (85–90%) can be managed by standard, non-operative techniques.

More than 50% of patients with thoracic trauma have associated injuries, most commonly of the head, abdomen, or an extremity.

The chest wall should be examined for bruising, wounds, and asymmetry of movement. The high compliance of a child's chest wall, however, allows ready transfer of energy to intrathoracic structures, and appreciable organ damage may be present with minimal evidence of chest wall injury.

If a *pneumothorax* (indicated by inequality of air entry) is under tension it requires immediate drainage. Classically this should be by needle thoracocentesis before placement of an intrapleural drain. The site should be lateral to the mid-clavicular line if the second anterior intercostal space is used, because of risk of injury to the great vessels and heart in the presence of significant mediastinal shift. In the older child, in experienced hands, the chest can be rapidly vented through a stab incision used for intercostal drainage.

The threshold for draining simple traumatic pneumo-thoraces should be low, especially if it is anticipated that the child will be ventilated, because of the risk of tension developing.

Open pneumothorax is unusual in children. It is initially managed by giving high flow oxygen, covering the wound on three sides with an air-tight dressing, thus creating a one-way outlet valve on the chest wall, and insertion of an intercostal drain.

Flail segments are also uncommon in children but require early treatment with chest drainage, intermittent positive pressure ventilation and positive end expiratory pressure, as these injuries are always associated with a severe pulmonary contusion. Gas exchange predictably deteriorates for 24–48 hours after injury associated with an increase in the work of breathing. Haemoptysis, subcutaneous emphysema, and a persistent air leak after drainage of a pneumothorax all suggest underlying lung damage.

Patients with *pulmonary contusion* present with tachypnoea, breathlessness, and hypoxia. The symptoms are often exacerbated by inhalation of gastric contents, especially if the abdomen has been compressed. If the child has undergone a garrotting injury tracheal rupture should be suspected, especially if there is subcutaneous emphysema in the neck. Noisy breathing and a persistent (massive) leak through the chest drain with failure to re-expand the lung suggests a tracheal or major bronchial tear.

As in adults, *diaphragmatic rupture*, most commonly on the left side, is often missed clinically, especially in ventilated patients, but should be suspected if the left side of the diaphragm is not clearly visualised on the chest radiograph.

Myocardial contusion is rare in children but is suggested by arrhythmias in a child who has sustained blunt trauma to the anterior chest wall. Continuous electrocardiography is essential for 24 hours.

Occult chest injuries in children

- Pulmonary contusion
- Pulmonary laceration
- Intrapulmonary haemorrhage
- Tracheobronchial tear
- Myocardial contusion
- Diaphragmatic rupture
- Partial aortic or other great vessel disruption
- Oesophageal tears

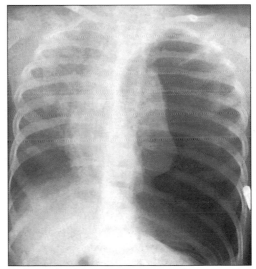

Radiograph of left tension pneumothorax causing deviation of the mediastinum to the right.

Indications for cardiothoracic surgical referral

- Large air leak or persistent haemorrhage following chest drain insertion
- Cardiac tamponade
- Disruption of great vessels

Cardiac tamponade caused by haemopericardium is also rare because penetrating injury is unusual in children. The signs are the same as in adults, and drainage using a 14 G intravenous cannula should be by the left subxiphoid route, ideally with monitoring via a precordial chest ECG lead and echocardiography.

Although mediastinal mobility in children means that there is a lower incidence of rupture of the great vessels than in adults, *aortic rupture* (which most commonly occurs close to the origin of the left subclavian artery) is suggested by a deceleration injury, widened mediastinum, fractures of the first or second ribs, and obliteration of the aortic knuckle in the chest radiograph. Displacement of a nasogastric tube to the right is also suggestive of this injury.

Clinical assessment of the signs of hypovolaemic shock should be frequently repeated to assess the response to fluid resuscitation.

Abdomen

The basic principle governing the evaluation of a child with a possible abdominal injury is to determine whether an operation is necessary, either for an acute abdomen or for controlling haemorrhage. As in thoracic injuries blunt trauma is most common. Penetrating wounds are rare but, when present, require an operation.

Early passage of a nasogastric tube of appropriate size is essential in children. Careful and gentle clinical examination of the conscious child will produce evidence of appreciable abdominal injury, which may be present despite minimal indications of trauma in the abdominal wall. The pattern and methods of clinical examination are the same as in adults.

As in adults the spleen and liver are the most commonly injured solid organs; a conservative approach is usually initially adopted as haemorrhage is usually self limiting. Splenectomy has significant long term health implications, leaving a child with lifelong vulnerability to overwhelming pneumococcal sepsis.

Rapid deceleration forces cause abdominal compression and may result in other injuries. Bowel perforation detected clinically or by computed tomography is an indication for immediate laparotomy. Pancreatic injury is usually treated conservatively unless it is complicated by late pseudocyst formation.

A renal injury should be suspected in every child with tenderness of the flank and haematuria. The injury can be well defined on a CT scan and again is usually managed conservatively unless there is uncontrolled haemorrhage. The lumbar spine, ribs, and pelvis are also commonly injured.

A full bladder is readily ruptured because of its intra-abdominal location in a child. Management is usually conservative with urethral drainage. Any clinical suspicion of urethral rupture must be confirmed by urethrography. Initial management is with a fine Silastic Foley catheter passed by an experienced urologist.

Assessment of the abdomen may be difficult in an unconscious child. Many trauma centres are increasingly using serial abdominal ultrasound studies in the resuscitation room, to look for free intraperitoneal fluid in children with persistent haemodynamic instability. This has helped to expedite the early transfer to theatre of children with uncontrolled intra-abdominal haemorrhage. Stable but multiply injured children are increasingly undergoing early rapid-spiral computed tomography to exclude occult intrathoracic or intra-abdominal injury.

Factors that suggest aortic rupture
- A deceleration injury
- A widened mediastinum
- Fractures of the first or second ribs
- Obliteration of the aortic knuckle in the chest radiograph.
- Displacement to the right of a nasogastric tube

Abdominal injuries caused by rapid deceleration forces
- *Duodenal*
  —perforation
  —obstructing haematoma
- *Pancreatic*
- Rupture of hollow viscera
  —at the ligament of Treitz
  —near the ileocaecal valve
- *Mesenteric avulsion*
- *Renal*
  —vascular
  —parenchymal
  —collecting system
- *Bladder*

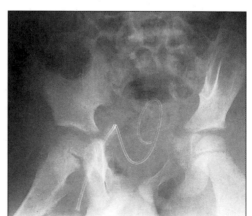

Radiograph showing fractured pelvis caused by a crush injury. A suprapubic catheter is in situ.

Diagnostic peritoneal lavage is now rarely performed in the UK unless there is no access to (or time to use) a CT scanner or abdominal ultrasound. The consultant surgeon responsible for the child's inpatient care should perform it.

Soft tissue and skeletal injuries

The principles of management of skeletal and soft tissue damage in children are the same as those for adults. In children the history of the injury is important. The radiological diagnosis of skeletal injury around the joints is more difficult in children because of the growth plate and lack of mineralisation of the epiphysis. Radiographs of the opposite side (if uninjured) may be helpful.

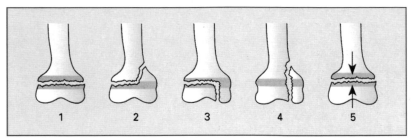
The Salter–Harris classification of epiphyseal fractures.

The pattern of fractures is different in children. They may be through the growth plate (Salter–Harris classification[1] types I–V), greenstick (through only one cortex of a long bone), or buckle (bony angulation without a fracture). Because of potential arresting of growth, malalignment of joints, and traumatic arthritis it is important to recognise any fractures involving the epiphysis and joint articular surfaces.

Supracondylar fractures at the elbow have a high incidence of associated vascular injury. The proportional blood loss after pelvic or long bone fractures in children is greater than in adults and may be an important cause of initial haemodynamic instability.

Old healed fractures should alert the medical team to the possibility of non-accidental injury.

Burns

Scalds from hot water are the most common cause of burns in children, and management does not differ appreciably from that of adult patients (see chapter 22).

The change in body proportions as children grow means that calculation of the percentage total body surface area burnt cannot be based on the adult "rule of nines". An accurate estimation of the percentage of the total body surface area burnt requires the use of detailed charts (Lund & Browder).[2] The surface of a child's hand approximates to 1% of the body surface area.

Crystalloid fluid replacement (in addition to maintenance fluid requirements) required in the first 24 hours can be calculated using the Baxter/Parkland formula:

$$4 \text{ ml} / \text{kg} \times \% \text{ burn}$$

The child should be given half of this requirement in the first 8 hours after the time of the burn. The adequacy of fluid replacement is monitored by ensuring that a urine output of at least 1 ml/kg/hour in children over 1 year of age and 2 ml/kg/hour in infants.

The indications for transfer to a regional burns unit include:
- 10% partial and/or full thickness burns
- 5% full thickness burns
- Burns to special areas (face, hands and genitalia)

If a burnt child presents with signs of hypovolaemic shock, then an additional source for blood loss should be urgently sought.

Clingfilm is the ideal emergency dressing for extensive burns and provides effective pain relief (protection from draughts). Topical sulphadiazine should be avoided in the first instance because it makes subsequent assessment of partial thickness burns more difficult.

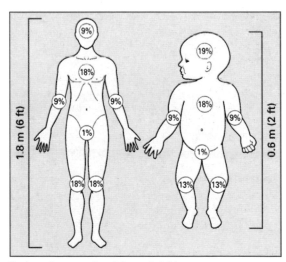
Body surface area in adults and children.

Pain relief in children

Adequate control of pain is humane and will improve a child's co-operation with diagnosis, investigation, and management. After initial fluid resuscitation a bolus of 50 µg/kg of morphine should be given intravenously. Further doses may be given at 10 minute intervals, titrated against the patient's response to just control pain.

In children with isolated extremity fractures, Oromorph at a dose of 200–400 µg/kg in combination with splinting of the fracture in a back slab cast will often produce rapid and satisfactory analgesia without the initial trauma of gaining intravenous access; topical anaesthesia can then be applied before peripheral venous cannulation.

Throughout the secondary survey the child's response to resuscitation and general condition should be constantly reassessed. Subsequent management depends on the expertise and facilities of the receiving hospital. If the anaesthetic, surgical, and intensive care services are not suited to the care of children a protocol for transfer to a designated paediatric centre should be an important part of the initial evaluation and management.

Control of pain

- After resuscitation give a bolus of morphine 50 µg/kg intravenously
- Titrate further doses of 25 µg/kg against the patient's response
- Narcotic drugs should be used with caution in patients with significant head injuries

Non-accidental injury

A wide variety of injuries can be caused by physical child abuse. Various points in the history and examination should suggest to the medical team the possibility of non-accidental injury.

Initial resuscitation and management of the battered child are the prime responsibilities of the emergency department medical team, but the need to inform the appropriate authorities must not be overlooked.

Careful recording (including photographs) of injuries is essential, and standard diagrams should be available for this purpose.

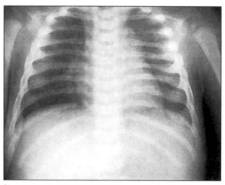

Chest radiograph showing multiple healing rib fractures after non-accidental injury.

Diagnostic criteria for non-accidental injury

- Delay in seeking medical advice
- Account of the accident is vague and inconsistent among parties
- Discrepancy between the history and the degree of injury
- Abnormal parental behaviour, with lack of concern for the child
- Abnormal interaction between child and parents
- Bruising caused by finger tips, especially over upper arms, trunk, sides of face, ears, or neck
- Bizarre injuries—e.g. bites, cigarette burns, rope marks
- Sharply demarcated burns in unusual areas
- Perioral injuries—for example, torn frenulum
- Retinal haemorrhage
- Multiple subdural haemorrhages
- Ruptured internal organs with no history of major trauma
- Perianal or genital injury
- Long bone fractures in non-ambulant children
- Previous injuries—e.g. old scars, healing fractures

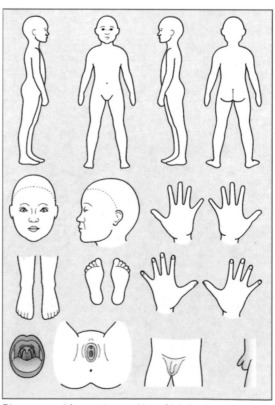

Diagram used for precise marking of injuries in a suspected case of non-accidental injury.

Should relatives be present in the resuscitation room?

Families must have open access to their children and must be given complete information about the child's condition and prognosis as soon as it is known. This information must be passed on in a sensitive but frank way.

Presence of relatives in the resuscitation room during attempted resuscitation is a controversial issue. A survey in 1994 (British Association of Emergency Medicine/Royal College of Nursing) revealed that less than one quarter of emergency departments allowed the relatives of children into the resuscitation room.

The view of many health care professionals, in contrast to the view of many relatives, is that the presence of relatives in the resuscitation room does more harm than good. There are few data to demonstrate any detrimental effect on the patient, relatives or staff of relatives' presence. Views among clinicians vary, with most emergency physicians and paediatricians in favour, and many physicians and anaesthetists against, often strongly so.[3]

Relatives perceive several advantages in being present in the resuscitation room. There are potential disadvantages: the reality of the resuscitation may prove distressing, particularly if the relatives are uninformed, and they may physically or emotionally hinder the staff's efforts at resuscitation; subsequently, relatives may be disturbed by the memory of the attempt, although there is evidence that fantasy is worse than fact. Current evidence suggests that for many it is more distressing to be separated from a family member during these critical moments than to witness attempts at resuscitation.[3]

In summary:
- Offer relatives the chance to be present during resuscitation
- Allocate a staff member to be with them at all times
- Make it clear that if they interfere they will have to leave
- Explain what is happening in terms that they can understand.
- Allow them to touch the child when it is safe to do so

Conclusion

The injured child must be systematically assessed and every life threatening emergency treated as soon as it is identified, following the "ABCDE" guidelines.

Those responsible for providing initial care for injured children must be familiar with the common patterns of injury and with their initial assessment, management and treatment. It is essential that good communication systems are in place so that the child can be assessed promptly by an experienced surgeon and, if necessary, transferred to a definitive paediatric care facility as soon as his or her condition is stabilised. Close liaison with the child and the family is essential for delivery of the highest quality of care.

- The paediatric resuscitation chart is by PA Oakley and was derived from the guidelines of the resuscitation council (UK). The radiographs were kindly provided by Drs B Kendall, D Shaw, C Hall, and D Hatch, Hospital for Sick Children, Great Ormond Street Hospital, London

Presence of relatives in the resuscitation room
Main fears expressed by staff
- The potential for increased stress for staff
- Increased distress in relatives
- Influence on the decision to abandon a resuscitation attempt
- Attempts by the relatives to interfere
- Impairment of staff's clinical performance

Advantages perceived by relatives
- They are saved the distress of separation from a loved one when they feel the need to be present
- They can see that everything possible is done
- They can provide emotional support to the conscious child
- They can speak to the child while he or she might still be able to hear them
- They can touch and speak to a child who has died while the body is still warm
- Grief may be more easily shared by those present
- The reality of death is more readily accepted, avoiding prolonged denial and contributing to a healthier bereavement

References

1 Salter RB, Harris WR. Injuries involving the epiphyseal plate. *Am J Bone Joint Surg* 1963; **45**: 587-622.

2 Lund CC, Bowder NC. The estimation of area of burns. *Surg Gynecol Obstet* 1944; **79**: 353-60.

3 *Should relatives witness resuscitation?* A report from a project team of the Resuscitation Council, October 1996.

Further reading

The Advanced Life Support Group. *Advanced paediatric life support — the practical approach* 2nd edn. London: BMJ Books, 1997.

Driscoll P, Skinner DV, eds. *Trauma care beyond the resuscitation room.* London: BMJ Books, 1998.

Skinner DV, Whimster F *Trauma. A companion to Bailey and Love's Short Practice of Surgery.* London: Arnold, 1999.

Walls RN. *Manual of emergency airway management. The airway course.* 3rd edn. Wellesley, MA: Airway Management Education Center, 1999.

20 Trauma in the elderly

Carl L Gwinnutt, Michael A Horan

The morbidity and mortality of older people is greater than that of any other age group, regardless of the severity of their injuries. However, the elderly are seriously injured less often than any other sector of the population. Fewer injuries are associated with motor vehicle accidents, falls being the main cause. This is because of changes in vision, vestibular function and proprioception, prolonged motor reaction time, and neurological and musculoskeletal diseases.

Until recently the outcome of trauma care for elderly people was poor but it has become increasingly clear that early and aggressive therapeutic intervention, accompanied by invasive monitoring, can considerably improve it. Age alone accounts for little of the variance in outcome in intensive care units; the underlying pathophysiology is the major determinant. Consequently, to maximise survival in the elderly, clinicians need to focus on detecting and correcting physiological and metabolic derangements that accompany major trauma.

Primary survey and resuscitation

Airway management with protection of the cervical spine

Many older patients are edentulous but some are not and may have loose, inconveniently situated or very carious teeth. Resorption of the mandible and lax cheeks may make maintenance of the airway more difficult.

Well fitting dentures may be left in place initially, but the doctor dealing with the airway should record this and inform the team leader. If dentures are removed, they must be inspected to ensure they are complete, particularly if they have been fractured. Airway adjunct must be used with care because the soft tissues of the oropharynx and nasopharynx are more prone to damage—particularly the turbinates, which may bleed profusely.

Intubation is generally straightforward, but beware of temporomandibular arthritis that may limit mouth opening. During all the manoeuvres to establish and maintain a patent airway, great care must be taken with the cervical spine because arthritis (osteoarthritis and rheumatoid disease) is the rule rather than the exception. Consequently, these trauma patients are particularly prone to cervical cord or nerve injury if subjected to excessive flexion or extension of the neck.

Breathing

Lung function in older patients is affected by changes in the chest wall, ventilatory muscles and lung parenchyma. The thorax becomes stiffer as a result of calcification of the costal cartilages, reduction in the intervertebral disc spaces and

> **It has been estimated that in the USA elderly people account for about one third of the cost of all trauma care**

Life expectancy of men and women at different ages

Age (years)	Active life (years) Men	Active life (years) Women	Dependent life (years) Men	Dependent life (years) Women
65	9.5	10.5	4.5	9.0
75	6.5	3.0	7.0	6.5
85	3.0	3.0	2.5	5.0

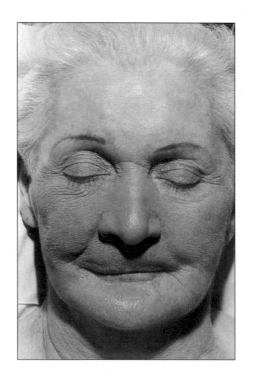

co-existing crush fractures of the vertebral bodies. Together, these produce an increase in the anteroposterior diameter of the chest and reduced rib excursion. The elastic recoil properties of the lung also decrease with age, which reduces the ease of ventilation and decreases compliance. In addition, there is an increase in the collapse of small airways during expiration, leading to non-uniform ventilation and air trapping. Collectively, these cause a small reduction in PaO_2. Such changes, together with an impaired mucociliary escalator, predispose elderly patients to atelectasis, pneumonia and hypoventilation.

For the reasons given above, it is often difficult to support ventilation with oxygen given by a facemask and hypoxia can develop rapidly. If there is any doubt about the adequacy of oxygenation, mechanical ventilation with 100% oxygen should be started early.

Pulse oximetry should be used routinely in all patients. Finger probes may give a poor reading in the elderly as a result of cold induced vasoconstriction and shivering. Probes designed for the nose and earlobe are often more reliable. All intubated, ventilated patients must have their end-tidal carbon dioxide concentration ($ETCO_2$) monitored. Under normal circumstances, $ETCO_2$ closely matches $PaCO_2$, with a gradient of 4–7 mm Hg (0.5–1.0 kPa). It can therefore be used as an indicator of the adequacy of alveolar ventilation and also as a disconnect alarm. In the elderly patient, however, the gradient is increased (because of a reduced $ETCO_2$), particularly in the presence of chronic obstructive pulmonary disease. Therefore the $ETCO_2$ should be checked against analysis of an arterial blood sample as soon as possible.

Pneumothoraces are produced more commonly in this age group, particularly in those patients with chronic lung diseases. The team leader should be constantly aware of this. In addition to frequent inspection of the chest for symmetry of movement, the development of surgical emphysema, equality of breath sounds, and in ventilated patients airway pressures, should all be monitored. Ventilation is adjusted to keep peak inspiratory pressures as low as possible to reduce the risk of barotrauma, particularly in emphysematous patients. In view of the serious potential problems that may arise in these patients, the help of an anaesthetist should be sought early.

Circulation and control of haemorrhage

The incidence of ischaemic heart disease increases with age but its prevalence in old age is unknown. Necropsy studies suggest a prevalence in those over 65 of about 60%, but in the living of similar age estimates vary between 10% and 30%.

Even in healthy people, advancing age is associated with cardiovascular changes. Increased stiffness of the arterial walls leads to an increase in systolic blood pressure and left ventricular hypertrophy. Resting cardiac output is maintained, but the ability to mount a compensatory tachycardia is reduced. Healthy old people compensate by increased venous return and raise cardiac output predominantly through the Starling mechanism. Consequently, reduction in intravascular volume may lead to a rapid reduction in cardiac output.

The initial fluid for resuscitation is warmed Ringer's lactate, but there must be continuous, accurate monitoring of the response in the elderly patient, because of the reduced tolerance of hypovolaemia or fluid overload. It is important to remember that measures of pulse rate and indirect measurement of blood pressure give only limited information about intravascular volume. Furthermore, the jugular venous pulse and fullness of peripheral veins can be difficult to assess in the elderly and should not be relied on. This is particularly true in

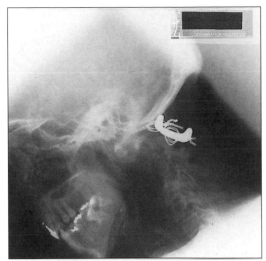

Lateral cervical spine radiograph showing severe degenerative changes.

All patients should be given 100% oxygen initially, regardless of whether they have chronic lung disease or carbon dioxide retention

It is the partial pressure of oxygen in arterial blood (PaO_2) that is maintaining respiratory drive, not the inspired oxygen concentration

Aging and ischaemic heart disease incidence (annual rate per 1000)

Age group	Men	Women
35–44	5	1
45–54	11	4
55–64	19	10
65–74	23	14
75–84	30	22
85–94	39	41

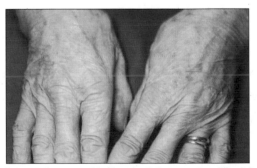

Intravenous access to the circulation may be difficult, especially in those with diabetes, obesity and connective tissue disorders.

patients with heart disease, indwelling pacemakers, and those taking cardiovascular drugs. Consequently, early consideration should be given to invasive monitoring. Initially, central venous pressure can be monitored, with trends being more informative than absolute values. However, even this may be misleading in those with significant pulmonary and heart disease. Ideally, a pulmonary artery catheter is required but this may not be easily achieved within the emergency department. Early consideration must therefore be given to moving such patients to a suitable environment, for example the intensive care unit.

Direct measurement of arterial blood pressure is informative and more accurate, particularly at extremes, than using non-invasive devices. It is also relatively easy to perform. The waveform that can be displayed gives an indication of the systemic vascular resistance and myocardial contractility. *A large artery, for example the femoral, is preferable for this purpose to the radial or dorsalis pedis,* but the groin must always be examined for signs of previous vascular surgery. The presence of an arterial cannula will also allow frequent sampling of arterial blood without the need for repeated aterial puncture.

The urinary bladder should be catheterised to measure urine output, and a strict aseptic technique must be ensured. Aging is usually associated with loss of renal cortical structures, a fall in the glomerular filtration rate, and decline in renal function by about 1 ml/min for each year after the age of 40 years. These changes make old people particularly vulnerable to incompetent fluid and metabolic management.

Cardiac dysrhythmias and conduction abnormalities are common, even in apparently healthy old people. Adequate oxygenation should be ensured and cardiac contusions excluded before they are discounted.

Dysfunction of the central nervous system

Most confused, ill, old people are not demented. Confusion can be a feature of almost any illness in the aged—particularly infection, fluid and metabolic derangements, head injury, and as a result of medications or their withdrawal. In addition, multiple sensory impairments may lead to disorientation and inappropriate responses and make assessment difficult.

Initial treatment is to ensure adequate cerebral perfusion with oxygenated blood, rather than to assume that confusion is the patient's normal mental state. In unconscious elderly patients, consider intracerebral haemorrhage as both the cause and effect of coexisting trauma.

Exposure

Patients must be completely undressed to ensure that all injuries are identified. It is, however, important to prevent the development or worsening of hypothermia. As soon as the examination is completed, the patient should be wrapped in blankets. Core temperature must be monitored rather than simply feeling the patient's peripheries to estimate body temperature. Infrared tympanic membrane thermometers are now widely available, but in the elderly patient it is important to ensure that the external auditory meatus is not occluded with wax.

Analgesia

Elderly people must not be denied adequate pain relief after trauma. Morphine is safe and effective provided that it is titrated in small doses (0.5–1.0 mg) intravenously. Intramuscular injections must be avoided as they are painful and absorption is unpredictable. Pethidine, buprenorphine (Temgesic) and non-steroidal anti-inflammatory drugs are less well tolerated and are

ECG abnormalities in apparently healthy old people
- Atrial ectopics
- Ventricular ectopics
- Atrial fibrillation
- Left anterior hemiblock
- First degree heart block

Direct measurement of arterial blood pressure is informative and more accurate than using non-invasive devices. It is also relatively easy to perform

Confusion is a common symptom in acutely ill old people. In its evaluation, consider withdrawal of psychotropic drugs (particularly benzodiazepines) and alcohol

Core temperature must be monitored rather than simply feeling the patent's peripheries to estimate body temperature

Elderly people must not be denied adequate pain relief after trauma

best avoided. If anti-emetics are adminstered the dose should be reduced accordingly to avoid unwanted extrapyramidal side-effects.

Local anaesthetic techniques are often ignored but are effective when used to supplement systemic analgesics. A femoral nerve block is easily performed and useful in patients with fractures of the neck or shaft of the femur. Intercostal nerve blocks may provide relief from the pain of fractured ribs, particularly for patients who have to be transported around the hospital. An axillary nerve block can be used for forearm fractures, but is usually best delayed until after a comprehensive assessment of neurological function.

> **Local anaesthetic techniques**
> - A femoral nerve block is useful in patients with fractures of the neck or shaft of the femur
> - Intercostal nerve blocks may relieve the pain from fractured ribs
> - An axillary nerve block can be used for forearm fractures, after asessment of neurological function

Secondary survey

Injuries arise from the transfer of energy at rates and in amounts that exceed the tolerance of tissues. In old people, particularly old women, bone strength may be appreciably reduced and fractures may occur after only modest transfers of energy. Age-related changes in other organs and tissues make them particularly vulnerable to injury, so a head-to-toe examination must be undertaken after even apparently minor injuries. This will also ensure the detection of coincident medical problems and the institution of appropriate treatment.

During physical examination care should be taken to maintain the usual anatomical position for the particular patient. It is particularly important to avoid producing traction and compression neuropathies (especially in the operating room) that may compromise rehabilitation. Extreme vigilance must be exercised during "log rolling", particularly if the patient is unconscious. The age-related changes described above make such patients vulnerable to iatrogenic damage to the cervical cord or nerve roots.

Consideration must also be given to the prevention of decubitus ulcers. Appropriate pressure-dispersing surfaces should be readily available and all patients with multiple injuries must be considered to be at high risk. Consequently, prevention must begin in the emergency department. Initial x ray examinations should include the standard three films of the cervical spine, chest and pelvis. Coexisting medical illness and disease of bone and joints may make interpretation difficult, and the advice of more experienced colleagues should be sought early.

> **Nerves at particular risk from compression or traction**
> - Axillary nerve
> - Radial nerve (in the spiral groove)
> - Common peroneal nerve

Head injuries

As the brain ages, its dura becomes tightly adherent to the skull, which makes epidural haematomas uncommon. A progressive loss of brain volume leads to an increase in the space around the brain that is thought to protect it from contusions, but makes subdural haematomas more likely.

Even mild head injuries, particularly in patients with pre-existing cognitive impairment, may lead to permanent neurological damage. If there is a skull fracture and an associated hemiparesis, a traumatic intracranial haematoma should be assumed and not a stroke. Similarly, confusion lasting more than 12 hours after head injury, even in a patient with no skull fracture, is an indication for computed tomography (CT). Any deterioration demands immediate action. A CT scan should be obtained in all patients who are unconsciousness for more than 5 minutes after head injury.

The outcome is extremely poor in elderly patients who have sustained head injuries sufficient to cause immediate coma that persists after correction of hypoxia and hypovolaemia. Neurosurgical intervention is not warranted for most of these patients.

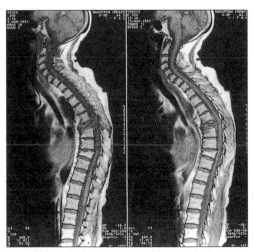

Magnetic resonance scan showing osteoporotic spine with collapse of T6 and T9.

Chest trauma

Rib fractures often complicate even mild blunt trauma to the chest in old people. Such fractures heal slowly and are often poorly tolerated. These patients must be watched carefully and the need for mechanical ventilation frequently reassessed. Those with more severe blunt chest trauma, such as those with penetrating injuries, are managed in the same way as younger patients.

Abdominal trauma

The principles of care for elderly patients with abdominal trauma follow those already outlined in chapter 9, but it must be remembered that old people are intolerant of shock and unnecessary laparotomy. Their assessment therefore demands a sense of urgency and a high degree of clinical acumen.

Those who have a history or clinical evidence of previous major abdominal surgery should have a CT or ultrasound scan of the abdomen rather than diagnostic peritoneal lavage.

Fractures

In old people with multiple injuries, fractures must be stabilised to permit optimal positioning and movement, both for immediate management and later rehabilitation. While isolated fractures of the humeral shaft are managed conservatively, there is no logic to such management in a patient with leg injuries who will need to use a walking frame or crutches for mobilisation. The aim of treatment should be to undertake the least invasive, most definitive, procedure with a view to early mobilisation as soon as other problems permit. Prolonged inactivity and disuse may seriously limit the eventual functional outcome.

AMPLE

A detailed history is particularly important and no source of information should be overlooked. The ambulance personnel will be able to give details of the immediate event and, when it occurred in the patient's home, may have brought medications with them. One member of the team should try to obtain hospital records and contact the general practitioner to find out about illnesses and medicines that may influence future management (see chapter 13). Sometimes the patient may be able to give information directly while those with diabetes, on anticoagulants, or on steroid hormones, may be carrying a medication card.

Communicating with deaf patients may be particularly difficult. Check that any hearing aid is working and switched on. Shouting tends to use high frequency sounds and may be counterproductive in patients with presbyacusis. The voice should be lowered and the patient, wearing spectacles if needed, should be in a position to watch the speaker's lips. Significant confusion can usually be assessed by checking that the patient knows where they are, what day it is and why they

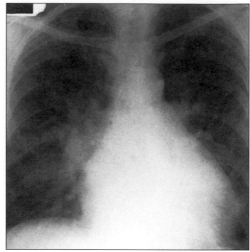

Cardiomegaly.

AMPLE history

Allergies

Medication

Past medical history

Last meal

Events leading to the injury

were brought to hospital. However, remember that even people who are not confused may not be able to cooperate because of pain and anxiety.

Conclusion

Elderly patients have a particularly high mortality rate and are extremely vulnerable to less than optimal management. A system of trauma care must be prepared to cope with this group of patients and their special needs. The trauma team must be aware of the anatomical and physiological changes that accompany aging and how these factors, together with the effects of coexisting illnesses and medications, make special demands on their skills. Oversights and thoughtlessness in initial management of patients may have serious adverse consequences on recovery and eventual hospital discharge.

Elderly patients should be informed of what is happening and, where possible, be encouraged to participate in treatment decisions. Not all old people are demented. This does not mean they should necessarily receive identical treatment to younger people; instead, they must be managed in a way that is appropriate to their needs in the light of the likely outcome.

21 Prehospital care

Carl L Gwinnutt, Alastair W Wilson

The principles of resuscitation are the same in the prehospital phase as in hospital, but the clinician faces greater impediments to success. Prehospital care may have been started by bystanders with a variable knowledge of first aid and continued by basic ambulance service personnel or paramedics, each of whom has a range of clinical skills and experience. Whatever the level of skills of those involved, the public will have great faith in the abilities of members of the emergency services. The hostility of the environment and the stress of working in unfamiliar surroundings, often with inquisitive and intrusive onlookers, should not be underestimated.

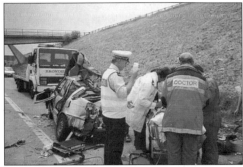
Scene of a road traffic accident.

Arrival at the scene

Safety
All accident sites are dangerous. At road traffic accidents for example, passing drivers may be distracted, causing secondary accidents by shunting cars in front; they may take a short cut via the hard shoulder, thereby endangering the rescuers. Training, appropriate clothing, correct equipment and common sense are therefore required by helpers at accident sites.

Personal safety begins with immunisation against tetanus and hepatitis. On arrival at the incident, if the emergency services are present, report to the most senior ambulance officer who will tell you about the type of incident, whether the scene has been declared safe by the police and fire services and how you can best help. You will be prevented from approaching the scene if you are inappropriately dressed or the environment is unsafe. Protective, high visibility clothing is therefore essential and should conform with the guidelines issued by the NHS Executive in HSG(94)52. Furthermore, when moving about accident sites, beware of jagged metal edges, glass, extrication equipment, rubble, and blood. Constant vigilance is required so that the risk of fire, electricity, sudden movement of heavy objects or cables snapping under tension, may be anticipated.

Reading the scene
A review of the accident scene, with analysis of the cause and nature of the incident, will give valuable clues to the type of injuries the victims may have sustained. This overview includes the number and type of vehicles involved, speed and direction of impact and whether a vehicle has rolled over. At a road traffic accident an inspection of the interior of the vehicles—to see the degree of intrusion, position of occupants and use of seatbelts—is also necessary. Although mechanism of injury is only 25% specific for serious injury, it should be part of the report that is given to the hospital with the patient. Polaroid photography of the scene greatly helps in providing this information.

The three tiers of safety
- Yourself
- The scene
- The patients

Minimum clothing requirements
- Warm underclothing
- High visibility jacket
  - —yellow and green
  - —fabric performance to BS 6629 (1985)
  - —appropriate identification; back and front, green on white, reflective
- Hard hat
  - appropriate material
  - —green on white identification
  - —polycarbonate visor
- Water and oil resistant footwear
- Latex gloves, for patient contact
- Heavy duty gloves (Firecraft type) for protection
- Ear defenders

Primary survey and resuscitation

All personnel involved in prehospital care must be familiar with the equipment they use; it should be checked daily for completeness and function and to ensure familiarity. Resuscitation is conducted using the ABCDE principles, but the patient's injuries and response to resuscitation often preclude completion of the primary survey before transportation.

Airway and cervical spine control

Total familiarity and competence with a wide variety of airway skills is essential for all personnel involved in prehospital care. Reduced levels of consciousness with positional airway obstruction require urgent attention and are frequently complicated by vomiting and facial injuries. If the patient is unable to maintain an airway, one must be created and secured urgently. Where access is difficult, simple adjuncts may have to be used initially. Endotracheal intubation requires free access and the administration of hypnotic and muscle relaxant drugs ("rapid sequence induction"). This requires continuing experience with anaesthetic techniques. The doctor should also be competent at creating a surgical airway. The prehospital environment is not the place to be using any of these skills for the first time. Alternatives to intubation are the Combitube or laryngeal mask airway, which can often be inserted even if only the victim's mouth can be reached. Both devices help prevent aspiration. However, they should be used only if the victim is deeply unconscious, to avoid provoking vomiting and a consequent rise in intracranial pressure.

If spontaneous ventilation is adequate, high concentrations of oxygen are given using a reservoir mask. If breathing is inadequate it must be supported as described below. The cervical and axial spine should be protected initially by manual immobilisation, best achieved with help from emergency personnel. As a rigid collar provides only limited immobilisation, it needs to be augmented with head blocks on a backboard or scoop stretcher. Beware of taping the patient's head to the backboard without securing the torso. In these cases, any movement of the patient on the board can result in the neck twisting.

Breathing

Underlying injury is often diagnosed by using tactile and visual observations. Breathing rates of less than 9 breaths/minute are always abnormal, but in the upper range, rates over 25 breaths/minute should also give cause for concern. Tracheal position, symmetry of chest movement, pain or crepitus may be the only clues to underlying chest wall and lung injury. Changes in percussion note may not be audible but can be felt. Surrounding noise often makes breath sounds impossible to assess by auscultation.

Inadequate ventilation in a patient with a patent airway requires ventilatory support. Initially this may be achieved using a bag-valve-mask technique, preferably using a two-person technique to deliver 100% oxygen. Alternatives are to ventilate the patient via a Combitube or laryngeal mask airway. These can then be exchanged, if necessary, under more controlled circumstances for a tracheal tube.

If tension pneumothorax is clinically diagnosed it should be treated immediately by needle thoracocentesis or, if the expertise is available, thoracostomy. A simple pneumothorax is more difficult to diagnose but if present will require drainage if positive pressure ventilation is to be instituted (see chapter 4). A haemothorax should be drained only if extrication is prolonged and there is difficulty maintaining adequate oxygenation.

Indicators of significant injury requiring a trauma team response by the receiving hospital

- Penetrating injury to the chest, abdomen, head, neck, or groin
- Two or more proximal long bone fractures
- Burns covering >15% of body area or burns to the face or airway.
- Evidence of high energy impact
  —falls of ≥ 6m (≥20 ft)
  —crash speed of ≥32 km/h (≥20 mph)
  —inward deformity of the car of 0.6m (2ft)
  —rearward displacement of the front axle
  —intrusion of the passenger compartment of 38 cm (15 in) on the patient's side or 50 cm (20 in) on opposite side
  —ejection of the patient
  —rollover
  —death of a car occupant
  —pedestrian hit at ≥32 km/h (≥20 mph)
  —abnormal values for physiological variables

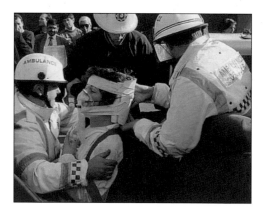

Cervical collar.

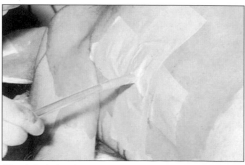

Chest drain in place.

Patients with severe head injuries (score 8 or less on the Glasgow coma scale) require early mechanical ventilation to ensure optimal oxygen delivery and avoidance of hypercarbia, cerebral vasodilation and the consequent rise in intracranial pressure (see chapter 6).

Pulse oximetry is a useful guide to oxygenation, but is often ineffective when the peripheral circulation is shut down. Remember, in the presence of a high inspired oxygen concentration, the oxygen saturation may be normal in spite of significantly reduced ventilation. Ideally, in all ventilated patients, the efficacy of ventilation should be monitored by measurement of end tidal carbon dioxide, using either an infrared analyser or a simple chemical indicator (see chapter 3).

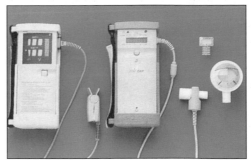
Pulse oximeter; infrared and chemical end tidal CO_2 analysers.

Circulation with haemorrhage control

If bleeding is visible and controllable, apply external pressure. If the patient is haemodynamically unstable and can be extricated rapidly and safely, do not waste time at the scene trying to insert large cannulae and infuse fluid. Rapid transfer for urgent surgical care is required and intravenous access can be attempted en route.

Where entrapment is prolonged, two large bore cannulae can be inserted, avoiding where possible veins lying over unsplinted joints or distal to fractures. Fluid resuscitation should aim at the restoration of a blood pressure that is compatible with stable clot formation and maintenance of cerebral perfusion.

Normotensive resuscitation encourages the administration of large fluid volumes, causing further bleeding, anaemia, a reduced oxygen delivery and a dilutional coagulopathy. Generally, a systolic blood pressure of 90–100 mm Hg is acceptable, although in a patient with a severe head injury, a higher pressure may be necessary to maintain brain perfusion. In prolonged entrapment, a blood sample, clearly marked, should be taken and sent ahead to the receiving hospital for cross matching.

All intravenous fluids given to patients should be warmed, particularly in winter or if the victim is already cold—for example, following a period of immersion. Heart rate, blood pressure and oxygen saturation must be monitored and recorded at regular intervals and the electrocardiogram displayed and recorded as necessary.

Fluid resuscitation should aim at the restoration of a blood pressure that is compatible with stable clot formation and maintenance of cerebral perfusion

Dysfunction

The Glasgow coma scale score and response of the pupils to light must be noted. If the patient is conscious, an assessment of spinal cord function can be made by asking the patient to move fingers and feet. If there is any doubt, assume that there is a spinal injury and immobilise the whole patient accordingly.

In the patient with a severe head injury who has had their airway secured and is being ventilated, the end tidal carbon dioxide concentration must be monitored, aiming for a value of 35 mm Hg (4.5 kPa). Extremes of hypocarbia must be avoided because of the risk of vasoconstriction causing cerebral hypoxia. Hypercarbia causes cerebral vasodilation, further elevating intracranial pressure

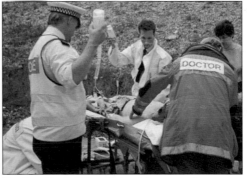
Road accident victim with two intravenous lines.

Exposure

Exposure and injury both cause patients to become hypothermic, particularly in wet and windy conditions or when they are trapped. Enough exposure is required to allow assessment and treatment of life threatening and debilitating injuries before extrication. Once this is achieved, the patient must be covered and kept warm and dry.

Protect emergency services personnel from medical "sharps"

Entrapment

Entrapment hinders resuscitation and the management of injuries. The fire service is responsible for extrication but it is important that there is close co-ordination of activity with the medical services to ensure the patient's safety. Doctors undertaking prehospital care must have an understanding of extrication techniques.

Throughout extrication ensure the ABCs are managed and protect endotracheal tubes, intravenous access and monitoring equipment. The patient must also be shielded from the effects of cutting equipment, broken glass, and impinging bodywork.

Adequate intravenous access is essential before the release of compressed limbs. Not only may this precipitate acute haemorrhage, but if a limb has been crushed and the circulation impaired for longer than 30–60 minutes, sudden restoration of the circulation may result in life-threatening hyperkalaemia and the release of myoglobin. These changes can result in a variety of deleterious effects, from sudden death to acute renal failure. Consequently, in these circumstances, the use of a high tourniquet or even amputation may be necessary before release of the damaged limb. Adequate fluid resuscitation will be mandatory to minimise damage to the vital organs in these patients.

In unconscious patients, or those in whom the mechanism of injury suggests spinal cord damage, adequate immobilisation is essential. Rigid collars (for example Stifneck, Vertebrace) help but only partially stabilise the cervical spine. A spinal immobilisation device—Kendrick Extraction Device (KED) or Russell Extraction Device (RED)—may improve immobilisation, but are slow to apply and difficult to remove. A careful manual extrication onto a long spine board may be safer and quicker. When the patient is trapped in a vehicle, the board can be placed behind the patient's back after the vehicle roof has been removed and the seat back lowered. The patient is then slid up the board in a controlled movement. Where rapid extrication is required, the patient can be rotated to sit across the seats and the board pushed under the buttocks. The patient is then lowered and slid up the board.

A spine board should be used for the shortest time possible to avoid the risk of pressure sores developing. These tend to occur where bony prominences meet the hard surface, typically at the occiput, scapulae, sacrum and heels. Remember, the spine has a number of natural curves and does not conform to the straight spine board, therefore the patient must be adequately padded. Care must also be taken to ensure that an unconscious patient is not left lying on hard objects within clothing, for example coins or keys in pockets. If a patient is likely to have to remain immobilised for any period of time, then this is best achieved using a vacuum mattress, which can be moulded around the patient, thereby distributing pressure more evenly.

Before the patient is moved, give a warning of what is about to happen. Ensure that intravenous lines remain secure and that the endotracheal tube is disconnected during extrication and reconnected again afterwards. If the patient is to be monitored properly, the doctor must not be involved with lifting.

Analgesia

Adequate analgesia is important in injured, trapped patients. Entonox (50% oxygen and 50% nitrous oxide) is useful for short procedures in spontaneously breathing patients. It has to be given without interruption, otherwise its analgesic action is lost. It must not be used in patients who are at risk of pneumothorax or if there is clinical evidence of a fractured base of skull. The application of traction splints to injured

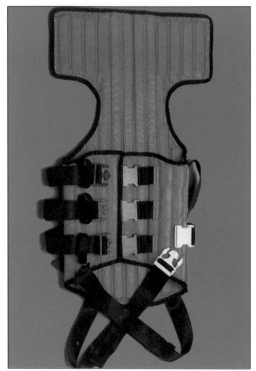
Kendrick extraction device.

A spine board should be used for the shortest time possible to avoid the risk of pressure sores developing

Anaesthesia is a useful prehospital technique, but should only be used by clinicians with appropriate training

limbs contributes significantly to reducing pain as well as reducing blood loss and the risk of neurovascular damage or fat emboli.

Opiates (morphine, or diamorphine) should be diluted and given intravenously, together with an anti-emetic, and the dose titrated against response. Contrary to popular belief, the use of opioids does not mask the development of either abdominal or intracranial pathology. Local anaesthetic techniques such as femoral nerve block for fractured femurs or intercostal blocks for fractured ribs, are of value, particularly if the patient faces a long journey to hospital.

Subanaesthetic or anaesthetic doses of ketamine will provide good analgesia to facilitate extrication. However, it should be preceded by a benzodiazepine to reduce the incidence of hallucinations during recovery, which may cause problems later, for example during transport to hospital.

Anaesthesia is commonly required to allow tracheal intubation in a patient who is not deeply unconscious or to prevent the rise in intracranial pressure in a patient with a head injury. The same techniques are used as in the hospital but particular attention must be paid to restoring circulating volume adequately before induction, because of the vasodilating and cardiac depressant effects of anaesthetics. For the same reasons, the dose and rate of administration will also have to be adjusted. Remember also that the use of muscle relaxants reduces the patients ability to splint fractures and that the axial skeleton is particularly at risk.

Records

Accurate written records of all procedures and response to treatment must be noted on a prehospital care chart. Vital signs, oximetry and capnography are best recorded automatically, to avoid an optimistic interpretation later. Drugs, dosages, route of administration and timing must also be noted. Injuries are recorded as they are identified in anatomical order. Ischaemic times and entrapment times are important.

Summary

With increasing frequency, accidents are being attended by medical practitioners who are trained in immediate care and experienced in prehospital resuscitation. Their aims are to treat the life threatening conditions using the same principles that are used in the hospital resuscitation room. They must also be able to recognise those patients who require rapid transfer to hospital for urgent surgical intervention, rather than delay at the road side simply to complete the primary survey. Transfer to hospital is not a therapeutic vacuum, and resuscitation and monitoring must be continued until responsibility is passed to the trauma team with a formal hand over.

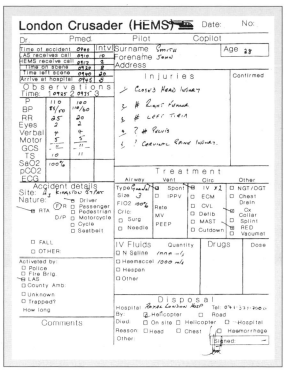

Record chart for the Helicopter Emergency Medical Service (HEMS).

Further reading

Bickell WH, Wall MJ, Pepe PE, Martin RR, Ginger VF, Allen MK, Mattox KL. Immediate versus delayed fluid resuscitation for hypotensive patients with penetrating torso injuries. *N Engl J Med* 1994; **331**: 1105–9.

Sampalis JS, Lavoie A, Williams JI, Mulder DS, Kalina M. Impact of on-site care, prehospital time, and level of inhospital care on survival in severely injured patients. *J Trauma* 1993; **34**: 252–61.

Podolsky S, Baraff LJ, Simon RR, Hoffman JR, Larman B, Ablon W. Efficacy of cervical spine immobilisation methods. *J Trauma* 1983; **23**: 461–5.

Criswell JC, Parr MJA, Nolan JP. Emergency airway management in patients with cervical spine injury. *Anaesthesia* 1994; **49**: 900–3.

Chestnut RM, Marshall LF, Klauber MR, Blunt BA, Baldwin N, Eisenberg MH, et al. The role of secondary brain injury in determining outcome from severe head injury. *J Trauma* 1993; **34**: 216–22.

22 Transfer of the trauma patient

Carl L Gwinnutt, Alastair W Wilson, Daniele C Bryden

The term primary transfer is used to indicate the movement of a patient from the scene of an incident to hospital. Secondary transfer refers to the movement of a patient between hospitals, usually for more specialised care such as neurosurgery or intensive care. Although the two types of transfer are very different, the fundamental principle "to do no further harm" should govern both.

Primary transfer

Primary transfer deals predominantly with prehospital emergencies. Timing, type of transport and destination are determined by the patient's injuries and their response to resuscitation. At the scene, time taken to secure the airway, institute effective ventilation, control external bleeding and splint the spine and limbs is time well spent. Such actions help to stabilise the patient before transportation by road or air ambulance to hospital. A "scene time" of 15 minutes is optimal to achieve hospital arrival times for definitive care well within the "golden hour". The "platinum 10 minutes", as used by the British Association of Immediate Care, is an even better target.

Failure to achieve haemodynamic stability at the scene, often because of uncontrollable bleeding, is an indication for transport by the fastest possible means. A doctor present at the accident scene can potentially undertake more interventions than a paramedic alone, but it is unnecessary to utilise every skill in an attempt to restore normal physiology. This is particularly true with uncontrollable bleeding, when a policy of extensive fluid replacement should be adopted. The greater interventional and diagnostic skills of a doctor should be employed to direct the patient to a hospital capable of dealing with the patient's injuries. This may not be the nearest hospital. There is considerable evidence to show that the selection of the right hospital at the beginning is extremely important for patient outcome.

Packaging and stabilisation

During any treatment, but particularly during primary transfer of the injured patient, all movement is potentially harmful. It encourages haemorrhage and worsens any cardiorespiratory instability. Movement of a fractured limb is painful and may result in neurovascular damage. Movement of the head, neck or thorax in the presence of injury to the vertebral column may cause or exacerbate injury to the spinal cord. Even in a fully immobilised patient, internal organs are at risk of further damage from forces of inertia when speeding ambulances brake, accelerate or corner. Significant secondary injury can also occur while stretchers are manhandled into and out of vehicles. From start to finish the journey should be as smooth as possible.

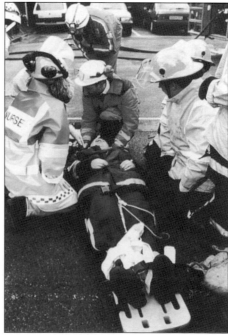

Patient immobilised on long spine board.

134

Managing the patient in the lateral position is inappropriate if a spinal injury has not been excluded. The whole spine must be protected. Consequently, most patients are placed in the supine position, usually on a long spine board or a Vacumat™ mattress, and loaded into the ambulance head first. This allows a patient to be tipped or turned if he or she starts to vomit, the risks of this can be reduced by inserting a nasogastric or orogastric tube. This is not a substitute for having suction immediately available for this emergency.

Patients with a known head injury should be positioned slightly head-up to help reduce intracranial pressure. This orientation can be difficult to maintain when entering or leaving an ambulance, but every effort must be made to ensure that they are not tipped head down. The greatest forces on the patient during transfer are those from deceleration under braking. Ideally the patient should travel in the ambulance feet first, because these forces will then be least damaging to the brain. This has practical implications, as equipment and the accompanying personnel are then concentrated at the rear of the vehicle.

Pregnant patients should be positioned in such a way as to displace the uterus to the left during transfer, to prevent supine hypotension syndrome (see chapter 18).

Confused, combative patients should only be transported once the cause of their state has been identified and treated, taking particular care to eliminate cerebral hypoxia. In head injured patients with a marked reduction in Glasgow coma score, controlled ventilation after anaesthesia with paralysis allows optimal oxygenation. Anaesthetic techniques should only be used by doctors familiar with in-hospital intubation and trained in the particular difficulties of applying these skills in the pre-hospital setting.

Any patient who is unconscious and tolerating an oropharyngeal airway, has airway burns, or has impending respiratory failure, should be intubated and ventilated before transportation. Remember, critically ill patients do badly if intubation has to be attempted during an ambulance journey. Therefore the airway should be secured before transfer.

The presence of a cervical spine injury is not a contraindication to intubation, but where difficulties are anticipated, remember the option of creating a surgical airway. Where these skills are not immediately available, the airway must be maintained using basic techniques, high flow oxygen administered and the patient transferred rapidly to hospital.

All intravenous cannulae must be secured. In the prehospital environment, they are often inserted in the antecubital fossa and an Armback splint will keep the arm straight and ensure the intravenous line continues to function. Although central venous access is seldom indicated at the scene of an accident, the external jugular vein is becoming increasingly used. All connections must be checked to prevent disconnection and the risk of lethal air embolism.

Limb splintage

The aim of splinting is to reduce blood loss, prevent soft tissue damage and provide pain relief. A variety of non-compromising traction splints are available that allow inspection of the limb and palpation of pulses. Conforming vacuum splints that can be moulded around limbs are helpful. Whole body splinting can, to some extent be achieved with the semirigid Vacumat. The Pneumatic Anti-Shock Garment (PASG) has been shown to be of little use for controlling haemorrhage, but may help to stabilise an unstable pelvic fracture. Its use remains controversial in seriously ill patients. When applied correctly it is almost impossible to examine the abdomen or do a diagnostic peritoneal lavage in the emergency room.

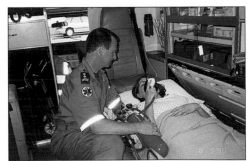
Interior of land ambulance.

Position patients with a known head injury slightly head-up to help reduce intracranial pressure

Position pregnant patients in such a way as to displace the uterus to the left during transfer, to prevent supine hypotension syndrome

Any patient who is unconscious and tolerating an oropharyngeal airway, has airway burns, or has impending respiratory failure, should be intubated and ventilated before transportation

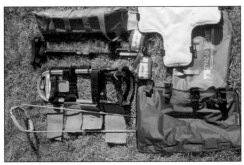
Variety of limb splints.

Transportation

The transport phase must not be regarded as a therapeutic vacuum. One of the most important tasks of the medical attendant during transportation is the continued assessment and monitoring of the patient to allow the detection and treatment of problems that develop with the patient or equipment.

On the way into hospital from the scene of an accident, monitoring is most commonly achieved using non-invasive devices to supplement clinical observation. Monitoring of respiratory rate, pulse oximetry, heart rate, blood pressure and electrocardiogram should be regarded as standard. The level of consciousness in the unsedated patient must be assessed regularly. If the patient is intubated and ventilated, end tidal carbon dioxide and airway pressures must also be monitored.

Ideally the patient should be positioned with the head next to the attendant's seat with enough room to gain access to the airway, to allow suction of the tracheal tube or, in an emergency, to perform intubation. It should be possible to identify and relieve a tension pneumothorax in a ventilated patient. Intravenous lines should be checked regularly and replaced when necessary. If there is cardiac arrest, cardiopulmonary resuscitation is almost impossible for a single operator. Two attendants allow effective therapeutic intervention.

> One of the most important tasks of the medical attendant during transportation is the continued assessment and monitoring of the patient

> The level of consciousness in the unsedated patient must be assessed regularly

Secondary transfer

Ideally, no patient should undergo secondary transfer. However, transfers do occur for specialised surgical care and investigations or for intensive care facilities. As all patients undergoing secondary transfer have had the benefit of medical intervention within hospital, there is no place for the transfer of an unstable patient. Treatment in the back of a moving ambulance is exceedingly difficult; therefore it is essential that the patient has been fully assessed, injuries treated and haemodynamic stability established before movement. Any intervention that may be required en route should be performed before departure. The decision to transfer a patient to another hospital must be made by senior medical personnel on the basis that the benefits to the patient outweigh any potential risks of the transfer.

The aim during secondary transfer is to provide the patient with the same standard of care that they would receive in an intensive care environment.

Before undertaking secondary transfer, it may be possible to rule out injury to the spine. If not, the patient should be fully immobilised using a long spine board, adequately padded with a semi-rigid collar and head blocks, or a vacuum mattress. Ventilation and gas exchange are optimised as demonstrated by arterial blood gas analysis. Heart rate, blood pressure, urine output and if available central venous pressure or pulmonary artery pressure are monitored to ensure cardiovascular stability. Inotropic support begun before departure will almost certainly have to be continued throughout the transfer. Despite the best preparations, the critically ill patient will be susceptible to the accelerative forces exerted during transportation, particularly at high speed, which can cause hypertension, arrhythmias and hypoxia. Aim to move these patients at normal road speed to minimise complications.

Patients who have been intubated will require controlled ventilation with an increased inspired oxygen concentration. Manual ventilation requires high flow oxygen at 12–15 litres/minute. If a portable mechanical ventilator is used, cylinder oxygen supplying the patient may also be used to power the ventilator. Consequently, small cylinders empty quickly. A size D oxygen cylinder will last approximately 20 minutes

Reasons for secondary transfers
- Specialised surgical care
    —neurosurgery
    —plastic or burns surgery
    —cardiac surgery
    —spinal surgery
    —paediatric surgery
- Specialised investigations
    —computed tomography (CT)
    —magnetic resonance imaging (MRI)
- Intensive care facilities
    —specialised organ support
    —lack of beds locally

> The aim during secondary transfer is to provide patients with the same standard of care that they would receive in an intensive care environment

during manual ventilation and 40 minutes during mechanical ventilation. Adequate reserves must be available. A disconnect alarm, such as the alarmPAC (pneuPAC) is an essential safety device. Humidification, using a HME device, should be provided on long journeys to reduce the risk of secretions blocking the tracheal tube. Patients with a needle thoracocentesis in situ or a simple pneumothorax or haemothorax, should have a large bore chest drain inserted and connected to a (non-fluid) drainage system before transport. Chest drains must never be clamped.

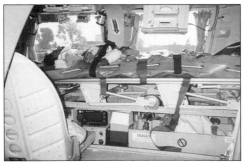

Interior of medical helicopter.

Pain control

Pain should be controlled with intravenous analgesics. Fractures should be immobilised in hospital before transfer, by applying external fixators or appropriate splintage. Where there is a fracture of the pelvis causing continuing bleeding, the application of an Exfix or C clamp will significantly reduce blood loss and make transfer of the patient much safer.

Once secondary transfer of a patient has been deemed necessary and the destination determined, arrangements should be made between the senior medical staff responsible for initiating and receiving the transfer.

Personnel and monitoring

The referring doctor is responsible for ensuring that the patient is stable and any treatment or investigations requested by the specialist have been performed.

Accompanying personnel must be adequate in number as well as skill and experience. Ideally there should be two attendants: one a doctor trained in intensive care and transportation with the skills to carry out resuscitation, ventilation and organ support, and the other a healthcare professional trained in intensive care procedures and familiar with the transfer equipment.

The referring doctor must fully brief the attendants and confirm that they have the patient's records (or a copy), with the results of all investigations, x rays and computed tomography scans, and any cross-matched blood that is available. Where possible, communication should be maintained between the transfer team and the receiving hospital: a mobile phone is recommended. Be clear about the destination in the receiving hospital. If the hospital is unfamiliar territory, arrange to have someone meet the ambulance at the hospital entrance or for the local ambulance service to act as guides. The final duty of the referring doctor is to ensure that the receiving hospital is aware of the estimated time of arrival, so that arrangements can be made to receive the patient.

Invasive monitoring of blood pressure is essential, and central venous pressure and urinary output are often monitored during secondary transfer. When indicated, intracranial pressure monitoring may be required. Hypothermia is a common complication of transfers and is easier to prevent than treat. All patients should have their temperature monitored, irrespective of how short the planned journey. In the intubated, ventilated patient, the adequacy of sedation, analgesia and muscle relaxation must be assessed regularly. The nasogastric or orogastric tube should be suctioned regularly.

Supplies

Provision should be made for all requirements during transfer, including adequate amounts of intravenous fluid, blood, supplementary drugs, oxygen and equipment for re-intubation and replacement of intravenous cannulae. Where drugs are administered by infusion pump, the rate, syringe volume and battery status should be checked regularly. Always take spares.

Equipment carried on medical helicopters

- Non-invasive blood pressure monitor
- Electrocardiograph and heart rate monitor
- Invasive blood pressure monitors
- Temperature monitors
- Pulse oximeter and pulse rate monitor
- Capnograph
- Defibrillator
- Syringe drivers and infusions pumps
- Ventilators
- Suction

Indications for helicopter transport

Primary transfer
- Need for specialist trauma centre care
- Long distances
- Obstruction to land transport by traffic
- Obscure or inaccessible accident sites
- Transportation of medical staff or equipment to accident scene

Secondary transfer
- Transfer for specialised surgery
- Long distances
- Transfer for intensive care

Contraindications

- Poor weather
- Difficulty in landing because of obstruction or poor lighting
- Patient's injuries do not warrant care in specialised unit
- Patient is violent or has psychiatric problems
- The incident is close to the hospital most appropriate for the patient's needs

Documentation during transfer

Adequate documentation is essential to provide the receiving hospital with a record of events during the journey. Ensure that all physiological parameters and significant events are recorded along with any drugs and fluids administered. This can be difficult to achieve in a moving ambulance but many modern monitors store the relevant data and allow subsequent retrieval. Prepared sheets are also useful, because they act as an aide memoire and allow subsequent audit.

Land ambulances

A compromise between speed and safety is required. The speed of an ambulance flashing a blue light is only marginally faster than its routine speed. Two tone sirens terrify patients, as well as passing motorists. Attempting to maintain a high speed in traffic may simply result in great acceleration and deceleration forces. These cause significant cardiovascular and respiratory disturbances in the patient and motion sickness in the attending personnel. Vertical forces from unevenness in road surfaces can be minimised by the use of a "floating" stretcher, but some conscious patients find this very nauseating. Space is at a premium in an ambulance, with few facilities for extra equipment. Care must be taken to secure all equipment, particularly oxygen cylinders. Everything must be within reach of the attendants, so that they do not have to remove their seatbelts and move around during the journey.

Most ambulances are inherently cold, but carry heating devices: one may simply need to ask for the heating to be switched on! Emphasis is placed on preventing heat loss by warming all intravenous fluids, using a heat and moisture exchanger (HME) on breathing circuits and minimising exposure of the patient.

Air ambulance

The designated medical helicopter is the most expensive part of the transfer armamentarium and should be used with care. The crew should be trained to the highest possible level and must act as the extended arm of the hospital. A helicopter can be used for both primary and secondary transfers, over long and short distances and therefore must be capable of allowing all monitoring facilities to be available during flight.

Helicopters that are not specifically designed for medical transportation (police or military aircraft) may have only minimal "carry-on" medical equipment. The use of monitoring and defibrillation equipment can interfere with aircraft avionics and only that which has been tested and found compatible should be used. Some helicopters are cramped, making management of the patient difficult.

Anticipating potential problems is even more important than during land transport and potential problems are best solved before lift off. Ensure that all the necessary equipment, and space to cope with emergencies, are available during flight.

Helicopters are noisy, making communication difficult and use of a stethoscope impossible. Headphones should be put on the patient's head to allow reassuring conversation. The patient must be kept warm and comfortable during the flight. If a long journey is expected an anti-emetic may be given to prevent air sickness and the stomach kept empty by gastric aspiration.

Communication and handover

Once the patient's transfer to hospital is underway, staff in the receiving hospital must be informed of the patient's impending arrival and condition by the ambulance staff or the accompanying medical attendant. In the light of this information, staff in the emergency department can prepare the resuscitation room and call the trauma team (see chapter 1).

Essential information given en route to the receiving hospital

- The number of patients
- Age and sex of the patients
- Mechanism of injury
- Vital signs at the scene
- Initial findings on assessment
- Procedures at scene
- Response to treatment given
- Estimated time of arrival

On leaving, collect all equipment

On arrival, details of the accident, the patient's initial condition, treatment given and response must be communicated to the designated member of staff. Of particular importance are details of any problems during transportation, along with any changes in vital signs in response to resuscitation. A structured handover should take place after all transfers, with a resume of the patient's history, investigations, results and treatment. All documentation should be handed over and equipment retrieved before leaving.

Summary

The underlying principle of any transfer is to do no further harm. Patient transfer from the scene of an accident to hospital must be accomplished with the minimum of delay and with resuscitation ongoing during transportation if necessary. Patients being transferred from a primary receiving centre to another hospital must be thoroughly resuscitated and stabilised before departure. The decision to transfer must be made by senior medical staff at both ends of the journey. The patient should be accompanied by staff trained and experienced in transferring critically ill patients. The aim should be to provide a level of care they would otherwise receive in the intensive care unit.

Further reading

Guidelines Committee of the American College of Critical Care Medicine; Society of Critical Care Medicine and American Association of Critical-Care Nurses Transfer Guidelines Taskforce. Guidelines for the transfer of critically ill patients. *Crit Care Med* 1993; **21**: 931–7.

Intensive Care Society. *Guidelines for transport of the critically ill adult.* London: Intensive Care Society, 1997.

The Neuroanaesthesia Society of Great Britain and Ireland and The Association of Anaesthetists of Great Britain and Ireland. *Recommendations for the transfer of patients with acute head injuries to neurosurgical units.* London: The Association of Anaesthetists of Great Britain and Ireland, 1996.

Morton NS, Pollack MM, Wallace PGM, eds. *Stabilisation and transport of the critically ill.* London: Churchill Livingstone, 1997.

Nicholl J, Hughes S, Dixon S, Yates D. *The costs and benefits of paramedic skills in pre-hospital trauma care.* London: Health Technology Assessment, 1998.

23 Management of severe burns

Colin Robertson, Oliver Fenton

At the scene of a fire, first aid procedures are often life saving. We begin this chapter with instructions for medical staff on preparing a victim for evacuation to a burns unit.

Evacuation from the scene

Under the direction of the fire service, and ensuring the safety of the rescuers, the patient should be removed from the scene of injury to a place of safety and fresh air.

Flames and heat track upwards, so keep the patient supine and rolled or covered with a heavy blanket, coat, or rug to extinguish any residual flames. Take care not to get burnt yourself, especially if dealing with petrol burns or self immolation.

If the clothing is still smouldering or hot, apply large amounts of cold water. Clothing saturated with boiling liquids or steam should be removed rapidly, but do not remove burnt clothing that is adherent to the skin. Cover burnt areas with clean (sterile if available) towels or sheets and ensure that the patient is kept warm. **Do not apply wet soaks or ice packs or use them during transit**, because this will not provide any pain relief for patients with full thickness burns and can cause profound hypothermia, especially in children.

Evacuate the patient to the receiving hospital as quickly as possible. In patients with severe burns, or those who have been exposed to smoke or fumes, high flow oxygen through a facemask should be given during transit. Alert the receiving emergency department by radio or telephone. Advise them of the number and ages of the patients, the severity of their burns, and the estimated time of arrival.

Reception and resuscitation

The primary assessment, investigation, and treatment of a patient with severe burns should be a continuous and integrated process rather than a stepwise progression. While assessment is being performed a member of staff must obtain the necessary information about the incident from the ambulance crew and other emergency services. This should then be conveyed to the senior doctor in charge of the patient.

Management of the airway
Rapidly examine the patient for clinical evidence of smoke inhalation and thermal injury to the respiratory tract (see box). In patients with one or more of the features described, respiratory obstruction from pharyngeal or laryngeal oedema may develop rapidly. Patients exposed to steam or hot vapours are at particular risk of damage to the upper airways. Stridor, difficulty in swallowing, and drooling of saliva are signs of

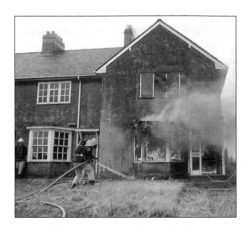

Necessary information about the incident

- Its nature (house fire, blast, release of steam or hot gas, etc)
- If possible, the nature of burning materials (furniture, polyurethane foam, polyvinyl chloride, etc)
- Was there any explosion?
- Was the patient in an enclosed space?
- For how long was the patient exposed to smoke or fire?
- The time elapsed from burn/injury/smoke inhalation to arrival in hospital

Clinical features indicating smoke or thermal injury to respiratory tract

- Altered consciousness
- Direct burns to face or oropharynx
- Hoarseness, stridor
- Soot in nostrils or sputum
- Expiratory rhonchi
- Dysphagia
- Dribbling, drooling of saliva

epiglottic swelling. In such patients examination and early endotracheal intubation performed by an experienced doctor with anaesthetic training is essential. Mucosal swelling of the oropharynx and epiglottis can be extremely rapid, and delay can render tracheostomy necessary.

If complete respiratory obstruction has already occurred or intubation unsuccessful, or both, immediate cricothyrotomy or "mini" tracheostomy is required, then formal tracheostomy. It should be emphasised, however, that in patients with severe burns the tracheostomy site is an important site of infection.

All patients suspected of having thermal or smoke injury to the respiratory tract should be given humidified high flow oxygen—an inspired oxygen concentration (FiO_2) of at least 40–60%—through a facemask. If bronchospasm is present give the patient a β_2 agonist (such as salbutamol or terbutaline) with an oxygen powered nebuliser.

Frequent repeated clinical assessment of the airway and ventilation is mandatory in patients with all types of injuries caused by fire, with further measurements of arterial blood gas tensions, carboxyhaemoglobin and, if the patient can comply, peak expiratory flow. Note that values for oxygen saturation measured by pulse oximetry may be erroneous in the presence of carboxyhaemoglobin.

Intravenous access

Establishing adequate intravenous access must not be delayed. Insert and secure one or more large bore (needle gauge 14–16) intravenous cannulas. If possible use 10–15 cm cannulas to reduce the risk of dislodgement. The normal and easiest sites for percutaneous insertion of intravenous cannulas are the forearms and antecubital fossae. Narrow bore cannulas inserted into small veins on the back of the hands are of little practical value. Occasionally, alternative sites such as the external jugular and femoral veins or the long saphenous vein at the ankle must be used, although the saphenous vein is prone to early occlusion.

Intravenous cutdown in the cubital fossa or on the long saphenous vein in the groin may be required if percutaneous intravenous access cannot be performed. This approach can be made through burnt skin, but do not attempt to suture the resulting gaping wound. If possible, before attaching the tubing of the intravenous drip take enough blood through the cannula for crossmatching and determining blood group, packed cell volume, and urea and electrolyte concentrations.

Intravenous fluid requirements

For rapid assessment the "rule of nine" is useful. Do not include areas of simple erythema in the estimate. The size of small burns can be judged roughly by considering the palmar surface of the patient's closed hand as about 1% of the total body surface area. Use your own hand to map out the burnt area, and then make allowances for the size of your hand compared with the patient's—for example, it would be three times the size of a 1 year old child's and twice the size of a 5 year old child's. The result can be cross checked by mapping the size of the unburnt area. In patients with very large burns it is simpler to measure the unburnt area and then subtract from 100.

Start treatment with intravenous fluids; the first 500 ml should be 0.9% saline. If colloid is then used—for example, 5% albumin, gelatin, or dextran solutions—the volume of fluid required for intravenous replacement treatment for the first 4 hours since injury should be judged roughly as the percentage of the body surface area of the burn multiplied by the body weight (kg) divided by two.

Patients with full thickness burns that cover more than 10% of the body surface area may need a transfusion of red blood cells in addition to fluid replacement. A blood transfusion is

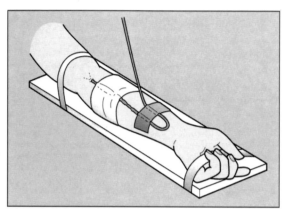

Intravenous cannulation.

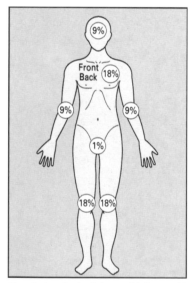

The "rule of nine" is useful for rapid assessment of the body surface area affected by burns.

Fluid replacement: example of calculation

Weight of patient who has sustained a burn = 70 kg

Body surface area covered = 35%

Volume of colloid required in first 4 h after injury = $(35 \times 70)/2$

= 1225 ml

given in place of the colloid requirement for that period. In major burns the blood is given during the resuscitation period; in smaller burns it can be given at the end of resuscitation.

Insert a urinary catheter and start hourly measurements of urine volume. Note the colour and consistency of the initial urine in patients with severe flame or high voltage electrical burns. The urine may be a treacly black, indicating haemoglobinuria or myoglobinuria, or both. This is of prognostic importance for subsequent renal function.

In elderly patients, patients with cardiorespiratory disease, and patients who have delayed presentation consider inserting a central venous pressure line if you are experienced in the technique. This can play an important part in subsequent restoration of volume in a patient with a severe burn. The risks of infection related to a central line are small in the early stages. With current methods of line management these risks are outweighed by the importance of the line for monitoring and access.

The rate of intravenous fluid replacement should be tailored by the above guideline and the clinical response of the patient in terms of haemodynamic variables and urine output. The aim in adults is to achieve a urine output of 0.5–1.0 ml/kg/hour.

Analgesia and reassurance

Severe burns cause both pain and distress. Analgesia and reassurance should be given as soon as possible. Treatment for pain in patients with severe burns must be tailored to the patient's individual requirements. Full thickness burns, if present, are pain free, but all patients will be frightened and distressed, and constant reassurance and communication are vital.

A mixture of 50% nitrous oxide and 50% oxygen (Entonox) given by an on-demand system with a tight fitting facemask can provide simple and effective analgesia, particularly before arrival in hospital. Subsequently, if required, an opioid such as Cyclimorph (cyclizine and morphine) should be given intravenously in aliquots of 1 mg at a dose carefully titrated to the clinical response.

Reassessment

The airway

Confirm that the patient's airway is secure and that ventilation is adequate. Repeat the measurements of arterial blood gas tensions and the analysis of carboxyhaemoglobin concentrations, which give an approximate guide to the amount of smoke inhaled; concentrations at the time of exposure can be predicted by using the nomogram. For example, if the carboxyhaemoglobin concentration is 30% at 1 hour after exposure the concentration at exposure would have been about 37%.

Clinical features of carbon monoxide poisoning correlate only moderately well with carboxyhaemoglobin concentrations but alteration of the conscious state should be regarded with suspicion. The so called "classic" feature of cherry red mucous membranes is a rarely seen, totally unreliable clinical sign.

Treatment with hyperbaric oxygen may be indicated in patients with carboxyhaemoglobinaemia, particularly if they are or have been unconscious, have cardiac or neurological symptoms, or are pregnant. Early consultation with local hyperbaric specialists is recommended.

Other toxic gases, such as hydrogen cyanide, hydrogen sulphide, and hydrogen chloride, are often produced in fires. They may cause local irritation to both upper and lower airways as well as acting systemically as direct cellular poisons. Few laboratories can provide cyanide concentrations in an emergency, but a severe metabolic acidosis, high lactate concentration, and an increased anion gap suggest cyanide

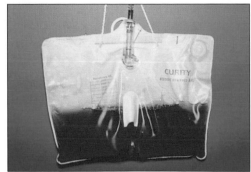

Urine from a patient with electrical burns that indicates haemoglobinuria.

Pain relief in patients with severe burns
- *Entonox*—for conscious, cooperative patients, especially in the prehospital phase
- *Opioids*—give intravenously in small aliquots titrated to the patient's clinical response

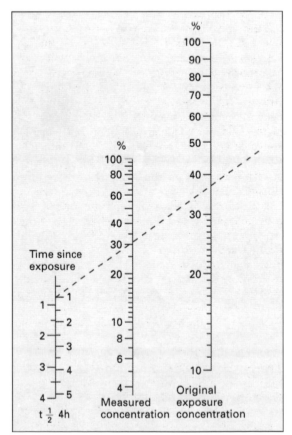

Nomogram for calculating carboxyhaemoglobin concentration at time of exposure.
Time since exposure is given in two scales to allow for the effects of previous oxygen administration on the half life of carboxyhaemoglobin (left scale assumes a half life of 3 h).

poisoning if there is an appropriate history of exposure. In these patients emergency resuscitation with assisted ventilation is required, and the use of cyanide antidotes—such as sodium thiosulphate with amyl nitrite (for enhanced distribution), and dicobalt edetate—should be considered. Ensure that deep circumferential burns of the thorax are not causing restriction in chest expansion and hence ventilation (see below).

Treatment with fluids

The rule of nine, used in the rapid assessment of burn injury, can result in overestimation of the extent of the burn. More accurate assessment can be made with Lund and Browder charts and the rate of fluid replacement adjusted accordingly.

Formulas for intravenous fluid requirements are only rough guides and need modification according to the patient's clinical state. Regular checks and recording of heart rate, blood pressure, central venous pressure (if indicated), urine output, packed cell volume and peripheral perfusion and the trends in these values provide additional guidance for adjusting the rate of infusion. Fluid replacement should not be limited in patients with burns and inhalation injury. Indeed, increased fluids are often needed to maintain the systemic circulation and optimise cardiac and renal function.

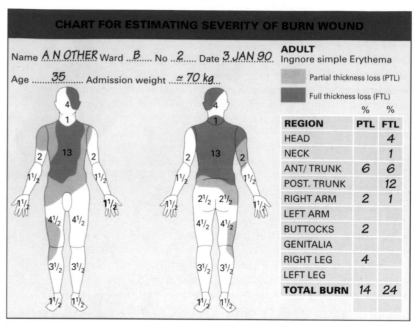

Lund and Browder chart.

REGION	PTL %	FTL %
HEAD		4
NECK		1
ANT/ TRUNK	6	6
POST. TRUNK		12
RIGHT ARM	2	1
LEFT ARM		
BUTTOCKS	2	
GENITALIA		
RIGHT LEG	4	
LEFT LEG		
TOTAL BURN	14	24

CHART FOR ESTIMATING SEVERITY OF BURN WOUND
Name A N OTHER Ward B No 2 Date 3 JAN 90
ADULT Ingnore simple Erythema
Age 35 Admission weight ≃ 70 kg
Partial thickness loss (PTL)
Full thickness loss (FTL)

The burns

Pending the patient's transfer from the emergency department to the ward or specialist burns unit the burnt area should be covered with a sterile, warm, non-adherent dressing. A layer of Clingfilm covered by a dry sheet and blanket is effective. Never transfer a patient in wet sheets or towels, because this can lead to hypothermia, with occasional fatal consequences.

Deep circumferential burns over the limbs, neck, and chest can produce a tourniquet like effect because the damaged skin is unable to expand as tissue oedema develops. If this occurs escharotomies (longitudinal incisions of the skin) are required to permit adequate circulation and ventilation. Escharotomy is also required if circumferential neck burns make intubation difficult. It is often necessary to do escharotomies before transfer. The affected part should be incised under sterile conditions on both sides, just as a plaster of Paris cast is bivalved. Ensure that the entire length of the constriction is released. In the hand, take the incisions right to the tips of affected digits.

If escharotomy of the chest is required, make vertical incisions along anterior and posterior axillary lines. If sufficient chest expansion does not occur further incisions in the midline and midclavicular lines and transverse incisions may be needed.

Escharotomy does not require anaesthesia as the burns are full thickness burns. If it does cause pain then escharotomy is probably not indicated. Failure to do an early escharotomy can lead to the loss of a limb; therefore if doubtful always err on the side of escharotomy. The incisions do not cause any additional scarring as the burns are full thickness. Substantial bleeding occurs from the wounds, and sterile absorbent dressings should be applied and, if necessary, blood replacement given. Ensure that the patient is adequately protected against tetanus.

Lethal burns

Improvement in the management of burns in intensive care is resulting in some patients surviving burns of more than 90% of the total body surface area. However, few patients survive full thickness burns of more than 70% of the total body surface area. As a rough guide, if the patient's age added to the

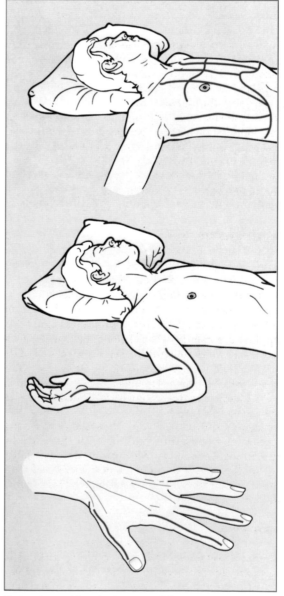

Escharotomy of the chest, arm, and fingers.

percentage of the body surface area of the burn exceeds 100 the chances of survival are less than 50%. Any decision not to treat a patient with a lethal burn aggressively must be taken by a consultant with experience in burns. If aggressive resuscitation is not to be instituted in a patient the other aspects of reassurance and analgesia are of even greater importance. Remember that even patients with 100% full thickness burns are usually conscious and sentient.

General aspects
Ask the patient and the relatives about preexisting medical conditions, especially if these may be relevant to the therapeutic intervention being performed—for example, obstructive airways disease and ischaemic heart disease. Consider the possibility of underlying medical conditions that may have led to the burn injury—for example, epilepsy, a cerebrovascular episode, hypoglycaemia, drug or alcohol overdose.

In elderly patients, patients with known ischaemic heart disease, and all patients with a carboxyhaemoglobin concentration greater that 15%, obtain a 12-lead electrocardiogram and attach a cardiac monitor. Myocardial ischaemia or infarction and arrhythmias occur commonly and often do not have their usual clinical features. Consider the possibility of non-accidental injury in children. Do not give prophylaxis with antibiotics or steroids. Depending on local policies, discuss the patient's management with the burns or plastic surgical receiving team.

If the patient is being moved within the hospital or to another referral hospital adequate intravenous fluids and analgesics should be transported along with him or her. All patients suspected of having inhaled smoke or requiring additional care of the airway must be escorted by an experienced anaesthetist with appropriate equipment. Make clear, concise notes, which must accompany the patient and should include the size of the burn; the weight of the patient; the time when intravenous fluids were started; which drugs were given for pain relief and at what dose and time they were given; the urine and fluids chart; and details of special problems.

Chemical burns

In an emergency all chemical burns can be treated with copious quantities of water and a bar of soap applied as soon as possible after the injury. Although there are specific treatments for certain chemicals (see below), these may be difficult to recall with accuracy in a confused environment and water and soap applied urgently in sufficient quantity for sufficient time will cover all eventualities. Running water should be applied for at least 20 minutes, and should be lukewarm rather than cold if possible. The soap is not always necessary, but will overcome difficulties with organic chemicals (such as phenol) that may not be soluble in water.

In most factories that deal with dangerous chemicals buffer solutions are available and procedures exist for neutralising specific agents. In some cases, however, these injuries may be first seen in an emergency department and some of those from more common substances will benefit from specific treatment.

Hydrofluoric acid
Hydrofluoric acid is used in the glass industry and for cleaning pipes and is both toxic and painful. It can be neutralised by calcium gluconate gel or, in more severe cases, the calcium gluconate may be injected as a 10% solution under the skin to prevent further tissue damage and relieve the pain.

> **Even patients with 100% full thickness burns are usually conscious and sentient**

Information required by burns unit
- Name, age, and sex of patient
- Percentage of body surface area covered by burns
- Depth of burns
- Any "special" areas affected, such as the face, head, and perineum
- Time of injury
- Presence of respiratory problems
- Associated injuries
- Medical history
- Treatment instituted and response

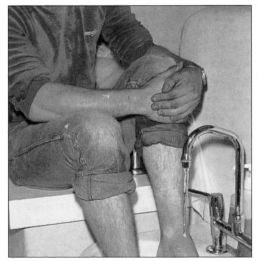
Chemical burn being copiously washed under a tap.

Phenol (carbolic acid)

Phenol is an organic acid so is not readily soluble in water, but it can be removed rapidly with ethylene glycol (antifreeze). Like hydrofluoric acid, phenol can not only cause local damage but is also a systemic poison, and as with many chemical burns the prognosis usually depends more on the systemic effects of absorption than on the surface area of the burn.

White phosphorus

White phosphorus is used in the manufacture of explosives, and continues to burn when in contact with air. Particles may become embedded in the skin and have to be covered with water to prevent further combustion. A dilute solution of copper sulphate added to the water will make the phosphorus go black, which makes it easier to identify and remove.

Electrical burns

A clear distinction should be made between flash and contact electrical burns.

Flash electrical burns result in a high dry air temperature for a brief period, which produces a superficial charring of the skin. This charring is almost always less severe than it looks and usually heals without the need for grafting unless there has been associated thermal injury from clothing that has caught fire.

Contact electrical burns are the result of an electric current passing through the tissues and damaging the tissue in its passage. These burns are almost always worse than they look because much of the damage may be in the deeper tissues in spite of a relatively minor injury visible on the skin.

Contact electrical burns are usually divided into low voltage and high voltage, the dividing point being 1000 volts. In practice this means the difference between household and industrial currents, and the distinction may help in deciding how severe an injury is likely to be. Lethal injuries do, however, occur at household voltages. Voltage is the only variable that may be gleaned from the history as density of current, resistance, and duration of exposure will not be known.

Alternating current (mains) can provoke a tetanic contracture of the muscles that makes it difficult to release the contact. Direct current (lightning) tends to throw the injured person away. In an emergency NEVER attempt to pull somebody off a current source unless you are CERTAIN that the current has been switched off or the person is pulled off with an insulated agent such as a dry wooden stake.

The passage of an electric current causes damage because of the heat it generates; the amount of heat is related to the density of the current, the resistance of the tissues through which the current passes, and the volume of tissue through which the current passes. Dry skin offers a high resistance and can therefore generate high temperatures, with obvious tissue damage. If the current passes through a large contact area both in and out of the body, there may be no visible skin injury; this is seen when a large contact plate is used in unipolar diathermy. Therefore, although an electrical contact will produce entry and exit points, it differs from a bullet wound in that the visible damage at either site will be related to the contact surface area.

An electrical current will follow the path of least resistance and will travel in the most direct line between the points of contact, of which there must be at least two (source and earth) to form a circuit. A current that passes from the palm to the dorsum of the same hand will not deviate to affect the

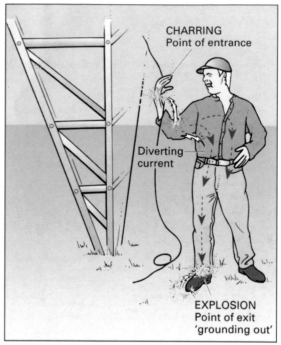

Worker receiving a high voltage electrical injury, entering

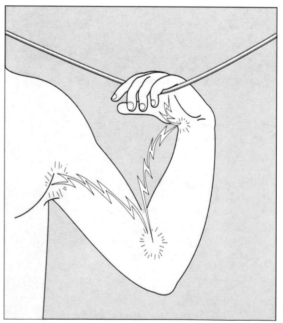

Arcing injury, between wrist, cubital fossa, and axilla.

myocardium or brain, but a current that passes from hand to hand or hand to foot will almost certainly affect the myocardium; this may produce arrhythmias that must be carefully monitored and treated if necessary. With high voltages arcing injuries may occur, in which the current will jump from forearm to upper arm or upper arm to chest causing thermal skin injuries at each site.

A current that is forced to travel through tissues of low cross-sectional area or volume (for example, a finger) or through tissues of high resistance (for example, bone) will generate temperatures of up to thousands of degrees Celsius and cause severe tissue damage, even though the overlying skin looks normal. Contact electrical burns should be treated with respect and usually the patient should be admitted to hospital for observation or treatment by appropriate staff. If there is any possibility of myocardial damage, and in all lightning injuries, patients should be monitored with an electrocardiogram because delayed arrhythmias may occur.

Conclusion

The initial management of severe burns can be intimidating for those who are unfamiliar with them. As with most major trauma, however, the management of burns is amenable to logical procedures, following the Advanced Trauma Life Support principles. The history can be as important as the physical examination in determining the likely severity of the burn and early consequences, such as airway impairment, chemical toxicity, electrical myocardial damage, etc.

Common mistakes are failure to:
● keep a patient with a major burn warm after the cause of the burn injury has been established
● assess the size of the burn properly, because of a failure to look at the whole patient
● carry out an early intubation in a patient with significant airway burns, especially if transport over any distance is contemplated. Emergency intubation in a moving ambulance must be avoided at all costs.

● The nomogram is reproduced with kind permission from Clark CJ et al, *Lancet* 1991; **i**: 1332–5.

Further reading

Settle J, ed. *Principles and practice of burns management*. Edinburgh: Churchill Livingstone, 1996.

Muir I, Barclay T, Settle J. *Burns and their treatment*, 3rd edn. London: Butterworth, 1987.

24 Chemical incidents

Virginia Murray

Recent experience at the Chemical Incident Response Service (CIRS) has given us cause for concern about the safety of emergency department staff when they find themselves managing patients contaminated during a chemical incident, and about the viability of emergency departments in the presence of contaminated patients.

We have therefore prepared guidelines entitled *Chemical incident management for accident and emergency clinicians;*[1] these cover many of the more detailed questions not dealt with in the present short chapter.

Common problems encountered

In a special CIRS study undertaken during October 1998, we found that nine health care facilities had been closed, in part or entirely, as a result of chemical incidents.

In the experience of CIRS, the main causes for such closures appear to be:

- contaminated patients arriving at emergency departments, with or without warning;
- spill or chemical release within the department, such as a leaking refrigerator or spillage of a pharmaceutical preparation;
- secondary contamination of air conditioning.

Major chemical accidents cause problems for emergency departments that are different from those recognized in other major incidents—for example, identification of the toxin, safety issues and the risk of cross chemical contamination of staff, and difficulties in patient management such as the need for specific antidotes. Particular attention should therefore be given to preparation and planning.

What is a chemical incident?

A chemical incident is the accidental or intentional release, or impending release, of a hazardous material. No definition of chemical incident is ideal; that currently used by CIRS is:

An unforeseen event, involving non-radioactive substances, that results in potential toxic risk to public health, or leads to the exposure of two or more individuals and results in illness or potential illness, or two or more individuals suffering from a similar illness that might be attributable to such an event.

Although this chapter is mainly concerned with the response by emergency departments to large scale acute chemical incidents, experience at CIRS has shown that equipment and training in some departments is sufficiently poor to make it difficult for them to manage even one or two chemically contaminated patients.

Contaminating substances that each caused the closure of an emergency department during October 1998

- Potassium cyanide
- Wood preservatives
- Contaminated soil containing chemicals such as solvents and polyaromatic hydrocarbons
- Fluothane anaesthetic agent

24-hour services provided by the Chemical Incident Response Service, London

- To respond to requests for information and advice from medical professionals managing chemical incidents
- To assess, as rapidly as possible, the nature of the chemical hazard, to assist in determining toxic risk, and to disseminate relevant toxicological information
- To provide advice on issues such as decontamination, treatment, analytical toxicology, case registration and follow up

---

For the purposes of an emergency department, a large scale chemical incident is any event where one or both of the following apply:

- The agent involved is present in large quantities or is potentially of high toxicity
- A large number of people are exposed or at risk of being exposed

How can emergency departments plan for chemical incident response?

Preparation, planning, availability of decontamination facilities and personal protective equipment are essential elements in developing an emergency department response. The NHS Guidance, *Planning for major incidents*,[2] includes a chapter on chemical incidents. It states that acute hospital trusts must ensure that satisfactory arrangements are in place for the provision of health care to casualties following a chemical incident.

What are the local chemical hazards?

A risk assessment by emergency departments is necessary under the new guidance. Departments may find it useful to strengthen their links with health authority public health departments, local emergency services, the fire brigade and local or county authorities, including the emergency planning officers.

Many of these agencies will have information on methods of assessment, control, and mitigation in the event of accidents, much of which concludes with "seek medical advice." Few of them have experience in acute medical toxicology, and as a result they rely on advice from emergency departments. The latter rely in turn on poisons centres, such as the National Poisons Information Service, London (NPIS,L).

How can the National Poisons Information Service help?

NPIS,L is one of six NPIS centres in the UK; the others are in Belfast, Birmingham, Cardiff, Edinburgh and Newcastle. The NPIS is a resource that provides information and advice on the diagnosis and management of cases of poisoning, from whatever cause. Most can also offer advice on the medical aspects of managing a chemical accident. Telephone numbers of the NPIS centres should be readily available in the emergency department.

Analytical toxicology services, such as the Medical Toxicology Unit at the Guy's and St Thomas' Hospital Trust, of which NPIS,L is part, can provide advice on appropriate collection of samples, testing and interpretation of the results.

Chemical Incident Provider Units

At the request of the Department of Health and others, every health authority in the UK is contracted to one of the five UK Chemical Incident Provider Units (CIPUs). These CIPUs, in collaboration with public health services, can provide additional support for investigation and epidemiological follow up. They may be able to provide on-site toxicological advice and support.

Where a significant chemical incident occurs, the local CIPU, with consent from the health authority, will notify the National Focus for Work on Response to Chemical Incidents and Surveillance of Health Effects of Environmental Chemicals. They will then cascade this information to the relevant government health department, if it is appropriate.

Essential actions in developing an emergency department's response to a chemical incident

- Preparing and maintaining plans
- Ensuring that staff are prepared and trained, and have access to the advice and expertise needed to provide medical care for the casualties
- Having carried out a risk assessment, providing the facilities and equipment necessary to provide a safe working environment, including decontamination facilities and personal protective equipment

---

Telephone numbers of National Poisons Information Service

London	0207 635 9191
Belfast	01232 240503
Birmingham	0121 507 5588/9
Cardiff	01222 709901
Edinburgh	0131 536 2300
Newcastle	0191 2325131

Chemical Incident Provider Units (CIPUs)	Regions covered
Chemical Incident Response Service, London	London, South East, Eastern, North West, Trent, South and West
Chemical Hazards Management and Research Centre, Birmingham	West Midlands
Chemical Incident Management Support Unit, Cardiff	Wales, Northern Ireland
Chemical Incident Service, Newcastle upon Tyne	Northern and Yorkshire
Scottish Centre for Environment and Health, Glasgow	Scotland

Health effects from chemical incidents

Initial symptoms usually relate to, but are not confined to, the route of exposure—inhalation will cause respiratory effects, and systemic effects may occur where the substance is absorbed. Most effects will appear within a few hours of exposure but some may be delayed. In particular, respiratory symptoms can be delayed for up to 48 hours after inhalation. Because effects may be delayed, it is important to identify and document as early as possible all those who were exposed, or are suspected of having been exposed. Individuals who do not initially require continuing hospital management can if necessary be recalled for further assessment.

Susceptible groups that are particularly at risk from a toxic exposure are the young, the old, pregnant women and their fetuses, and those who have chronic illnesses. The route of exposure is an important factor in predicting which illnesses will result in increased susceptibility: for example, patients with emphysema are particularly sensitive to respirable gases.

Multiple hazards such as fire may present a complicated picture with both trauma and toxic effects.

What emergency facilities are required?

Facilities for triage, resuscitation, decontamination, investigation and treatment, and also short and long term follow up of those exposed, should be provided. The facilities for decontamination are often inadequate. Other equipment should include suitable personal protective clothing. In addition, adequate training and rehearsals in the use of equipment and facilities are essential. After reading this chapter, you should check your own emergency department.

Actions

To allow early assessment of the toxic hazard, the emergency department must obtain as much information as possible about:
- chemical(s) involved
- type of incident
- route(s) of exposure
- type(s) of initial clinical effects.

It is important to identify and document everybody who has been exposed to chemicals. Some who are initially symptom free may develop symptoms or become concerned about the effects of exposure at a later date.

Reports received at CIRS over the past 4 years indicate that few emergency departments have sent medical teams to chemical incidents. The need for a mobile medical team is likely to arise only where patients who have been exposed to chemicals are also injured. If undertaking on-site support, the following section deals with important factors that should be considered.

On-site support
At the site of an incident, protection of the mobile medical team is essential, though there is no single set of protective clothing suitable for protection against every hazardous chemical. To minimise the risk of injury, the fire service usually has responsibility for control of the incident, with the site being divided into "dirty", "contamination reduction" and "clean" zones.

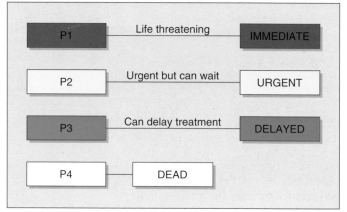

Triage categories.

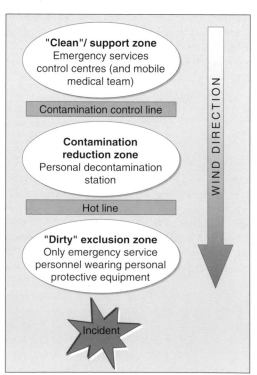

Control lines at the site of a chemical incident.

The principles of management of walking or stretcher patients include initial rescue, triage, and strip to remove contaminated clothing, decontamination and resuscitation and evacuation. The emergency services control centres should advise the mobile medical team when it is safe to provide medical aid or triage and should stay in communication. Preferably only decontaminated casualties should be attended. (Decontamination facilities are provided only for fire brigade staff but may be used for other casualties at the fire brigade's discretion. These are usually suitable only for walking patients, and provide only cold water decontamination.)

The management of physical injuries follows the routine already described. For the benefit of the casualty and emergency responders, all contaminated clothing should be removed, bagged, labelled and sealed in double clear plastic bags—preferably at the incident site—and stored in a secure area away from staff and patients. Consider removing valuables and storing them separately. In addition to medical equipment, consider taking surgical gowns or other clothing for casualties.

Chemical contamination of the skin, eyes and wounds may require prolonged irrigation or even immersion of the affected part—the solution to pollution is dilution.

At the emergency department

The above principals also apply to casualties arriving at the hospital. Early notification of an incident and of any casualties allows final preparation of hospital decontamination facilities and protective clothing by senior staff to minimize any spread of contamination hazard inside the hospital.

Preparation for triage assessment of chemical exposure and toxic risk assessment will probably require support from the NPIS or a CIPU or both. In addition, the medical staff may find it helpful to seek advice from other experts on and off the incident site, including public health staff. A list of such contacts should be held ready for use.

Arrangements should be made as early as possible to obtain antidotes, if appropriate, and to provide facilities for supportive care. Collection of blood, urine, vomit, and other relevant biological samples is valuable for confirming exposure and dose received, and should be carried out as soon as possible after an incident in consultation with the NPIS or a CIPU.

When discharging patients who have attended the emergency department, it is important not to return any patient to a previously contaminated environment without checking that it is safe to do so.

Conclusion

Although the management of injuries sustained in a chemical incident is the same as that of injuries from any other cause, special precautions must be taken by mobile medical teams attending such an incident and by the receiving emergency department. These should be taken in conjunction with the public health department of the health authority and the emergency services. Remember that the NPIS and Chemical Incident Provider Units can provide invaluable information and advice.

Management of walking or stretcher patients after a chemical accident

- Initial rescue
- Triage
- Strip to remove contaminated clothing
- Decontamination and resuscitation
- Evacuation

The solution to pollution is dilution

References

1 Fisher J, Morgan-Jones D, Murray V, Davies G. *Chemical incident management for accident and emergency clinicians* London: Stationery Office, 1999.

2 NHS Executive. *Planning for major incidents: the NHS Guidance.* London: NHS Executive, 1998.

25 Blast and gunshot/missile injuries

Nigel Rossiter, Tim Hodgetts, Jim Ryan, David Skinner

Injuries from explosions and bullets are common throughout the world. Here we discuss the mechanisms of injury, the management at the scene of a bomb or a shooting, and the treatment of individual casualties.

Explosions

An explosion may be the result of a domestic accident (for example, household gas), or an industrial accident (for example, mining), but the principal cause outside a war zone is a terrorist bomb. Multiple casualties ranging from a handful to several hundred can be expected.

At the scene of an unexploded bomb the police will take charge. If doctors and nurses are deployed before the bomb explodes and can see the device, they are clearly standing in the wrong place—it is not a firework display. Secondary devices are common after one explosion, and the scene should not be approached until it is declared safe by the police. If people are to be moved from one area to another it is important to have the area cleared for a secondary device. Radio silence should be maintained initially to avoid triggering a radio-controlled bomb.

A bomb has six distinct mechanisms of causing injury:
- the blast wave
- the blast wind
- fragmentation
- flash burns
- crush
- psychological.

> **Police role at the scene of an unexploded bomb**
> *Remember the four Cs*
> - Confirm that there is a suspect device
> - Clear the area of people
> - Cordon to protect the scene
> - Control the incident

Blast wave

The blast wave is a front of overpressure formed by the compression of air at the interface of the rapidly expanding sphere of hot gases. The size of the overpressure falls off rapidly, and in proportion to the inverse of the distance cubed.

With conventional "high" explosives such as trinitrotoluene (TNT) or Semtex the blast wave will last only a few milliseconds. A "low" explosive is petrol or gunpowder, which must be highly contained before it will explode.

Injury is produced mainly by a combination of initial body compression, causing contusion of underlying solid organs, followed by the disruption of tissues at air/tissue interfaces—particularly in the lungs. Shearing forces then occur at tissue interfaces of different density causing subserous and submucosal haemorrhage, particularly in the abdomen, and implosion of gas filled organs causing acute perforation of intestine or tympanic membrane.

> **Blast injury is produced mainly by a combination of initial body compression, causing contusion of underlying solid organs, followed by the disruption of tissues at air/tissue interfaces**

> **A ruptured ear drum indicates exposure to an appreciable blast load:**
> - Is the patient deaf?
> - Is the patient bleeding from the ears?

The size of the overpressure can be multiplied several times over when the incident pressure is reflected by solid objects such as ceiling or walls; the pressure wave will be attenuated by water.

If air enters the pulmonary circulation as a result of disruption of the alveolar membrane, fatal coronary artery or cerebral artery air emboli may occur, possibly without external evidence of injury.

Rupture of the eardrum is a useful clinical indicator that the patient has been exposed to an appreciable blast load. The converse is not true if the drum is intact, because the angle of the blast wave against the ear drum is thought to be critical.

The blast wave can produce two distinct patterns of lung injury (see box). The common feature is intra-alveolar haemorrhage. There may be associated pneumothoraces and non-fatal air emboli that may cause central nervous system signs, which may be seen in the retinal vessels. Although pulmonary injury is important, this "blast lung" is rare in those surviving to reach hospital (less than 1%). The second pattern of pulmonary injury is an adult respiratory distress syndrome, which may be seen 48 hours from injury.

By contrast, ischaemia of the bowel from subserous and submucosal haemorrhage can result in perforation delayed up to 5 days, which is usually heralded by abdominal pain and tenderness. Laparotomy should be reserved for patients with clear signs of perforation, such as localised peritonitis or free air in the abdominal x ray film, because of the anaesthetic risk from the inevitably associated pulmonary injury.

Blast winds

Blast winds are the rapidly moving displaced columns of air that follow the blast wave. They can be powerful enough to disintegrate and dismember anyone close to the point of the explosion. People who are further away or partly protected may sustain traumatic amputation of a limb. This sort of amputation, unlike a guillotine amputation, is usually unsuitable for reimplantation.

The blast wind may also throw people against solid objects, resulting in impact fractures or deceleration injuries. Debris of stone, glass, or broken street furniture carried in the wind will produce fragmentation missile injuries.

Fragmentation missiles

Most injuries after an explosion will be caused by fragmentation. They are caused by momentum resulting in fractures and contusions, laceration, and penetration with high or low energy transfer.

Flash burns

Flash burns are usually superficial and of exposed skin. The possibility of smoke inhalation with upper airway involvement should always be considered.

Crush injuries

An explosion indoors may collapse the building on to the people inside, resulting in crush injuries.

Psychological injuries

Psychological injuries are the main objective of the terrorist. There will be short term panic and fear, and long term post-traumatic stress disorder. Many more will have psychological scars than will sustain physical injuries, and symptoms of stress should also be watched for in carers at the scene and at the hospital (see chapter 27).

Patterns of lung injury (blast wave)

- Immediate respiratory failure, usually fatal, from massive pulmonary contusion
- Diffuse lung damage producing adult respiratory distress syndrome (hypoxia, reduced lung compliance, widespread pulmonary infiltrates in x ray film). This may be delayed for up to 48 hours

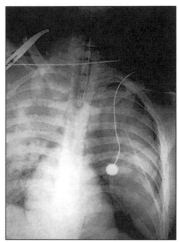
Radiograph of blast lung.

Missiles following fragmentation

Primary

- Missiles arising from the bomb
  —natural: parts of the bomb casing
  —preformed: nails, nuts, bolts packed around the explosive

Secondary

- Missiles arising from the environment
  —stones, glass, wood

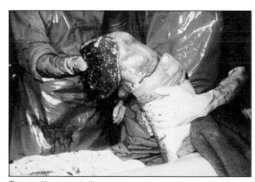
Traumatic amputation.

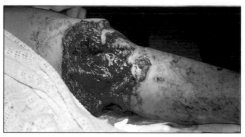
Shotgun injury injury to the knee—a high energy transfer wound.

Penetrating missiles

Missiles include the primary and secondary fragments that follow an explosion, and bullets. Missile injuries from a bomb are often multiple, but the mechanism of injury and the management are the same whatever the cause. The key is to treat the wound, not the weapon.

The degree of injury that a missile produces depends on how much energy it imparts to the tissues. This in turn depends on how much energy the missile had to start with and how much it is retarded by the tissues. Because kinetic energy is the product of half the mass multiplied by the square of the velocity, a missile travelling at high speed will maximise available energy. The density of the tissue and the type and stability of the missile will regulate the degree of retardation and therefore the energy transferred to the tissues.

Low energy transfer injuries

Missiles have traditionally been divided into "low velocity" and "high velocity" and the arbitrary division is the speed of sound. More important, however, is the distinction between whether there has been high or low energy transfer to the wound. Either is possible with either missile.

Clinically this can be assessed by assessing the wound itself. If the sum of the diameter of the entrance and exit wounds (if present) at their widest points is less than 10 cm, this is likely to be a low energy transfer wound. If the sum of the entrance and exit wound diameters is greater than 10 cm, or two fingers can easily be introduced into either wound (indicating that cavitation has occurred—see below), or both, the wound is likely to be high energy transfer.

Nevertheless, low energy missiles, such as from a handgun, or large irregular fragments from an explosion, tend to produce injury only along the wound track by crushing and laceration, producing a permanent cavity, with little damage away from the track. Death is likely only if a vital organ is damaged. Large irregular fragments are more readily retarded, and consequently will give up more energy.

High energy transfer injuries

High energy transfer missiles such as military rifle bullets also produce a permanent cavity, but the devastating injury seen in high energy transfer wounds can be a result of the temporary cavity that develops when the tissues continue to move away from the wound track after the missile has passed through. This produces a large cavity for a few milliseconds which then collapses and oscillates, and sucks in contaminated debris from the wound surface at either end. Solid, semisolid, and abdominal hollow viscera can be disrupted. Microscopically there are large areas of heterogeneous tissue damage, vascular instability, and some reversible ischaemia. If bone is struck there is a higher energy transfer and pieces of bone or broken missile can act as secondary missiles.

Management of injuries

Safety is paramount at the scene of a bomb or shooting incident. In the emergency department always consider that the person who has been shot may also be carrying a gun. A hypoxic and confused patient with a gun is clearly a danger.

Resuscitation

Resuscitation of the injured follows the standard protocol of airway, breathing, and circulation. Ventilatory support may be needed for patients with blast lung, but this must be balanced

---

Missile and bullet injuries

Important points:

- If chest penetration is possible, suspect and exclude tension pneumothorax
- Could the missile have injured the abdomen? If so, the prognosis is compromised and surgical exploration is usually essential. Administer broad spectrum antibiotics and tetanus prophylaxis early
- Wounds may be multiple, and patients may not be aware of all their injuries. Perform a thorough examination
- Suspect that minor wounds may contain foreign bodies. Perform radiography

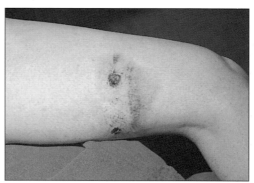

Low energy transfer wound.

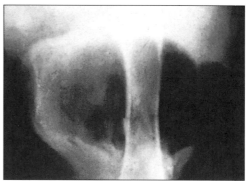

High energy transfer wound: radiograph showing cavitation.

In the resuscitation room

- Ensure safety. *Check* the patient for weapons
- Treatment priorities are airway, breathing, and circulation
- Bag, seal, and label all of the patient's clothing and personal belongings. Secure these until handed to the police (to ensure continuity of evidence)
- Label any missile fragments found and hand them directly to the police
- If the patient is stable make notes of the position and size of all wounds (and retain a personal copy)

against the theoretical increased short term risk of producing an air embolism. This can occur with intermittent positive pressure ventilation but is more likely with positive end expiratory pressure. Rapid transfer to the operating theatre for control of haemorrhage may be important with penetrating injuries.

Contamination

All missile wounds are contaminated. With high energy transfer wounds, clothing can be disrupted into minute fragments and spread widely along tissue planes up to 20–30 cm distant from the wound track. These wounds are particularly susceptible to anaerobic infection with clostridia (tetanus and gas gangrene). With low energy wounds the plug of clothing is often closely associated with the missile.

High energy transfer wounds require aggressive surgery to remove dead tissue and foreign material and to ensure that no tension develops in the wound. This typically involves wide excision and fasciotomy.

Immunity to tetanus must be ensured with immuno-globulin, or toxoid, or both.

In high energy transfer wounds antibiotics help in preventing or delaying infection if given early. Benzylpenicillin is the antibiotic of first choice to cover for beta-haemolytic streptococcal and clostridial infection. If a fracture is also present the risk of penicillin resistant staphylococcal osteo-myelitis as a long term sequel is significant and flucloxacillin should be added. However there is no substitute for adequate surgery and radical debridement of the wound.

In low energy transfer wounds the need for antibiotics in civilian practice is debatable.

Surgical management

There is no substitute for surgery. Techniques for debridement are outlined in chapter 11. Soft tissue damage and the risk of infection are the two critical factors determining outcome in patients with serious open injuries and fractures. The management in the first few hours can make the difference between complete recovery and lifelong disability. The infecting organisms may be the contaminating ones and samples for culture should therefore be obtained at the outset. The priorities are to clear contamination and devitalised tissue and so reduce the potential culture medium and size of an infecting inoculum.

In a multiply injured patient with reduced oxygen delivery and an anticipated rise in tissue pressure, wound hypoxia and an increased susceptibility to infection are inevitable. Closure of a wound is therefore rarely indicated.

Wound debridement is often inadequate. Debridement should be performed by the orthopaedic surgeon in conjunction with the plastic surgeon who may subsequently be required to provide tissue cover. Surrounding skin is shaved and the wound and surrounding area scrubbed with a brush. The wound is extended in the long axis of the limb to facilitate examination, and fasciotomies performed if required. All non-viable muscle, fascia and fat is carefully but radically excised. Large volumes of irrigation fluid—in excess of 4 litres should be used—as stated in the previous chapter, "the solution to pollution is dilution".

The most commonly used irrigant is physiological saline, although Hartman's solution and mild antiseptics can be used. There is evidence that Hartman's solution in large quantities may cause less postoperative wound oedema. No evidence supports use of antibiotics in the lavage fluid. Pressurised pulsed lavage systems are advantageous, but it is the rate and volume of flow that are important rather than the pressure.

Skin flaps of dubious viability are best dealt with by taking a split skin graft from the flap surface. This will serve to delineate

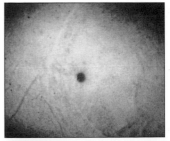

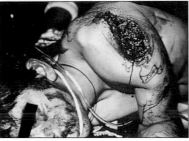

Shoulder wound caused by bomb fragment. Energy deposit damage and contamination (left) was found on exploration of what seemed to be a simple wound (above).

Management of blast injuries

- ### Suspect

If exposed to appreciable blast, even if no injury is apparent, observe the patient for 48 hours

- ### Examine

Initially follow standard ABC examination protocols, but also look for these specific injuries associated with exposure to a blast:

Chest

—examine for signs of respiratory failure and pneumothorax

—do a chest *x* ray (is there evidence of a pneumothorax? free gas under the diaphragm? signs of developing adult respiratory distress syndrome?)

Abdomen

—is there evidence of local peritonitis?

Central nervous system

—look for abnormal neurological signs (secondary to air emboli)

Funduscopy

—look for air emboli

Ears

—are the tympanic membranes perforated?

Olfactory function

—the blast wave can produce anosmia through direct damage of the olfactory nerve endings. This has medicolegal consequences

- ### Treat

Confine the patient to a chair or bed to prevent exertion

Give high flow oxygen through a tight-fitting mask with reservoir

Maintain ventilation if there is respiratory failure, but balance this against the risk of embolism

If intermittent positive pressure ventilation is needed, consider prophylactic chest drains

Treat other injuries (amputation, missiles, burns) as necessary

Do laparotomy in cases of definite perforation

the margin of viability, as the dead area will show no capillary bleeding. The harvested graft may be applied later if necrosis of the flap occurs. Remove loose fragments of bone.

Most open fractures are unstable. Stabilisation will promote tissue healing. This should be done using the most appropriate method for the fracture, the soft tissues, the unit in which the procedure is undertaken, and in consultation with plastic surgeons if their services are required for soft tissue cover.

The debrided wound should initially be left open and covered with a dry dressing such as fluffed gauze. Wet dressings should be avoided except over large areas of exposed tendon or bone or both where there is no viable soft tissue that can be used to cover. The wound is ideally inspected again at 48 hours. Early closure of the soft tissue wound, when the wound is suitable for closure with an appropriate method and no tension, reduces the rate of infection and non-union rate of a fracture.

Non-surgical management

There is *in some instances* a role for non-surgical management of penetrating wounds and fractures in low energy transfer wounds. However this should *only* be undertaken with the direct participation of a trauma surgeon experienced in the management of ballistic injuries. If there is any doubt, the safe management is by operative exploration of the wound.

A decision making sequence is outlined in the flow diagram.

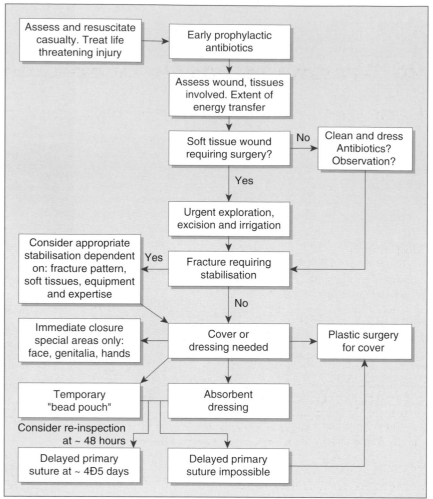

A decision-making sequence in the management of limb injuries.

Conclusion

Gunshot and blast injuries are common world-wide, and an understanding of the mechanisms of injury is important in predicting clinical problems.

Priorities in management are safety, airway, breathing and circulation, before considering injuries specific to bombs or bullets.

26 Trauma in hostile environments

Chris Cahill, Vanessa Lloyd-Davies, Katherine Hartington

Most trauma in the UK is managed in a controlled environment, such as an emergency department or an organised pre-hospital care system. The trauma team leader, in most circumstances, will be able to take control of the situation in the knowledge that he or she possesses appropriate equipment and expertise within the team, and can ensure rapid evacuation to a definitive care centre. In a hostile environment, however, this is not always the case.

In a war zone, the aftermath of an earthquake or in a remote area, limited equipment, inclement working conditions and uncertain evacuation will be coupled with the inherent dangers of the particular situations.

The conditions will undoubtedly affect patient presentation. A knowledge of the history of injury and the environment is therefore of even more importance and will modify the management plan. It may be necessary to improvise according to the equipment available.

It must be emphasised that the priorities for patient assessment, triage and treatment remain the same as set out in earlier chapters: A, B, C, D, E. In a hostile environment, however, E also encompasses evacuation. Full exposure may be impractical, dangerous or both, and evacuation appropriate before the secondary survey.

In this chapter we aim to highlight some particular situations and give guidelines to assist in meeting the difficult challenges they present.

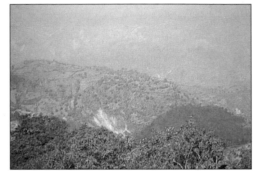
Foothills in eastern Nepal.

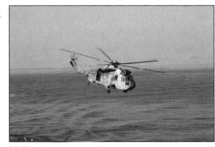
Helicopter rescue at sea.

General guidelines for hostile environments

You may find yourself in a hostile environment unexpectedly; however, if you are able to pre-plan the following additional ABCDE will assist in preparing yourself and your team.

A—Anticipation
Planning is the key. A thorough knowledge of the area and the conditions are essential. Ideally, use local knowledge, ensure you have up to date and accurate maps and think of all the likely and unlikely scenarios. The "unexpected" will happen. Ask yourself if you really need to go into the area of risk. For example, tourists and "go it alone saviours" are not welcomed in disaster zones because they risk becoming casualties themselves.

B—Back-up
Ask yourself who is going to get you out if it all goes wrong. Make sure that your back-up team know where you are going to be and when you should be back. Do you have the

ABCDE of resuscitation
- Airway and cervical spine
- Breathing
- Circulation and control of haemorrhage
- Dysfunction of the central nervous system
- Exposure

The hostile environment:
- Will modify patient presentation
- Will affect your management
- Will necessitate improvisation
- But does not alter the priorities: "ABCDE"

appropriate clearances or approvals and have you linked with other agencies involved in the same area and activities? Their expertise and experience might be essential to your success.

C—Communication

Poor communications often contribute to failure and disaster. Careful planning, appropriate equipment and training must be considered. More than one method is desirable to minimise risks. The press, if present, can make useful allies but remember that their priorities are different.

Technology is advancing rapidly; satellite communications and portable computers make telemedicine, potentially, available world-wide. However advice from afar is no substitute for planning and preparation, and technology is fickle—*if it can go wrong, it will.*

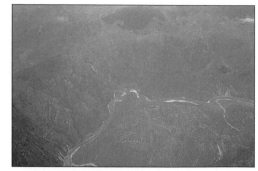
Mountainous territory, Nepal.

D—Danger

It is essential to assess the known risks and balance these against the benefits that you and your party can offer to a situation. Appropriate safety equipment is essential, as is training and knowledge. The aim is to avoid becoming a casualty yourself. Be self sufficient in all regards to prevent becoming a burden to others.

E—Equipment

Keep it simple: the less technical equipment is, the more likely it is to work. Plan the packing so that you can get to an item when you need it.

Spread your resources evenly around your team to minimise the effect of losing part of your kit. Stores should be broken down to reduce packing materials to a minimum and quantities should reflect your expected length of stay plus a reserve for emergencies. Remember, at all times, that you have to be able to carry or transport your stores.

Improvisation is essential and relatively easy; for example, outlines of semi-rigid neck collars can be drawn onto sleeping roll-mats before departure to be cut out when required, and sandbags can be made from socks filled with earth, etc.

Classical ATLS teaching was formulated for the hospital environment. In hostile environments modification of the protocols and a flexible, pragmatic approach is required. Nevertheless, the priorities and underlying principles remain the same. The following are examples of modified approaches within the framework.

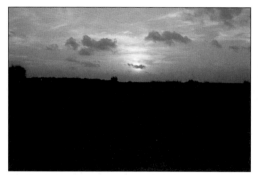
Sunrise in the desert.

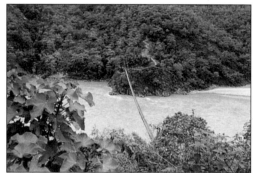
Tropical rain forest.

Airway with cervical spine protection

If you suspect spinal injury from the history and mechanism of injury then immobilise the spine, but needless immobilisation makes casualty handling and evacuation more difficult and could endanger your patient.

A naso-pharyngeal airway may be better tolerated than an oro-pharyngeal one and therefore require less supervision. Cricothyroidotomy may be more appropriate than intubation, because oral or nasal intubation is only possible if the patient is deeply unconscious. Sedation, paralysis, or both, may be difficult to accomplish and attempted nasal or oral intubation will raise intracranial pressure in a conscious patient.

The technique of cricothyroidotomy is simple and requires little equipment, but appropriately sized tubes (size 5/6) are necessary.

Airway
- Open
- Maintain
- Secure
- Cervical spine immobilisation as appropriate
- Nasopharangeal airway
- Cricothyroidotomy

Breathing and ventilation

Oxygenation is essential, but remember that oxygen therapy may be a limited resource or unavailable, because portable cylinders are heavy and last only a short time at high flows. Patient selection and conservation of valuable stocks is crucial. Give oxygen only when it is absolutely necessary. Consider using oxygen concentrators, if available, to conserve bottled gas.

Remember to secure all tubes with sutures and tapes. *If a tube can fall out, it will fall out!* Under water seal drainage is not practical and flutter valves (for example, Portex Emergency drainage bags) should be used, while being alert to the possibility of blood clot blocking these devices.

Manual or mechanical ventilation may be necessary but should be avoided if possible, bcause without adequate monitoring there is a risk of hyper- or hypocarbia. If possible, spontaneous respiration is preferable.

Breathing
- Assess thoroughly
- Identify life threatening conditions
- Place and secure appropriate drains
- Conserve oxygen supplies
- Avoid under and over ventilation
- Reassess frequently

Circulation with haemorrhage control

In hostile environments a casualty is likely to have been exerting himself or exposed to extreme conditions before injury, and therefore will almost certainly be fluid depleted. A rapid overall assessment must be performed, taking into account this and the mechanism of injury, before estimating fluid requirements.

Only minimal monitoring may be available, but clues can be obtained from simple observation, examination and frequent re-assessment; for example, a palpable radial pulse indicates a systolic blood pressure sufficient to achieve at least basis periphcral tissue pcrfusion.

Supplies of intravenous fluids will almost certainly be limited, so conservation of those fluids must be a significant consideration. Immediate surgery to "turn off the tap" may not be an option. Complete control of external haemorrhage is essential to avoid pouring in fluids only to have them lost from a bleeding wound. "Hypotensive" resuscitation should be considcred. This aims to maintain vital organ perfusion and hencc oxygcnation without increasing blood pressure to a point where further haemorrhage may result from loss of clot haemostasis (see chapter 5).

Colloid vs crystalloid
Blood is obviously the best fluid to replace blood loss but stored blood is unlikely to be available. Consider grouping your team before departure to provide a source of blood for transfusion, although this requires the equipment to bleed them to be carried too.

It is suggested that a mixture of crystalloid and colloid be carried to provide a variety of responses to blood and fluid loss. Colloid takes up less space, stays in the circulation longer and is required in lower volumes. However, it is not appropriate for replacing simple fluid and electrolyte losses and may precipitate at low temperatures (below 4°C).

Oral fluid can supplement intravenous fluids to cover basic requirements. Every fluid loss should be monitored and recorded, if possible, to help in estimation of requirements.

Circulation
- Assess carefully
- Limit haemorrhage
- Conserve intravenous fluids
- Consider hypotensive resuscitation
- Monitor response
- Remember preinjury losses

When are intravenous fluids required?
Class I haemorrhage (less than 15% loss)
- Oral fluids may be enough
- Make every effort to control blood loss

Class II haemorrhage (15–30% loss)
- Give oral fluids and monitor carefully
- Intravenous (IV) access is essential and IV fluids may be required
- Make every effort to control blood loss

Class III haemorrhage (30–40% loss)
- Intravenous fluids essential but with every effort to control blood loss
- An improved level of consciousness, a palpable pulse and urine output are your indicators of success

Class IV haemorrhage (more than 40% loss)
- The casualty is in trouble and unless immediate evacuation and surgery are available your fluids may be better conserved for others

Disability

Major head injury in isolated and hostile environments carries an appalling prognosis, because life saving surgical intervention is unlikely to be an option. Unless immediate evacuation is available, signs of rapidly increasing intracranial

Disability
- Assess level of consciousness
- AVPU/Glasgow Coma Score
- Reassess and record frequently
- Rapidly increasing intracranial pressure requires immediate evacuation

pressure presage death and probably little can be done. Diuretic therapy with mannitol will only delay the inevitable unless help is close at hand. Amateur neurosurgery is not recommended. Good management of the ABCs, with simple measures such as head up positioning, is the mainstay of controlling intracranial pressure and preventing secondary brain injury.

Environment and evacuation

Each hostile environment presents its own problems and no list can be exhaustive. Nevertheless, we have indicated types of problem that can occur in various settings and make trauma care a serious challenge.

Evacuation requires careful pre-planning and preparation. It is the wrong time to be organising your way out when catastrophe has occurred.

Physiological problems of hostile environments

The above summaries reveal that many hostile environments superimpose abnormal physiological stresses on the "normal" problems of trauma. The whole situation is often compounded by geographical isolation, limited resources and minimal support. The exact stresses depend on the nature of the hostile environment and can change from hour to hour in a particular location or situation. The following generic notes are aimed at stimulating thought to facilitate pre-planning.

Dehydration

Dehydration is a problem common to most, if not all, hostile environments. The tendency is to underestimate fluid requirements and fluid losses. This is particularly so in cold environments, where losses through sweating may be less apparent. Heavy physical effort is frequently the norm in these challenging situations and will result in increased fluid losses. It is also easy to underestimate losses resulting from gastro-intestinal illness, and to ignore low fluid intakes as a result of scarce clean water and preoccupation with other activities.

Pre-existing dehydration compounds the effects of hypovolaemia caused by haemorrhage and depletes valuable intravenous fluid resources if resuscitation is required. Minimise dehydration problems by raising awareness and teaching simple monitoring of urine output. All urine must be pale yellow in colour; if it darkens then fluid intake is inadequate. Checking that individuals carry enough drinking water and organising regular refreshment breaks will help ensure adequate hydration.

Hyperthermia

Hyperthermia or heat stroke (deep body temperature above 40°C) is a risk in environments with ambient temperatures above 32°C at high humidity, or temperatures above 43°C in dry air. Temperature, humidity, radiant heat, air movement and levels of physical activity all contribute to the development of hyperthermia, and all need to be considered. The key is prevention rather than cure. Consider monitoring the environment, planning work patterns, ensuring good hydration and active cooling.

Problems likely to be encountered in various environments

Environment	Features	Likely problems
Desert	Dry, with extremes of temperature (hot and cold)	Dehydration, lack of water supply, heat, cold, dust
Disasters	War, earthquakes, famine, flood	Self-preservation, lack of food and clean water; easy to become a drain on others' resources
Jungle	Wet, hot	Dehydration, lack of food and clean water, endemic diseases
Arctic	Dry, cold, wind chill	Dehydration, hypothermia, freezing cold injury
Altitude	Dry, wet, cold, low atmospheric pressure	Dehydration, exhaustion, altitude sickness (hypobaric hypoxia), freezing cold injury
Sea	Wet, cold	Dehydration, hypothermia, motion sickness, non-freezing cold injury

Environment
- Preplanning
- Good communications
- Appropriate transport
- Appropriate personnel
- Appropriate receiving facility
- Stabilise the patient
- Secure all lines and tubes

Physiological problems of hostile environments
- Dehydration
- Hyperthermia
- Hypothermia
- Freezing cold injury
- Non-freezing cold injury
- Altitude sickness

Hypothermia

Defined as a deep body temperature below 35°C, hypothermia considerably worsen the outcome after major trauma. The condition results when normal thermoregulation is overwhelmed by extreme cold, or from exposure to moderate cold in the presence of disordered thermoregulation.

Trauma adversely affects the normal thermoregulatory response to cold and greatly increases the risk of hypothermia. Hypothermia modifies the physiological response to trauma, making monitoring and treatment difficult. The onset may be insidious and prevention is easier than correction, particularly in field conditions. The mainstays of prevention are adequate protection by thermal insulation and shelter from wind.

Freezing cold injury

Freezing cold injury or frostbite results from freezing of peripheral tissues. The formation of ice crystals in the cells destroys them, resulting in tissue necrosis. Sub-zero low temperature environments, especially when exposure to wind results in wind chill, predispose to freezing injury. Low perfusion states such as hypovolaemic shock also predispose peripheral tissues to freezing. Shelter, insulation and external warmth are essential in prevention and thawing of already frozen parts. Protection from mechanical injury is essential if tissue loss is to be minimised.

Non-freezing cold injury

Non-freezing cold injury is peripheral tissue damage or necrosis caused by prolonged exposure to low temperatures above freezing. Cell metabolism is disordered and ultimately cells die. Cold, wet conditions and poor tissue perfusion predispose to the development of this type of tissue injury. Avoidance is the best prevention, because once damage has occurred re-warming leads to debilitating pain and swelling with severe immobility.

Altitude sickness

Oxygen partial pressure falls with ascent to height leading to hypoxia, with a haemoglobin oxygen saturation of 90% at 3000 m. Almost all villages in the Alps of Europe are at below 2000 m, but in the Andes of South America a long term acclimatisation allows people to live at 5500 m, which is the limit of human habitation. There the haemoglobin oxygen saturation is 73% and there is a compensatory polycythaemia. Mountain sickness can occur in individuals at lower altitudes, and the best treatment, apart from emergency diuretics and oxygen, is to descend quickly to a lower level.

The summit of Mount Everest, at 8000 m, has been climbed without supplementary oxygen by well acclimatised mountaineers. Some acclimatisation occurs within 24 hours, and it is usually done best in short, repeated spells. Tourists trekking in Nepal are always at risk in these high altitudes even if they have climbed in the Alps, where the highest peaks are in the 4000 m range.

Hypoxia can cause a reduced level of consciousness and the physiological response of tachycardia and tachypnoea confuses monitoring of vital signs in trauma. In addition, high altitude pulmonary and cerebral oedema can potentially compound the situation. Prevention is by planned acclimatisation and appropriate training. Treatment is with oxygen, portable compression devices and early rapid descent.

Conclusion

The key elements required to successfully meet the challenge of trauma care in a hostile environment are a sound understanding of the principles of trauma care, anticipation and, above all, a flexible response.

27 Psychological trauma

Martin P Deahl

More than 60% of us suffer potentially traumatising events at some point in our lives. For those who go on to suffer long-term psychological sequelae the aftermath is often undetected, untreated, and yet may be more disabling than any physical injury. This is particularly the case when there are concomitant physical injuries; these may mask psychological symptoms, yet paradoxically increase the likelihood of long-term psychological disorder. After road traffic crashes, for example, more than 20% of patients attending the emergency department go on to suffer post-traumatic stress disorder (PTSD) that may be a social handicap and persist for years, despite having made a satisfactory physical recovery.

A variety of disorders often occur after traumatic incidents whether or not physical injuries are present. Clinicians involved in trauma care should be able to identify and manage common psychological reactions following trauma, and know when to refer for a specialist psychiatric opinion.

> After road traffic crashes more than 20% of patients attending the emergency department go on to suffer post-traumatic stress disorder (PTSD). Driving phobias and major depressive disorders are also seen in 10–20% of survivors. These may be a social handicap and persist for years, despite the patient having made a satisfactory physical recovery

Psychological responses to trauma

Immediate emotional reactions to trauma
A wide range of emotional reactions are seen after physical or psychological trauma. Many individuals show little or no immediate emotion. However, an absence of emotional distress does not mean that an individual is immune to subsequent disorder. Emotional reactions may be delayed or precipitated by secondary events such as media coverage, inquests and police investigations. Intense fear, anxiety and distress is generally short lived and responds well to reassurance, empathic concern and practical support. However, brief courses of hypnotic and anxiolytic drugs may be needed for more severe reactions.

Adjustment disorders
Several patients experiencing stress or significant life-change (for example as a result of illness or disability following trauma) develop psychiatric symptoms which, although a handicap, are insufficient to meet diagnostic criteria for any other specific psychiatric disorder. These adjustment disorders generally develop within a month or so after significant life-change and resolve within 6 months. Various clinical features are recognised but most patients typically manifest depressive or anxiety symptoms.

These disorders may respond to simple reassurance and supportive counselling specific, but symptom targeted treatment with psychotropic drugs or cognitive–behavioural psychotherapy may be indicated in more severe cases.

> **Psychological responses to trauma**
> - Immediate emotional reactions to trauma
> - Adjustment disorders
> - Acute stress disorder (ASD)
> - Post-traumatic stress disorder (PTSD)

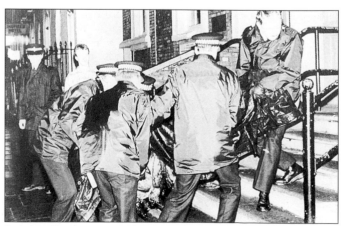
Body handling is a stressor that can make victims out of rescuers.

Acute stress disorder

Acute stress disorders (ASD) are defined in DSM-IV as occurring within 4 weeks of a life threatening traumatic event, lasting for at least 2 days and resolving within that 4-week period. Symptoms include intrusive phenomena (nightmares, flashbacks, etc.), avoidance of reminders of the trauma, hyperarousal, and dissociative symptoms such as emotional numbing and depersonalisation. It is important to distinguish ASD from normal "understandable" distress. Although the condition often resolves spontaneously, it identifies a group of patients at high risk of going on to develop long-term disorders and requiring careful follow-up. As many as 75% of patients suffering ASD after traumatic events will suffer from clinically significant post-traumatic stress disorder 2 years later.

Post-traumatic stress disorder (PTSD)

PTSD is a common and potentially disabling condition affecting all age groups; it may, if untreated, run a life-long relapsing course. Diagnostic criteria for PTSD are operationally defined (see table), although many individuals experience symptoms of PTSD that themselves are insufficient to meet the full diagnostic criteria—so-called "partial PTSD". Intrusive symptoms such as flashbacks and avoidance symptoms are a normal part of the stress response after trauma and are considered pathological only when they become excessive in frequency, duration, or intensity.

The point prevalence of PTSD in the population is at least 1–2% and lifetime prevalence figures for the full-blown PTSD syndrome may exceed 10%. Between 30% and 50% of survivors of combat, man-made and natural disasters (including rescue workers), and well as personal tragedy such as torture, accidents, abuse and rape will go on to suffer from PTSD. Compared to the rest of the population individuals with PTSD are much more likely to make negative life-course decisions. Teenagers with PTSD are less likely to succeed academically or complete secondary or higher education. The unemployed are less likely to obtain stable employment and those in work are more likely to become unemployed. Single people with PTSD are less likely to marry, and those in stable relationships are more likely to divorce. The indirect socioeconomic costs of PTSD are therefore incalculable.

Vulnerability to PTSD—Whether an individual develops PTSD or other psychiatric disorders after traumatic events depends upon an amalgam of the event itself, its context and the emotional significance attributed to it by an individual. In addition, several predisposing factors have been identified. These include the emergence of an acute stress disorder (ASD) after the trauma, a past history of psychiatric disorder, a "neurotic" anxiety-prone personality, exposure to previous traumatic experiences, including childhood abuse, and perceived threat to life and personal safety at the time of a traumatic event. Important gender differences have been noted; for example, women are more likely than men to develop PTSD after interpersonal, and specially sexual, violence. The presence of premorbid vulnerability factors also increases the likelihood of persisting, long-term PTSD and the development of comorbid psychopathology, particularly affective disorder and substance misuse.

Comorbid disorders and behavioural sequelae of PTSD—A "pure" PTSD syndrome is unusual, and the condition is often complicated by concurrent affective disorder, particularly major depression, generalised anxiety and panic disorder, alcohol and drug misuse. Pre-existing psychiatric disorders may also be significantly exacerbated following psychological trauma. Dysfunctional behaviour often coexists and may be

> **Symptoms of acute stress disorder (ASD) include intrusive phenomena (nightmares, flashbacks, etc.), avoidance of reminders of the trauma, hyperarousal, and dissociative symptoms such as emotional numbing and depersonalisation**

"Core" diagnostic criteria for post-traumatic stress disorder

A A life-threatening event outside normal human experience

B Re-experiencing the trauma
  —intrusive memories
  —dreams/nightmares
  —flashbacks: a sense of reliving the event
  —distress at exposure to events resembling trauma

C Avoidance of stimuli associated with the trauma

D Evidence of increased arousal
  —sleep disturbance
  —irritability
  —hypervigilance
  —exaggerated startle response

E Duration beyond 1 month

Post-traumatic stress disorder: important facts

- PTSD may present with dysfunctional social behaviour such as the breakdown of previously stable relationships and antisocial behaviour

- Other psychiatric disorders such as depression, alcohol and drug misuse are often associated with PTSD

- No single intervention effectively treats PTSD, and combinations of treatment are usually necessary

- Families may suffer as much as the patient and should always be involved in treatment

Factors predisposing to the development of post-traumatic stress disorder

- Emergence of an acute stress disorder (ASD) after the trauma

- Past history of psychiatric disorder

- "Neurotic" anxiety-prone personality

- Exposure to previous traumatic experiences, including childhood abuse

- Perceived threat to life and personal safety at the time of a traumatic event

the only presenting feature of an underlying PTSD. Occupational instability, antisocial behaviour and the break-own of previously stable relationships occur frequently and should raise the possibility of PTSD in any individual following traumatic events.

The biology of PTSD—Several enduring biological abnormalities have been identified in individuals with PTSD. Abnormalities of the hypothalamo–pituitary–adrenal axis (HPA) include hypo-cortisolaemia and enhanced adrenocorticoid sensitivity to the effects of dexamethasone suppression ("supersuppression"), which is proportional to the clinical severity of PTSD. It has been suggested that central glucocorticoid receptor hyper-sensitivity occurs in PTSD. Other neurochemical findings include evidence of increased central catecholamine activity, particularly noradrenaline and 5HT, both neurotransmitters that play a part in the encoding and retrieval of memory.

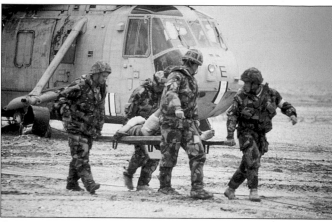

Our understanding of post-traumatic stress disorder is based upon studies of combat veterans. It is unclear to what extent their experiences can be generalised to civilian trauma victims.

Management of psychological responses to trauma

Primary prevention (prophylaxis)

True prevention means reducing trauma by measures such as improving safety in the workplace, on the roads and in the home, crime prevention and preventing war. Specific measures include the preparation of emergency service workers, soldiers and others routinely exposed to traumatic events, to help them cope with anticipated trauma. Thorough recruit selection to "screen out" vulnerable individuals, realistic training and establishing "tightly knit" cohesive teams can all mitigate against the effects of trauma. "Stress-inoculation" pro-grammes are increasingly used in training; these programmes include the exposure of prospective body-handlers to human remains and postmortem examinations, and educational briefings before combat that explain the likely effects of trauma to servicemen.

Secondary prevention

After traumatic events a variety of general and specific measures are used to reduce immediate emotional distress and help reduce the incidence of post-traumatic illness such as PTSD. General measures ("tea and sympathy") may seem intuitively obvious but can be easily overlooked in a busy department, particularly after major incidents when staff are preoccupied with major trauma rather than the minor physical injuries. Paradoxically, in the immediate post-trauma period, the psychological needs of the patient are inversely proportional to the extent of any physical injury; consequently, those with minor injuries often require proportionately more psychological support.

The patient should be made as physically comfortable as possible as quickly as possible—for example, by expediting physical and forensic examinations, and allowing the patient privacy and the opportunity to remove wet or soiled clothing and wash themselves. Allocating a specific staff member to supervise the patient facilitates a therapeutic relationship and provides an opportunity for the patient to discuss their experience and feelings should they wish to do so. Simple support is not only a matter of kindness but also allows staff to make a brief mental state assessment. After major incidents telephones should be made available for patients to contact friends and family, to let them know they are safe and make arrangements to be collected. Neither distressed patients nor those with marked emotional numbing or other dissociative symptoms should be allowed to leave the department

> **In the immediate aftermath of trauma the patient needs a sympathetic ear, and practical advice from someone who has time to listen—mental health workers are neither necessary nor desirable**

Goals of psychological debriefing

- Ensure participant's basic needs are met and adequate information provided
- Explore the symbolic meaning of loss
- Normalise feelings and reduce the sense of uniqueness of the individual
- Provide group supports, enhance peer social support and improve group cohesion
- Explain normal and abnormal stress reactions
- Encourage, teach and reinforce coping skills
- Teach anxiety reduction techniques
- Facilitate return to pre-incident functioning and routine
- Identify "high risk" participants with acute stress reactions. Ensure follow-up and refer for professional assistance where necessary

unescorted. Chaplains and agencies such as the Salvation Army should be enlisted to provide comfort and immediate psychological support following major incidents with multiple casualties. In the immediate aftermath of trauma the patient needs a sympathetic ear, and practical advice from someone who has time to listen. Mental health workers are neither necessary nor desirable.

Specific measures designed to reduce long term psychiatric morbidity after trauma include various forms of acute intervention including "critical incident stress debriefing" (CISD) or "psychological debriefing" (PD). Originally designed for groups of emergency service workers, debriefing allows victims of psychological trauma to be able to both cognitively and emotionally process their experience. It also has an important educational function explaining the nature of post-traumatic stress reactions, what normal and abnormal symptoms occur, and when and where the patient can seek help. The earlier debriefing occurs, the less is the opportunity for maladaptive and disruptive cognitive and behavioural patterns to become established. The effectiveness of these techniques in preventing PTSD is unclear.

Although victims generally appreciate it at the time, inappropriate and ill timed interventions may serve only to accentuate symptoms of stress. Furthermore recent randomised controlled trials have failed to demonstrate any long-term benefit of debriefing, although all have methodological shortfalls. It is generally accepted that debriefing or any other form of "stand alone" acute intervention is in itself inadequate. Consequently the best long term psychological outcome is likely to be achieved when debriefing is used as one element of an integrated "stress management" package which includes immediate support, practical help and adequate follow-up to identify those who go on to develop long-term disorders.

Treatment of established PTSD

A variety of psychological interventions and drug treatments have been shown to relieve at least some PTSD symptoms. The diversity of available treatments is an indication that none in isolation is particularly effective and an eclectic approach combining psychotherapy, drug treatments and social support is most likely to succeed. PTSD victims can be difficult to engage and are often reluctant to discuss symptoms or seek help. Time should be taken to establish a good therapeutic relationship with the patient before embarking on specific therapies. The therapist should also be prepared to be proactive and include facilities for community outreach. PTSD creates secondary victims among families and it is important to involve significant others wherever possible in any treatment programme.

Psychological therapies—A variety of psychological treatments have been advocated in the treatment of PTSD. Group based therapies may be particularly useful when dealing with the victims of a shared trauma such as combat or in disaster rescue workers. Cognitive techniques and exposure based behavioural interventions are popular and have proven efficacy. Anxiety management programmes used alone are probably less effective. Audiotape desensitisation is an effective and commonly used technique based on the principle of "imaginal" exposure. The patient writes a detailed script, describing not only events but also the feelings, sights, sounds and smells of the trauma. These are then recorded onto audiotape. Repeated exposure to the audiotape using a "personal stereo" often reduces symptoms of hyper-arousal to tolerable levels within 2–3 weeks. Eye movement

---

The seven stages of psychological debriefing

Introduction
- Purpose of the meeting, confidentiality, ground rules

Facts
- Chronolological account of events by each group member

Perception and thoughts
- Sights, smells, other sensory impressions and thoughts about what happened

Emotional reactions
- Feelings, regard of self, victims, colleagues and managers during and after trauma

Symptoms
- Review of symptoms and signs of distress
- Description of the normal trauma response, demonstrating universality and normalising the feelings of group members
- Challenge of inappropriate feelings of guilt and responsibility

Education
- How to deal with similar situations in the future
- Going home and coping with family and friends
- Coping strategies to deal with post-traumatic psychological symptoms
- When, where, how and under what circumstances to get further help if necessary
- Supplementary written information

Re-entry and disengagement
- Summary, discussion of outstanding issues
- Additional advice where appropriate

Individual factors influencing the debriefing process

Trauma exposure
- Multiple (type II) versus single (type I)
- Perceived life threat
- Concomitant physical injuries
- Losses

Participants
- Training, experience and acceptability of debriefers
- Prior trauma exposure
- Support networks
- Gender

Group factors
- Group cohesion
- Size
- Debriefing environment
- Timing of debriefing after trauma

desensitisation and reprocessing (EMDR) is a popular but controversial technique, in which the patient relives traumatic memories while the therapist induces saccadic eye movements, that is claimed to produce rapid symptom relief in PTSD. Its mechanism of action is uncertain but is almost certainly due in part to exposure. Despite the current popularity of EMDR, randomised controlled trials are urgently required to evaluate its effectiveness.

Drug treatment—although drugs alleviate some of the symptoms of PTSD, they are not generally as effective as psychological treatments and should always be combined with psychotherapy. Drug treatments tend to be most effective following acute PTSD and are of particular benefit in reducing "positive" symptoms such as nightmares and intrusive thoughts. Comorbid depression and other psychiatric disorders are also indications for drug treatment.

Drugs acting on central serotonergic transmission appear to have the most beneficial effects on the symptoms of PTSD. These include selective serotonin inhibitors (SSRIs) such as fluoxetine. Doses considerably in excess of those used to treat depression are commonly required and treatment maintained for 2 months or more before the full therapeutic effect is observed. Although benzodiazepines are occasionally useful in reducing symptoms of hyperarousal they should generally be avoided, particularly if there are concurrent problems with alcohol and other substance misuse.

A variety of other drugs have been used to some effect, including more sedative antidepressants acting primarily on 5HT systems such as nefazadone, tricyclic antidepressants, monoamine oxidase inhibitors (MAOIs) and non-psychotropic drugs such as clonidine that act by reducing central noradrenergic activity. The 5HT antagonist cyproheptadine is occasionally useful in preventing nightmares.

Conclusion

Psychological trauma is common and disabling. Stigma, shame and the avoidance symptoms associated with PTSD mean that patients all too often suffer in silence or present with dysfunctional social lives and a variety of diverse and seemingly unrelated difficulties. Many cases go undetected and a high incidence of clinical suspicion is required, particularly in high risk groups such as emergency service workers, participants in combat and rape and accident victims, to enable them to have access to treatment and therapeutic facilities. Health professionals are not immune to the psychological effects of trauma. They are also more likely to deal with their difficulties by self-medicating with drugs and alcohol than face the stigma and professional opprobrium associated with seeking help.

Public attitudes towards psychological trauma are ambivalent and at times downright hostile ("...after all, they're lucky to be alive", "...they're malingerers only after compensation"). Contrary to popular opinion, when litigation follows trauma a successful resolution for the plaintiff seldom brings about any significant clinical improvement. In the aftermath of traumatising events psychological symptoms are easily disregarded.

There can be no room for complacency and symptoms should not be dismissed merely because they are understandable in the context of trauma. Any patient with significant psychological distress more than 6 months after a traumatic event, or whose symptoms are socially handicapping, should be referred for a psychiatric assessment. The earlier the treatment of psychological trauma the more

Elements of successful debriefing
- Cohesive group with shared experience
- Experienced debriefers accepted by group
- Proximity
- Immediacy (48–72 h)
- Expectancy (of full recovery)
- Simplicity
- Combine debriefing with practical support and adequate follow-up

What not to do in debriefing
- Enforce mandatory debriefing on unwilling subjects
- Use outside debriefers alien to the group (especially mental health workers)
- Be complacent — fail to make efforts to detect subsequent psychopathology in group members
- Fail to arrange adequate follow-up and inform primary care physicians that patient has been a victim of trauma and a recipient of debriefing

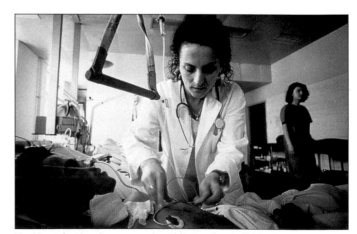

Health professionals are as vulnerable as other individuals to the psychological effects of trauma, yet often receive little or no support.

effective it is and trauma victims should not have to wait for a crisis before receiving help. Follow-up should be offered to all trauma victims seen in the emergency department.

Major incident planning must include provision to inform the general practitioner of all patients involved in an incident, including those sustaining only minor injuries. The report should include brief details of the incident, information about the possible sequelae of psychological trauma, and how and where the GP can obtain specialist advice. Most importantly the GP should review the patient 6 months to 1 year after the incident, to assess the patient's mental state and lifestyle pre and post-incident. A significant change in personality, or deterioration in relationships and social or occupational functioning, excessive alcohol or substance misuse, in addition to obvious signs of psychological disorder should alert the GP to the possibility of an underlying post-traumatic illness, This should trigger a more detailed examination and specialist referral if necessary.

Information for the GP
- Brief details of the incident
- Possible sequelae of psychological trauma
- How and where the GP can obtain specialist advice

Signs of post-traumatic illness
- Significant change in personality
- Deterioration in relationships and social or occupational functioning
- Excessive alcohol or substance misuse
- Obvious signs of psychological disorder

Further reading

Wilson JP, Raphael B, eds. *International handbook of traumatic stress syndromes.* New York: Plenum Press, 1993—the definitive text book on PTSD; comprehensive and the best reference source available.

Black D, Newman M, Mezey G, Hendriks JH, eds. *Psychological trauma: a developmental approach.* London: Gaskell Press, 1997—a small but comprehensive work covering all aspects of traumatic stress throughout the life-cycle. The first book on PTSD to be written from a British perspective.

O'Brien LS. *Traumatic events and mental health.* Cambridge: Cambridge University Press, 1998—a useful, well referenced and easy to read book that describes many of the controversies surrounding PTSD, including the medicolegal aspects. The author emphasises that PTSD is only one of several stress response syndromes that have been relatively neglected by researchers.

Raphael B, Meldrum C, McFarlane AC. Does debriefing after psychological trauma work? *Br Med J* 1995; **310**: 1479—an excellent editorial describing the limitations and problems associated with psychological debriefing.

28 Major incidents

Tim Hodgetts, Stephen Miles

An incident is described as "major" when the number, severity, and type of live casualties or the location of the incident require extraordinary arrangements to be made by the NHS. Natural incidents (floods, hurricanes, tidal waves) still account for most of the deaths worldwide, but man made incidents that result from technological or other human interaction are more common. The potential for a man made incident exists whenever a large number of people gather together.

Preparation

Preparation for a major incident involves planning, training, and acquisition of equipment. Every hospital that may receive casualties must have a major incident plan that details the organisation and actions of staff both in hospital and at the scene. When making a major incident plan, reference to *Planning for major incidents: the NHS guidance* will be useful.[1]

The doctor in charge at the scene is the medical incident officer; doctors and nurses sent to treat patients at the scene under his direction are termed mobile medical teams. Doctors who may take on the role of medical incident officer at the scene must be given supplementary training in command and communications as well as gaining experience in prehospital care, in addition to training for their individual responsibilities. Any doctor at the scene is not necessarily better than no doctor at all. The Prehospital Emergency Care Certificate and the Diploma in Immediate Medical Care provide standards for training, but doctors should also take a specific course in the medical management of a major incident. Doctors and nurses who are members of the mobile medical team should also be trained in prehospital care and should understand their roles and the organisation of the scene.

Equipment

Protective clothing should meet British standards and the current recommendations of the Ambulance Policy Advisory Group. For example, the helmet should be Kevlar composite, green with white lettering, with a visor and chin strap; jackets must be high visibility (motorway standard) and should be clearly labelled in green "DOCTOR" or "NURSE." National standardisation will help recognition at the scene and facilitate control.

Medical supplies are best carried in rucksacks with partitions clearly dividing them into "airway," "breathing," and "circulation." Other rucksacks or boxes that contain only disposable items (airways, dressings, cannulae, and fluids) can be used for resupply. A checklist on the wall of the major incident room will remind team members not to forget important analgesic or anaesthetic drugs from the controlled drugs

---

Major incident definition

Major incidents can be
- Simple or compound
- Compensated or uncompensated
- Natural or man made

Most incidents are
- Simple (environment intact)
- Compensated (patient load less than capacity available)
- Man made

Suggested staff training requirements

Medical Incident Officer
- Diploma in Immediate Medical Care (Royal College of Surgeons of Edinburgh) or Prehospital Emergency Care Certificate

and

- Major Incident Medical Management and Support (MIMMS) course (3 days) *[other major incident training courses available]*

and

- Advanced life support instruction (Advanced Trauma Life Support/Prehospital Trauma Life Support)

Member of mobile medical team
- Prehospital Emergency Care course

and

- Major Incident Medical Management and Support (MIMMS) course (first 2 days only)

and

- Advanced life support instruction (ATLS/PHTLS)

cupboard or the refrigerator. Specialist operations such as amputations are rarely required and the necessary equipment will not be part of the standard response bag. Consequently it should be stored in a separate mobile surgical team bag with the equipment needed by the assisting nurse, and kept at the base hospital until needed.

The initial response

A hospital is usually alerted to a major incident by ambulance control, who may contact the switchboard or speak directly to the emergency department. Standard phrases are used to avoid confusion. "*Major incident, stand by*" is used to warn of a potential incident—perhaps an aircraft about to land with engine trouble. Generally only senior staff such as the duty consultants in accident and emergency, general surgery, and intensive care need to be told, together with the senior accident and emergency nurse, the duty manager, and the duty nurse administrator. It is wise if these people assemble and establish a *control centre*. Depending on the perceived threat, members of the mobile medical teams can be nominated, change into protective clothing, and check their equipment. When a major incident has been confirmed a full hospital response is initiated by the phrase "*Major incident declared, activate plan*". The response can be terminated at any time by "*Major incident cancelled*" or "*Stand down*".

There will not always be adequate warning from the ambulance service, and it may be the emergency department that activates the plan. In these circumstances ambulance control should be informed.

When a "Major incident declared" message is received the following should be established:

- When the accident occurred (time)
- Where it is (including grid reference if known)
- What sort of accident (derailment, aircraft crash, chemical)
- What are the estimated number and severity of casualties
- What medical response is required

The ambulance incident officer should request a doctor to go to the scene as medical incident officer, together with one or more mobile medical teams. It is not advisable to draw these teams from the hospitals nominated to receive the first casualties. The major incident plan will specify whether the medical incident officer is supplied by a hospital or by a local BASICS (British Association for Immediate Care) scheme. This group of doctors works voluntarily with the emergency services, particularly at road traffic accidents where people are trapped, and their experience may assist with the smooth running of the scene.

Site organisation

Command and control

The overall control of the scene is the responsibility of the police, who will place a secure cordon around it. A second, inner cordon may also be established round the immediate incident if it is necessary to control people moving into a hazardous area. Each emergency service will appoint a commander or incident officer, usually a senior officer. Incident officers will be found near their emergency control vehicles, which should be the only vehicles at the scene that do not switch off their coloured beacons. The incident officers can be regarded as forming "silver command" and their chief officers (who will meet remote from the scene) as "gold command". Forward incident officers will be appointed to control the rescue work at the heart of the incident. If the incident is spread over a large area it will be broken into sectors, each of which will have its own set of forward incident officers referred to as "bronze commanders".

Personal protective clothing for staff on site at a major incident
- Warm underclothing
- Fire-retardant suit
- High visibility jacket marked "DOCTOR" or "NURSE"
- Hard hat with visor
- Gloves (robust and latex pairs)
- Ear defenders

Additional essential equipment
Everybody
- Personal identification and money
- Notebook (ideally plasticised with water-resistant pen)
- Action card

Medical Incident Officer
- Radio and spare battery
  Optional:
    —aide memoire
    —camera
    —dictaphone
    —cellular telephone

Initial information to be passed from the scene
Exact location
Type of incident (road? rail? aircraft?)
Hazards (present and potential)
Access to the scene
Number and severity of casualties (estimate)
Emergency services present and required ("ETHANE")

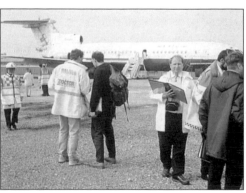
Training for medical command.

The police

In addition to securing the scene the police will clear routes in and out of the incident, control the public and volunteers, liaise with the media, activate the voluntary societies (such as the Women's Royal Voluntary Service, the Salvation Army, the St John's Ambulance Service, and the Red Cross), set up a casualty bureau to collate information about the casualties and the dead, identify the dead and organise their removal from the scene, and protect the forensic evidence.

The fire service

If there is a fire or chemical hazard the senior fire officer will assume control of the immediate scene and is responsible for the rescue of any casualties. The fire service also provides specialist equipment and skills to release trapped casualties, as well as emergency lighting and heavy lifting gear.

The ambulance service

The ambulance incident officer will liaise closely with the medical incident officer throughout. It is important that those with specialist paramedical skills are identified and given appropriate tasks. There are several key roles for ambulance personnel including a loading officer (to record the destination of casualties), a primary triage officer (to sort the casualties into priorities when they are first found), a casualty clearing station officer (to set up the clearing station), a safety officer (to identify hazards and check personal protective equipment), and a communications officer. It is the ambulance incident officer's duty to nominate the receiving hospitals and arrange provision of the medical incident officer and the mobile medical teams.

The medical service

The medical incident officer is responsible for all medical resources at the scene. Discipline is essential and all members of the mobile medical teams or individual doctors (no matter how senior) will take their instructions from him. As doctors arrive they will be appointed to key roles including triage officer (who may initially be sent forward, then withdrawn to the clearing station), casualty clearing station officer in charge, treatment officers (based at the clearing station), forward medical incident officer, and mortuary officer.

When more than one mobile medical team with nurses is present, a nursing incident officer may be appointed who is responsible to the medical incident officer and who oversees the welfare of the nurses. Members of each mobile medical team must report to the medical incident officer on arrival to be given their jobs. It is usual to concentrate those doctors and nurses used for treatment at the clearing station and send them forward only for specific tasks; otherwise command and control is lost.

Responsibilities of the medical incident officer

The medical incident officer has seven principal areas of responsibility (see box).

Command and control

This is the cornerstone of efficient management. It can be greatly simplified by reference to the Prehospital Emergency Management Master, a waterproof scene guide that doubles as the incident log.[2] A log is essential to compile the report after the incident.

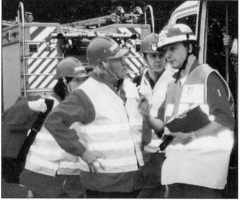

At the scene of a major rail crash (rail disaster at Clapham, London).

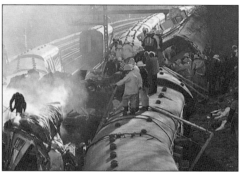

Medical incident officer briefing mobile medical team.

Medical Incident Officer's responsibilities

Command and control

Safety

Communications

Assessment

Triage

Treatment

Transport

"Control Spells Calm And Time To Treat"

Safety

Always consider your own safety first—are you correctly dressed? Next think of the safety of the scene—is it safe to approach and is my team safe? The medical incident officer is responsible for preventing access by any doctor or nurse inappropriately dressed (if they have not already been spotted by the ambulance safety officer). Finally, think of the safety of the casualties.

Communications

Communications are the weakest link in the major incident response. All the incident officers must liaise regularly, but the ambulance and medical incident officers should be almost inseparable. The medical incident officer must also relay information to the receiving hospitals.

The radio is the usual tool of communication and a knowledge of radio voice procedure will be assumed. At the least you must know how to start and finish a message and how to spell using the phonetic alphabet. Do not forget the value of a runner, particularly when the radio is busy and difficult to get to. Use written messages to avoid "Chinese whispers": "I need Entonox" could become "I need an empty box".

Assessment

Assessment of the scene for hazards to your team and estimation of the number and severity of casualties allows an appropriate early medical response.

Triage

Triage is the sorting of casualties into priorities for treatment and specifically those who need immediate treatment (for example, tension pneumothorax), urgent treatment (for example, fractured femur),

> **Communications are the weakest link in the major incident response. All the incident officers must liaise regularly**
>
> **Do not forget the value of a runner, particularly when the radio is busy and difficult to get to**
>
> **Use written messages to avoid confusion**

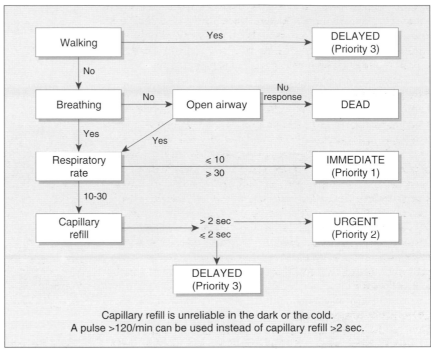

Capillary refill is unreliable in the dark or the cold.
A pulse >120/min can be used instead of capillary refill >2 sec.

The triage sieve.

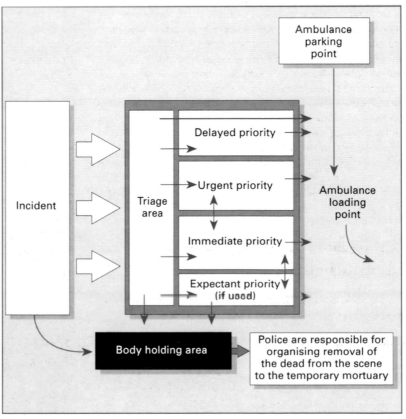

Triage label.

Organisation at the site of a major incident.

those whose treatment can be delayed (for example, sprained ankle), and the dead. These priorities are colour coded red, yellow, green, and white, respectively. The triage officer must not stop to treat individual patients. As priorities can change after or while awaiting treatment, triage must be constantly repeated. Colour coded folding labels enable this to be done quickly. The task will be delegated, but supervised, by the medical incident officer.

When dealing with a large number of casualties the aim is to do the most for the most. Consequently there will be a few who are identified as likely to die. Attending to these patients will distract resources from those who are likely to live, and they are given minimal treatment initially. They are termed "expectant". Their colour code is green (some use blue), but with the card endorsed "expectant".

An initial rapid assessment, perhaps taking only 30 seconds, is known as the triage sieve. This is followed by a more detailed assessment (usually done at the clearing station) known as the triage sort, for which the triage revised trauma score is used. This gives a score of 0–4 for each of its three components—systolic blood pressure, Glasgow coma scale, and respiratory rate. Triage priorities can be assigned depending on the total score, which ranges from 0 to 12.

Treatment

Treatment is always delegated by the medical incident officer and usually will take place in the casualty clearing station. The temptation to delay movement of untrapped casualties to the clearing station, where the procedures can be done more easily, should be avoided. Priorities for treatment follow the rules of airway, breathing, and circulation. Those needing only minor treatment may not receive it at the scene.

Transport

The ambulance service is responsible for transporting injured patients to hospital. To decide the most appropriate transport, the medical incident officer should consider its capacity, availability and suitability, such as access to difficult terrain. Before the patient is loaded into the ambulance it should also have been decided which hospital is most appropriate (can the patient go directly to a specialist centre?), what observations and treatment will be needed on the way, and if the patient should be escorted.

In addition to these seven areas of responsibility the medical incident officer will monitor the medical response to ensure that it is adequate and that there is a continuing supply of equipment. He will observe team members for signs of fatigue, and organise relief staff—usually every 4 hours. A debrief of all medical personnel involved at the scene should be held within 24 hours.

Hospital organisation

The key to successful hospital management of a major incident is, once again, command and control. It depends on early establishment of an effective control centre staffed by senior hospital medical, nursing, and administrative coordinators with appropriate support staff. All should be of the most senior rank possible—(for example, a consultant, a senior nursing officer, and a senior administrator—and thoroughly familiar with the major incident plan.

Other personnel should also be aware of their roles in the response to a major incident, but to anticipate a lack of familiarity and assist junior staff everybody should be issued with an "action card" when they report for duty. These cards are distributed according to clinical need, and not personal choice.

Patient transport

When choosing the transport think of:

Capacity (a bus may be suitable for large numbers of 'delayed' priority casualties)

Availability (save the emergency ambulances for the seriously injured)

Suitability (do you need a wheeled or a tracked vehicle? Is a helicopter more suitable?)

("CAS")

When you have loaded a patient:

Move to the appropriate hospital (are you going straight to a specialist centre?)

Observe in transit (what equipment do you need?)

Verify the treatment before departure (do you have enough oxygen, fluids, or analgesia?)

Escort if necessary (doctor, nurse, or paramedic?)

("MOVE")

Actions on receiving "Major incident—stand by"

Medical, nursing and administrative coordinators meet and establish the control centre. They then:

- Liaise with the ambulance service about the details and status of the incident
- Nominate the medical incident officer and dispatch him or her to the scene, if appropriate
- Start to prepare the accident and emergency department for the reception of casualties
- Warn theatres, the intensive care unit, and outpatients about the possible disruption of activities
- Establish an accurate bed state

Actions on receiving "Major incident declared—activate plan"

Coordinators meet and establish the control centre, if no prior warning. They then:

- Dispatch the medical incident officer to the scene
- Establish whether mobile medical teams are required; collect the teams, ensure the members are properly clothed and equipped, and dispatch them to the scene
- Establish a triage point
- Clear the emergency department of existing casualties and prepare for the reception of casualties
- Inform theatres and outpatients that normal activities must be suspended; ask the intensive care unit to clear beds if possible
- Designate a ward for the reception of admitted casualties and start emptying it of existing patients
- Organise staff as they arrive
- Arrange facilities for the police, relatives, and the media

Medical coordinator

The immediate priorities of the medical coordinator are to clear the emergency department, dispatch the medical incident officer if requested from that hospital, and organise the mobile medical teams, ensuring that they are appropriately dressed and equipped and have transport to the scene. The medical coordinator should check that the switchboard operators are calling in appropriate staff from home and the hospital residences, and he must nominate a senior doctor to be *chief triage officer*. This doctor receives casualties at the ambulance entrance and reassesses their treatment priority before allocating them to a treatment area within the department.

The clinical activity is supervised by the surgical triage officer (usually the duty consultant surgeon) and where needed the medical triage officer (the duty consultant physician or intensive care specialist). Surgical triage must take account of not only which patient has priority, but what operation has priority for each patient; those that are life saving should be done first.

The medical coordinator (or a deputy, the team coordinator) will form doctors and nurses into either treatment or transfer teams, and allocate them to appropriate areas of the department. Many of the staff in the emergency department will be drawn from other areas in the hospital. It is important that regular emergency staff can be identified by tabards to help the unfamiliar staff find equipment and supplies.

With the help of the nursing coordinator an accurate tally of bed state, including intensive care beds, must be maintained, together with available operating theatre resources. Staff welfare must be monitored and refreshments ordered. At intervals the medical coordinator may be requested by the administrators to address a press conference.

Nursing coordinator

The nursing coordinator will recruit nurses to go with the mobile medical teams and to attend patients in the emergency department. One nurse should be provided for each stretcher patient although up to four may be required for the resuscitation of a critically ill patient if resources allow. The nursing coordinator should liaise closely with the medical coordinator.

Administrative coordinator

Successful running of a hospital's major incident response requires a great deal of documentation and record keeping; firstly to keep track of patients (particularly if they are to be discharged); secondly, to provide the police with information for their documentation team (one of whom is sent to each receiving hospital to report to the central casualty bureau); and thirdly, to answer questions from relatives who arrive at the hospital. The administrative coordinator must: allocate a room for the police documentation team, ideally with a telephone and facsimile machine; and organise a media centre remote from the emergency department where the press can be briefed at regular intervals.

Porters and security staff must be organised to ensure expeditious transport of patients and to keep unwanted people out of the treatment areas. Space for relatives must be set aside, and a room allocated in which staff can talk to the bereaved.

The aftermath

When the medical or ambulance incident officer reports that the last casualty has left the site, and when all patients have been admitted to or discharged from the emergency department, the medical coordinator will declare a "stand down" of the major incident procedure.

> **Control centre equipment**
> - Stationery, including triage labels and prenumbered patients' notes
> - Staff control board, with a list of staff roles and allocations
> - Patient control board, with the names of casualties, their triage priority and disposal details
> - Telephones for internal hospital use, plus a line to the press room and police documentation team
> - Signs to direct staff, relatives and the press

> **Duties of the administrative coordinator**
> - Place clerical staff in the triage area to collect information as the patients arrive
> - Organise security and portering staff to direct relatives, the public and the press away from the treatment area, and organise the erection of signs
> - Organise an area for the police documentation team and the press, and equip these areas with a telephone and facsimile
> - Designate other administrative staff to act as press officer, patient information officer, and police liaison officer
> - Check that switchboard is coping with the overload of calls, and that the callout of off-duty staff is proceeding smoothly
> - Ensure catering, pharmacy, and supply needs are met

Debriefing is essential. An "emotional" debriefing should be organised within 24 hours so that all the departmental staff have a chance to express their feelings. If proper opportunities are not given to staff for debriefing and counselling some are likely to develop symptoms of post-traumatic stress disorder. Heads of departments should prepare formal reports that can be the basis for improvements to the Major Incident Plan.

● Photograph of Clapham rail disaster from Frank Spooner Pictures.

References

1 NHS Executive. *Planning for major incidents: the NHS guidance.* London: NHS Executive, 1998.
2 Hodgetts TJ, McNeil I, Cooke MW. *The prehospital emergency management master.* London: BMJ Publishing Group, 1995.

Further reading

Hodgetts TJ, Mackway-Jones K. *Major incident medical management and support: the practical approach.* London: BMJ Publishing Group, 1995.

Index